Essential Immunology

Essential Immunology

Editor: Avery Steele

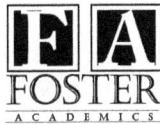

FA
FOSTER
ACADEMICS

www.fosteracademics.com

www.fosteracademics.com

FA
FOSTER
ACADEMICS

Cataloging-in-Publication Data

Essential immunology / edited by Avery Steele.
    p. cm.
Includes bibliographical references and index.
ISBN 978-1-63242-688-8
1. Immunology. 2. Clinical immunology. 3. Immunologic diseases.
4. Serology. I. Steele, Avery.
QR181 .E87 2019
616.079--dc23

Foster Academics,
118-35 Queens Blvd., Suite 400,
Forest Hills, NY 11375, USA

ISBN 978-1-63242-688-8 (Hardback)

Contents

Permissions

List of Contributors

Index

Preface

This book has been an outcome of determined endeavour from a group of educationists in the field. The primary objective was to involve a broad spectrum of professionals from diverse cultural background involved in the field for developing new researches. The book not only targets students but also scholars pursuing higher research for further enhancement of the theoretical and practical applications of the subject.

Immunology is a branch of biology, which is concerned with the study of the immune system. The malfunctions of the immune system cause immunological disorders such as immune deficiency syndromes, hypersensitivities and transplant rejection. Immunological disorders fall into the broad categories of immunodeficiency and autoimmunity. In an immunodeficiency disease, the immune system fails to provide an adequate response. Some examples of immunodeficiency diseases are primary immune disease and chronic granulomatous disease. In autoimmune diseases, the immune system attacks its host's body such as in Hashimoto's disease, systemic lupus erythematosus, myasthenia gravis and rheumatoid arthritis. Different approaches, evaluations, methodologies and advanced studies on immunology have been included in this book. There has been rapid progress in the understanding of immunological disorders, their diagnoses and treatments, which have been included in this extensive book. It is an essential guide for both academicians and those who wish to pursue this discipline further.

It was an honour to edit such a profound book and also a challenging task to compile and examine all the relevant data for accuracy and originality. I wish to acknowledge the efforts of the contributors for submitting such brilliant and diverse chapters in the field and for endlessly working for the completion of the book. Last, but not the least; I thank my family for being a constant source of support in all my research endeavours.

Editor

Effect of cryopreservation on delineation of immune cell subpopulations in tumor specimens as determined by multiparametric single cell mass cytometry analysis

Elma Kadić[1], Raymond J. Moniz[2], Ying Huo[1], An Chi[3] and Ilona Kariv[1]* ⓘ

Abstract

Background: Comprehensive understanding of cellular immune subsets involved in regulation of tumor progression is central to the development of cancer immunotherapies. Single cell immunophenotyping has historically been accomplished by flow cytometry (FC) analysis, enabling the analysis of up to 18 markers. Recent advancements in mass cytometry (MC) have facilitated detection of over 50 markers, utilizing high resolving power of mass spectrometry (MS). This study examined an analytical and operational feasibility of MC for an in-depth immunophenotyping analysis of the tumor microenvironment, using the commercial CyTOF™ instrument, and further interrogated challenges in managing the integrity of tumor specimens.

Results: Initial longitudinal studies with frozen peripheral blood mononuclear cells (PBMCs) showed minimal MC inter-assay variability over nine independent runs. In addition, detection of common leukocyte lineage markers using MC and FC detection confirmed that these methodologies are comparable in cell subset identification. An advanced multiparametric MC analysis of 39 total markers enabled a comprehensive evaluation of cell surface marker expression in fresh and cryopreserved tumor samples. This comparative analysis revealed significant reduction of expression levels of multiple markers upon cryopreservation. Most notably myeloid derived suppressor cells (MDSC), defined by co-expression of $CD66b^+$ and $CD15^+$, $HLA-DR^{dim}$ and $CD14^-$ phenotype, were undetectable in frozen samples.

Conclusion: These results suggest that optimization and evaluation of cryopreservation protocols is necessary for accurate biomarker discovery in frozen tumor specimens.

Keywords: Mass Cytometry (MC), CyTOF™, Flow cytometry (FC), Tumor samples, Tumor microenvironment (TME), Tumor infiltrating lymphocytes (TILs), Immunophenotyping, Cryopreservation, ViSNE

* Correspondence: Ilona_Kariv@merck.com
[1]Department of Pharmacology, Cellular Pharmacology, Merck and Co. Inc, 33 Avenue Louis Pasteur, Boston 02115, MA, USA
Full list of author information is available at the end of the article

Background

Cancer represents a multifaceted disease characterized not only by extreme genetic and epigenetic heterogeneity of the transformed cells, but also by clonal progression of treatment-resistant tumors as a result of targeted therapies. In addition to molecular resistance, tumor-mediated suppression of the self-immune system is thought to contribute to tumor evasion from effector cells [1]. Early efforts to modulate immune system's anti-tumor functionality has resulted in only marginal therapeutic efficacy [2, 3]. However, to date, more than 10 antibody (Ab)-based therapies are available in the clinic [4]. Most recent are targeting two immuno-checkpoint receptors; CTLA4 (cytotoxic T-lymphocyte-antigen 4), PD-1 (programmed cell death 1) and its ligand PDL1, and show a remarkable efficacy against certain tumors, through re-activating cytotoxic T (Tc) cell mediated tumor killing [5, 6]. These positive clinical outcomes support further investment in targeting additional immunomodulatory receptors on T-cytotoxic (Tc) cells, and expanding these approaches to other immune cells. For example natural killer (NK) cells can be recruited to kill tumor cells, without potential concern for causing acute cytokine storm or long-term auto-immune responses [7, 8], while suppression of T-regulatory (Treg) cells can be used to enhance immune response against tumor cells [9].

In order to accelerate the delivery of immunomodulators from the bench to the bedside, it is imperative to have a toolbox of biomarkers that can be used for in-depth understanding of the complexity of disease-underlying biology, and refine translational validity between preclinical efficacy and the highly diverse patient response [10–12]. To address this, a greater emphasis on the use of clinical specimens for discovery of disease relevant biomarkers has been placed for diagnosis, prognosis, assessment of treatment efficacy and patient stratification strategies [13, 14]. Today, the collection of patient samples, such as core-needle biopsies and blood, for genetic and other analyses has become common practice, offering accurate determinations from limited clinical tissues [15]. However, effective bioanalytical tools that encompass complex immune- and tumor cells interactions in a clinical trial setting have been lacking [16, 17].

For the past several decades multiparametric fluorescent cytometry has been used in research and clinical laboratories to significantly advance biomarker discovery by immunophenotyping highly heterogeneous tumor samples [18–20]. However due to spectral overlap of fluorophore conjugated to detection antibodies, and inherent high sample auto-fluorescence, practical detection is currently limited to 12–18 simultaneous independent markers [21–23]. The recently developed mass-spectrometry (MS) based technology, or commonly referred to as cytometry by time-of-flight (CyTOF™), has enabled multiplexed cellular analysis of up to 100 parameters. Mass cytometry has overcome many limitations seen with FC, by utilizing metal conjugated antibodies coupled with atomic MS detection [24]. The use of rare-earth transitional metals as detection tags provides a clear advantage over fluorescent labels as these are not naturally occurring within the human body, and the added advantage of MS resolution capabilities of single mass differences, allows for quantification of signals without cellular background interference or significant signal spillover, thus making CyTOF™ well suited to for multi-dimensional single cell analysis of limited clinical specimens [25, 26]. Furthermore, integration of highly multiplexed detection on a single cell level with an advanced statistical analysis allows for the unbiased delineation of the cellular subsets that can be easily overlooked by trying to assemble several detection Ab panels utilized by flow cytometry [27]. In the short period of time since the introduction of this technology several break-through studies demonstrated the potential of this platform to interrogate complex mechanistic and biomarker networks [28–30]. Moreover, recent studies of tumor samples demonstrated that MC could greatly improve knowledge of the complex cellular milieu of acute myeloid leukemia (AML) by utilizing 35–40 simultaneous detection markers [31]. While findings like these have highlighted the advanced analytic capabilities of MC, the use of this platform to develop a fit-for-purpose immunophenotyping analysis of tumor specimens from clinical trials remain to be evaluated in the context of clinical sample handling logistics.

In this study, MC detection stability was first evaluated by nine independent experimental runs of a well-characterized single PBMC lot utilizing 14 cell surface markers. After establishing optimized MC throughput, detection and data analysis protocols, we expanded on previous publications [32, 33] by further validating applicability of the comprehensive immunophenotyping of PBMCs and clinical tumor samples as compared to measurements obtained using conventional FC. The cumulative findings of these studies confirmed that the CyTOF™ platform supports comprehensive multiparametric biomarker discovery, as evidenced by the analysis of 39 simultaneously detected markers.

While assessing accuracy of the high multiparametric analytical potential of MC detection, this study further evaluated the impact of cryopreservation on the immune cell markers by comparing fresh and subsequently cryopreserved human tumor specimens. Due to concerns about clinical sample stability during shipment and in an effort to standardize analysis conditions across many specimens, the samples are commonly cryopreserved shortly after collection [34], and analyzed at a later time as a single batch to minimize technical and systems variability. However recent publications have raised questions about sample integrity and reliability of these specimens [35, 36]. Results of our study showed a significant reduction in expression levels of most myeloid markers such as CD11B, CD14, CD15, CD16, CD66, CD86, CD80, and CD56 as well as immunoregulatory receptors (IMRs) upon cryopreservation. Most notable was the complete loss of detection of myeloid derived suppressor cells (MDSC). These results strongly caution the use of cryopreserved tumor samples for biomarker discovery and merit further studies to identify advanced cryopreservation protocols.

Methods

Fluorescent and mass cytometry detection antibodies

Sample sourcing

PBMCs were purchased from SeraCare Life Sciences Inc., (Milford, MA). Frozen dissociated tumor cells (DTC) and normal adjacent tissue (NAT) were purchased from ConversantBio (Huntsville, AL). The frozen samples were shipped on dry ice and stored in liquid nitrogen. Dissociation and cryopreservation of tumor tissue specimens, resected in 2010 and 2012, were performed by the vendor by applying tissue specific protocols that employed both enzymatic and mechanical dissociation. Fresh human tumor specimens were properly collected with all necessary approvals, consents and/or authorizations for the collection, use and/or transfer of such human tissues through Neurologica Cognitiva Research LLC DBA Boston Biosource (Newton, MA). Tumor samples were stored in AQIX® media (AQIX LTD, London, UK), a formulation optimized to maintain pH levels and mimic the intestinal fluid layer while preserving genetic and histological profiles of excised tissue for up to 72 h following removal from patients [37]. The samples were shipped and stored at 4 °C, and tissue processing occurred within 12 h of surgical removal.

Frozen sample recovery

Cells were rapidly thawed in a 37 °C water bath, and diluted in pre-warmed complete medium: Roswell Park Memorial Institute (RPMI) 1640 medium supplemented with 10% fetal bovine serum (FBS), (both LifeSciences, Carlsbad, CA). Residual dimethyl sulfoxide (DMSO) was removed by centrifugation at 400 g for 5 min and pelleted cells were resuspended in growth media and allowed to recover for 30 min at 37 °C and 5% CO_2 prior to subsequent procedures [38].

Fresh tissue dissociation

Dissociation of fresh renal cell carcinoma and colorectal tumor tissues was performed according to manufacturer's instructions for the human tumor dissociation kit (Milteny, Auburn, CA); briefly the tissue samples were cut up into smaller pieces and subjected to enzymatic and mechanical dissociation using the vendor supplied enzyme cocktail and the GentleMACS™ dissociator (Miltenyi, Auburn, CA). The mechanical dissociation protocol employed variable blade rotation speeds for 60 min at 37 °C. After tissue dissociation, red blood cells (RBC) were lysed using Ammonium-Chloride-Potassium (ACK) buffer (Life Sciences, Carlsbad, CA) for 5 min at RT. The samples were washed twice with complete medium by pelleting at 400 g for 5 min and the cell count was determined using Vi-Cell (Beckman Coulter, Indianapolis, IN). The resulting single sell suspension was stained for immediate analysis by FC and MC while residual cells were cryopreserved.

Cryopreservation of dissociated tumor cells (DTC)

The cells were cryopreserved in four different freezing media at concentrations ranging from 2×10^6 to 5×10^6 cells/mL. The following cryopreservation media (CM) were tested; CM1: 90% FBS (Gibco, Grand Island, NY) and 10% DMSO Hybri-Max™ (Sigma-Aldrich, St. Louis, MO); CM2: 50% AQIX® media, 40% FBS and 10% DMSO Hybri-Max™; CM3: 90% AQIX media and 10% UltraPure™ Glycerol (Invitrogen, Carlsbad, CA); CM4: CryoScarless DMSO-Free media (BioVerde, Kyoto, Japan). The freezing media was added gently to the cells and transferred to sterile Nalgene® cryogenic vials (Sigma-Aldrich, St. Louis, MO). CoolCell® alcohol-free cell freezing containers (Biocision, San Rafael, CA) were used to limit rate of freezing to a −1 °C to −3 °C per minute temperature drop. After 24 h incubation at −70 °C, the cryovials were transferred to −140 °C liquid nitrogen for long term storage. Two cryovials from each cryomedia formulation were recovered after 28 and 56 days for immunophenotyping analysis.

Flow cytometry staining and acquisition

Cells were stained for FC via traditional methods. Briefly, cells were re-suspended in Dulbecco's Phosphate Buffered Saline (DPBS) (GE Healthcare, Logan, UT) and stained with cell viability dye (Life Technologies, Carlsbad, CA) for 15 min on ice. Cells were washed twice by pelleting at 400 g for 5 min, using standard FC buffer (1% BSA (w/v) in DPBS). The samples were then treated with human Fc Block™ (BD Biosciences, Franklin Lakes, NJ) for 15 min at a concentration of 2.5 μg per 1 × 10^6 cells in FC buffer. The samples were washed once, and incubated for 60 min on ice with the antibody cocktail prepared in FC buffer. Following incubation the samples were washed twice with FC buffer and analyzed using LSR Fortessa SORP (BD Biosciences, Franklin Lakes, NJ). Compensation was performed using AbC™

bead kit (Invitrogen, Carlsbad, CA) and fluorescence minus multiple (FMM) controls were employed to benchmark sample background and signal-spillover. A high-throughput sampler (HTS) module was used for sample acquisition.

Mass cytometry staining and acquisition
The cells were stained as previously described [28]. Briefly, in preparation for staining with Lanthanide-conjugated antibodies, the samples were resuspended and incubated for 30 min at 37 °C with Cell-Staining-Medium (CSM) and 1X ^{103}Rh DNA Intercalator (both Fluidigm, San Francisco, CA) at a concentration of 1×10^6 viable cells/mL. The samples were pelleted by centrifugation at 400 g for 5 min at RT and incubated for 20 min at RT with 10 μl of human TruStain FcX™ (BioLegend, San Diego, CA). A mixture of antibodies, using vendor specified concentrations as well as concentrations determined by single stain titration (data not shown), in CSM, was added to a final volume of 100 μl/well. The samples were incubated with staining antibodies for 60 min at 4 °C with gentle vortexing. The samples were washed twice and incubated for 60 min at 4 °C with Fix/Perm buffer containing 1x ^{191,193}Ir DNA Intercalator (both Fluidigm, San Francisco, CA), and then again twice with DPBS and resuspended in Milli-Q® water (Millipore, Billerica, MA). The samples were acquired using CyTOF™, with upgraded mass channel range (CyTOF™ 2, Fluidigm, San Francisco, CA), as previously described [24, 29]. Metal minus multiple (MMM) control samples were used to define positive signals and determine spillover, if any. Daily maintenance and tuning was performed according to manufacturer's instructions [39]. In addition to internal vendor-set calibration procedures, Europium beads were incorporated into daily operation before and after sample analysis, enabling inter-run normalization.

Data analysis
Flow cytometry samples were analyzed using FCS Express 4 Flow RUO (De Novo Software, Glendale, CA). CyTOF™ data was analyzed using Cytobank (Cytobank, Inc., Mountain View, CA) as previously described [40]. Briefly doublets and debris were excluded from analysis using previously described gating schemes [41], and manual gating on bivariate plots allowed for identification of populations of interest using published phenotypes [42]. Similarly exclusion of doublets and debris from FC data was performed using traditional methods in published literature. Positive signals were identified using FMM and MMM controls as well as anti-CD3/CD28 activated PBMCs overexpressing immunoregulatory receptors (IMRs) (data not shown). Pearson product moment correlation (PPMC) was used to compare FC

and MC data sets, with a two tailed p value (GraphPad Software V.6, La Jolla, CA). The data sets were compared using median intensity values measured for common antibodies. Non-hierarchical, clustering of tumor samples was performed using viSNE [43]. Briefly, high-dimensional biological data generated by mass cytometry is reduced to two dimensions using the Barnes-Hut implementation of the t-SNE algorithm [44], and visualized as a traditional scatter plot. Between 10,000 and 40,000 cells were sampled and live singlet cells were used as the parent population, subsequent clustering was performed using markers included in the panel. Expression levels were displayed as median intensities in all viSNE plots.

Results
Determination of mass cytometry inter-run reproducibility
A commercially sourced lot of frozen PBMCs from a single healthy donor were used to optimize CyTOF™ protocols, and to establish inter-assay variability for mass cytometry as assessed by measurements of well-defined immune cell subsets. For all experiments a total of two-million cells were stained per sample. Due to cell loss during sample preparation and CyTOF™ sampling [45], on average 300,000 to 500,000 cells were acquired per run. By adhering to published guidelines for rare-event analysis [46] we chose to exclude subpopulations consisting of less than 100 cellular events. The gating scheme used to identify major cellular subsets is shown in Fig. 1a. Dead cells and doublets were excluded from analysis using previously described methods for MC and FC [41, 47, 48]. CD45 positive cells were used as the parent population for the initial bivariate plot identifying T-cells (CD3+) and B-cells (CD19+). The T-cell compartment was further delineated into helper T-cells (CD3 + CD4+) and cytotoxic T-cells (CD3 + CD8+), whereas B-cell were identified by co-expression of CD19+ and CD45RA+. The CD3-CD19- double negative population was used to identify monocytes (CD14+) and NK-cells (CD14-CD16+), while the dendritic cell (DC) phenotype was characterized by the absence of CD16- and CD14- expression, and positive co-expression of CD11c and HLA-DR. The Log_{10} radial plot (Fig. 1b) summarizes the distribution of these cellular subsets across nine independent assays. Average values for helper-T-cells, cytotoxic-T-cells and NK-cells represented 38.1 ± 3.2, 20.0 ± 3.4 and $16.3\% \pm 3.1\%$ of CD45$^+$ cells respectively, while B-cells, monocytes and MDCs made up a smaller fraction of PBMCs with 7.4 ± 2.1, 10.3 ± 2.5 and $4.1\% \pm 1.0\%$ respectively. This data confirms significant inter-run correlation using MC detection, across nine independent runs.

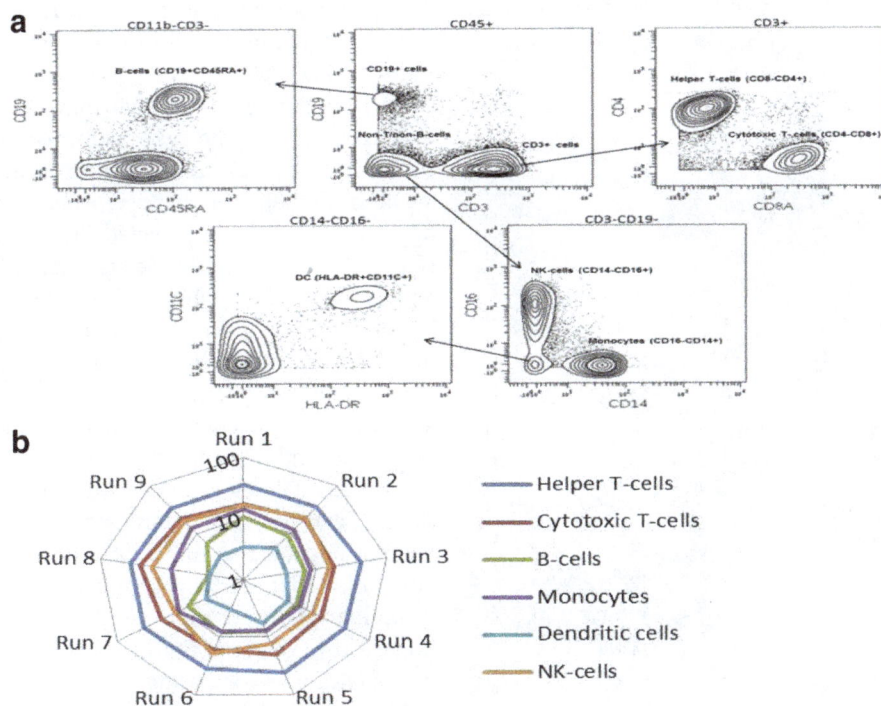

Fig. 1 Determination of inter-run reproducibility of mass cytometry platform (CyTOF2™). **a** Representative gating scheme applied to identification of immune subsets in PBMCs from a single donor. **b** Longitudinal analysis of major immune subsets in CD45+ cells ($N = 9$). Data is expressed as percentage of CD45+ cells on $\log_{10}$ scale

Comparison of MC and FC for frozen PBMC and DTC sample analyses

To further confirm accuracy of mass cytometry detection as compared to flow cytometry, we used the same lot of frozen PBMCs to compare frequencies of cellular subtypes, as determined by both detection methods. The PBMC samples were stained for common cell surface markers, with clonally matched Abs whenever possible for both platforms (Table 1). The number of detection markers was limited to one panel of 15 Abs due to the FC detection limitations [21]. The percentage of positive cells on the bivariate plot of CD45+ and markers common to both platforms was measured in three independent experiments (Fig. 2a). The results obtained using FC and MC detection were compared using PPMC analysis (Fig. 2b), and data indicated a statistically significant agreement in percentage distributions across both platforms as evident by the correlation coefficient (r) value of 0.96 ($p < 0.0001$). These findings are in agreement with previously published reports indicating comparable results between fluorescent and mass cytometry for PBMCs [31, 33].

In order to determine if the correlation between MC and FC observed in a single donor PBMC lot extends to significantly more heterogeneous tumor samples, comparison experiments were conducted using five frozen commercial DTCs. Upon thawing cell suspensions were split for FC and MC analysis, and subsequently further split into staining and control panels. The frequency of positive cells was measured on bivariate plots of CD45+ and markers common to both platforms, as detailed in the gating strategy for PBMC analysis (Fig. 2a). For the FC analysis, samples were subdivided into four panels; myeloid, lymphoid and corresponding FMM panels, while MC samples were split into a control MMM panel, and a single staining panel. Due to limited sample availability, only one comparison experiment was feasible for each tumor sample, with acquired cell numbers ranging from 13,000 to 500,000 on either platform (Fig. 3b). The distribution of ratios of percentages of positive cells determined by FC over MC, for each of the 19 common markers, is summarized in Fig. 3a. The correlation between FC and MC detection varied between specimens, with r values ranging from 0.34 to 0.86. The greatest agreement was observed for the ovarian tumor sample with frequency distribution within two-fold of each other, and the corresponding r of 0.86 and $p < 0.0001$ values confirming significant correlation across both detection platforms. The greatest discrepancy in measurements was apparent for the stage I thymus sample, with the FC/MC ratios of the measured populations being greater than three-fold, $r = 0.34$. A detectable difference in percentage of measured populations was also observed between MC and FC analysis for the lung sample

Table 1 Antibody Panels for Flow and Mass Cytometry Analyses

Antibody	Clone		Conjugate for detection		Vendor	
	FC	MC	FC	MC	FC	MC
CD3	UCHT1	UCHT1	BUV737	170Er	BD	FL
CD4	RPA-T4	RPA-T4	PerCPCy5.5	145Nd	BL	FL
CD8a	RPA-T8	RPA-T8	AF 700	146Nd	BL	FL
CD11b	ICRF44	ICRF44	APC-Cy7	144Nd	BL	FL
CD11c	Bu15	Bu15	AF 488	147Nd	BL	FL
CD14	HCD14	M5E2	BV 737	160Gd	BD	FL
CD15	W6D3	W6D3	BV 605	164Dy	BD	FL
CD16	n/a	3G8	n/a	148Nd	n/a	FL
CD19	HIB19	HIB19	AF 800	142Nd	BL	FL
CD25	2A3	2A3	PE	169Tm	BD	FL
CD27	L128	L128	BV 510	155Gd	BD	FL
CD33	n/a	WM53	n/a	158Gd	n/a	FL
CD38	n/a	HIT2	n/a	167Er	n/a	FL
CD44	n/a	BJ18	n/a	166Er	n/a	FL
CD45	HI30	HI30	BUV395	154Sm	BD	FL
CD45RA	n/a	HI100	n/a	143Nd	n/a	FL
CD45RO	n/a	UCHL1	n/a	149Nd	n/a	FL
CD56	HCD56	HCD56	PE-Cy7	176Yb	BL	FL
CD62L	n/a	DREG-56	n/a	153Eu	n/a	FL
CD66b	G10F5	80H3	AF 647	152Sm	BD	FL
CD66	n/a	CD66a-B1.1	n/a	171Yb	n/a	FL
CD80	L307.4	n/a	BV 510	n/a	BD	n/a
CD86	2331	IT2.2	BV 510	156Gd	BD	FL
CD107a	n/a	H4A3	n/a	151Eu	n/a	FL
CD127	A019D5	A019D5	BV 605	165Ho	BL	FL
CD152	n/a	14D3	n/a	161Dy	n/a	FL
CD183	n/a	G025H7	n/a	156Gd	n/a	FL
CD185	n/a	51,505	n/a	171Yb	n/a	FL
CD194	n/a	205,410	n/a	158Gd	n/a	FL
CD196	n/a	G034E3	n/a	141Pr	n/a	FL
CD197	n/a	G043H7	n/a	159 Tb	n/a	FL
CD223	n/a	874,501	n/a	150Nd	n/a	FL
CD273	MIH18	24 F.10C12	BV 711	172Yb	BD	FL
CD274	29E.2A3	29E.2A3	BV 421	175Lu	BL	FL
CD279	EH12.2H7	EH12.2H7	BV 786	175Lu	BL	FL
CD357	621	In-house	PE	159 Tb	BL	FL
TIGIT	MBSA45	n/a	AF 647	n/a	eBio	n/a
KI-67	n/a	Ki-67	n/a	168Er	n/a	FL
HLA-DR	L243	L243	PerCPCy5.5	174Yb	BL	FL
HLA-ABC	G45-2.6	W6-32	PE-Cy7	141Pr	BD	FL
FOXP3	259D	PCH101	AF 488	162Dy	BL	FL

The antibodies used in both fluorescent and mass cytometry were
commercially sourced

Abbreviations: *MC* mass cytometry, *FC* flow cytometry, *AF* Alexa Fluor, *BV*
Brilliant Violet, *BUV* Brilliant Ultra Violet, *FL* Fluidigm, *BL* BioLegend, *BD* BD
Biosciences, *eBio* eBiosciences

($r = 0.77$), with percentages for CD15, CD86 and GITR showing between 4 and 6-fold difference in calculated ratios between platforms.

Further analysis indicated that samples with high correlation across the two platforms also had a greater percentage of viable cells, and this correlation was also significantly better in samples where starting cell numbers were similarly detected by both FC and MC (Fig. 3b). While viability determination by FC employed amine reactive dyes, which are added prior to fixation and permeabilization [49], MC utilized two distinct DNA intercalators; one which is added prior to permeabilazation (^{103}Rh), and a second DNA intercalator ($^{191/193}$Ir) which is added in a buffer containing paraformaldehyde and saponin [50]. Although fixation and permeabilization after cell surface staining is a standard procedure for immunostaining and has minimal consequences to epitope binding, it is possible that tumor cells, already subjected to enzymatic and mechanical dissociation as well as cryopreservation are more sensitive to membrane effects imposed by even brief exposures to detergents [51]. Previous publications comparing FC-based detection of sample viability and cellular enumeration to other methods, reported that poor specimen quality and low cellularity samples generally result in inconsistencies across different methodologies [52, 53]. Thus a combination of both limited cell numbers available for analysis and the inherent differences in cell viability determination methodologies between FC and MC in these samples can partially account for discrepancies in detected positive cell percentages.

Validation of multiparametric MC analysis for biomarker discovery

Consistent results from MC and FC in reproducibility studies using the same sample indicate that both platforms perform similarly in quantifying common leukocyte lineage markers in both PBMC and tumor samples. However, increased multiplexing potential of the MS detection can significantly facilitate the discovery of specific immune cell subsets involved in mediating anti-tumor activity [54, 55]. Applicability of this platform to biomarker discovery and its translational value was evaluated next. A representative example of an in-depth cell population analysis of a fresh renal carcinoma (RCC) tumor enabled by MC detection was performed using a 39 surface marker CyTOF™ panel (Additional file 1). Data in Fig. 4 illustrates median expression levels of selected surface markers in tumor infiltrating lymphocytes (TILs) and identifies distinct subpopulations (Sp) in tumor cells in the RCC sample. Approximately 40,000 single nucleated cells were evaluated by a viSNE analysis [43], using CD45, CD19, CD11B, CD4, CD8A, CD11C, CD34, CD66B,

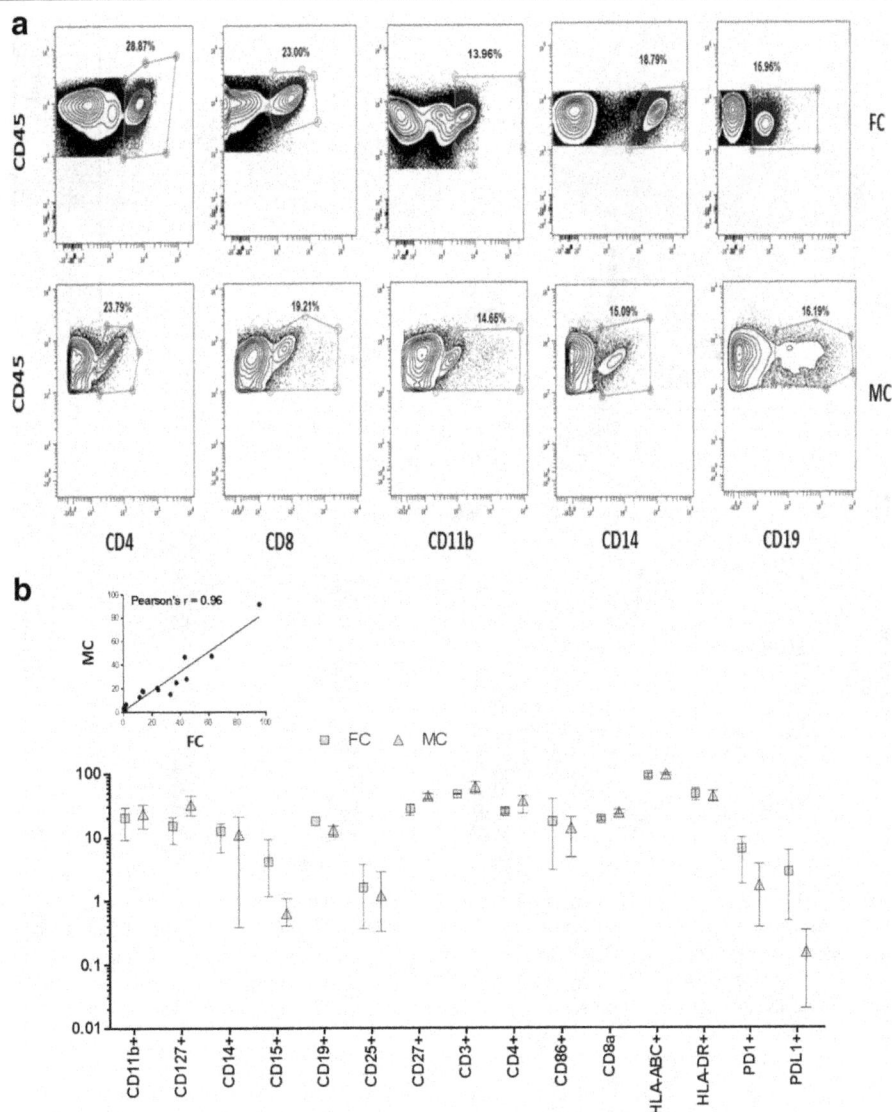

Fig. 2 Detection of cellular subsets in PBMC samples by mass and fluorescent cytometry. **a** Representative gating scheme identifying major immune cell populations in PBMCs by FC and MC. Singlet cells, deemed viable by a Live/Dead marker (FC) or DNA intercalator (MC) were used as the parent population for cell surface marker analysis. Percentage of positive cells on a bivariate plot of CD45 and markers common to both platforms were compared. *Markers* included in analysis: CD11b, CD127, CD14, CD15, CD19, CD25, CD27, CD3, CD4, CD86, CD8a, HLA-ABC, HLA-DR, PD-1 and PD-L1. **b** Comparison of population percentages quantified by FC and MC. Percentages of cells positive for CD45 and *15 common markers* were quantified by both platforms. Data represents $\log_{10}$ (average) ± standard deviation (SD) ($N = 3$) of percent positive cells. Correlation between FC and MC was determined by Pearson Product Moment Correlation (PPMC) ($r = 0.96$, $p < 0.0001$)

CD14, CD15, CD3 and CD56 markers for the cell population clustering. We performed a typical immunophenotyping analysis (Fig. 4a) in which first distinct leukocyte (CD45+) populations are identified, and subsequently expression of both inhibitory (marked by a -) and stimulatory (marked by a +) checkpoint receptors [56] are evaluated on these subsets. Data demonstrates that T-and NK cell subsets comprise a large percentage of TILs, and indicates that inhibitory check point receptors are predominantly co-expressed by CD56 and CD8 positive cells. Our findings are in agreement with other published reports [57–59] and can be used not only in the biomarker discovery, but also benchmarking responsive patient population in the clinical settings. While immunophenotyping of solid tumors is not unique to MC, and has been reported using FC both in the research and clinical settings [19, 60], the maximum number of analytes by FC still remains well below of total of 39 markers used in our studies, as well as reported by others [61], Taking advantage of all the markers in our panel beyond identifying leukocyte phenotypes we extended

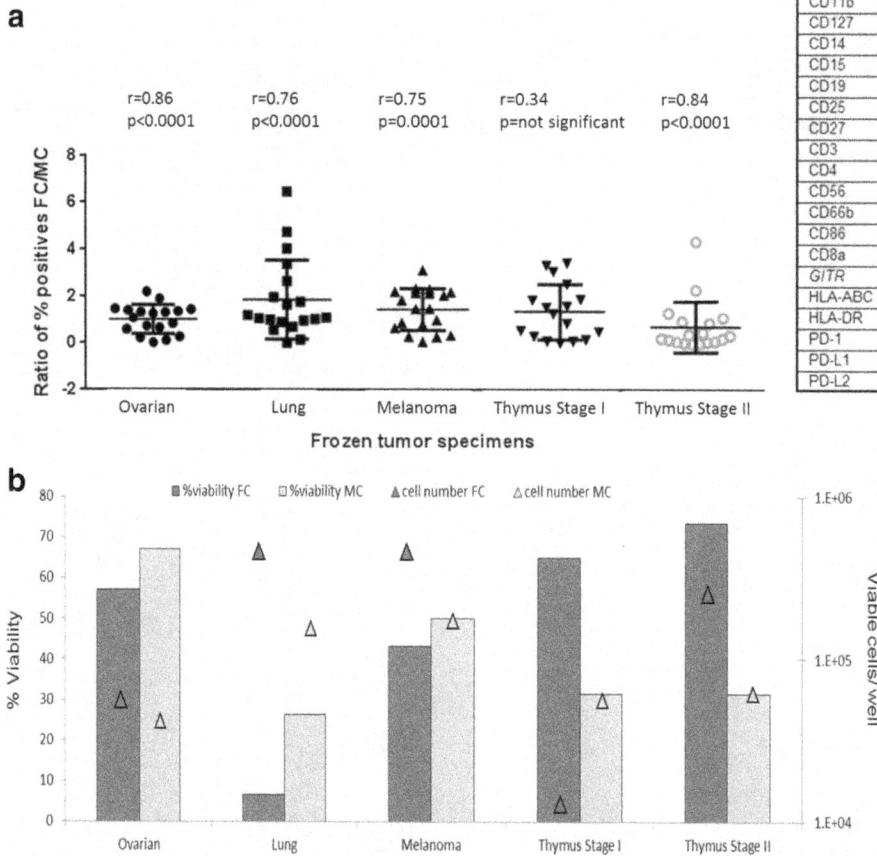

Fig. 3 Comparison of FC and MC detection of immunophenotyping markers in frozen primary tumor samples. **a** Ratio of percent positive cells detected by FC over MC for 19 common markers. Correlation between FC and MC was determined by Pearson Product Moment Correlation (PPMC). **b** Cell number and viability measurements. Viability and cell number as determined by FC analysis using an amine-reactive dye. Viability and number of acquired events as determined by MC analysis using ^{103}Rh and $^{191/193}$Ir DNA intercalators. Cellular counts are expressed on a $\log_{10}$ scale. Data indicate that the viability and cell number differences acquired using FC and MC were major contributing factors in divergence of detected cellular frequencies in tumor samples

this analysis to the tumor cells (Fig. 4b). Sp1 cells were marked by expression of CD34, CD107a (LAMP-1) and HLA-ABC, while Sp2 cells expressed CD199 (CCR9), PD-L2, CTLA, CD56 (NCAM), PD-L1 and PD-L2. Sp1 and Sp2 made up 39.59 and 22.44% of the tumor cells respectively. These data indicate that analysis of fresh clinical specimens using high multiplexing capabilities of CyTOF™ can provide insights into tumor cell microenvironment, thus enabling in-depth studies of complex interplay between tumor cells and infiltrating immune cells, and potentially elucidating novel targets for immunotherapy. This analysis was also applied to fresh colorectal carcinoma (CRC) specimen (Additional file 2) with similar findings.

Effects of cryopreservation on cell viability, and lymphoid and myeloid cell lineages detection in tumor samples

The effects of cryopreservation on clinical specimens resulting in loss and/or alteration of multiple cell surface and intracellular marker detection, has long been a

challenge for accurate sample immunophenotyping on different detection platforms, potentially hindering determinations of immune cell subpopulations relevant to patient stratification [62]. These changes might be due to decrease in either receptor expression levels or modifications in epitope conformation rendering these no longer accessible to detection antibodies. With the emergence of high-multiplexing detection of 50 or more markers by mass cytometry, the overall effect of cryopreservation can be now effectively interrogated on a single cell level.

In order to determine cryopreservation effects associated with long-term storage of tumor samples, an immunophenotypic analysis of fresh tumor specimens immediately after tissue dissociation was performed and compared to the samples analyzed on day 28 (T1) and 58 (T2) after cryopreservation. For this analysis fresh primary RCC and CRC were obtained and processed within 12 h after surgical removal. The tumor specimens

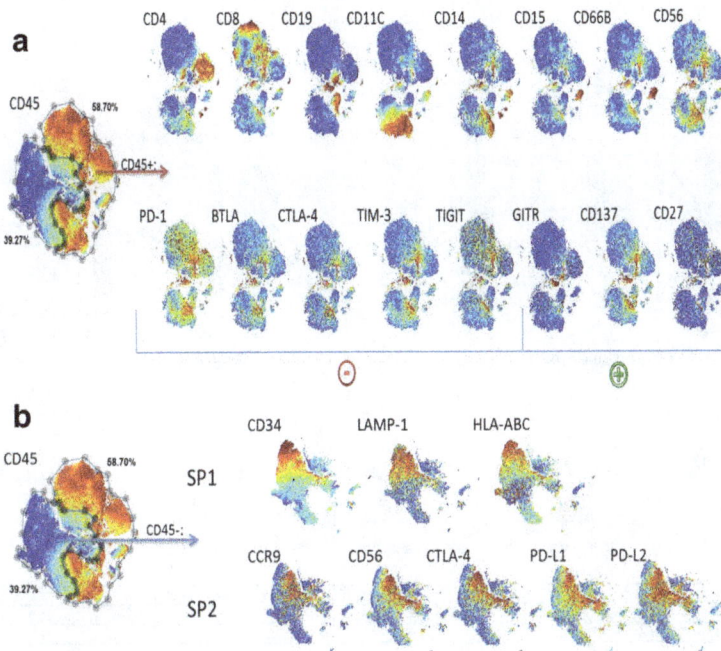

Fig. 4 MC analysis of expression patterns of immunomodulatory and disease prognostic biomarkers in immune and tumor cell subsets. ViSNE analysis of fresh renal cell carcinoma performed using single nucleated cells as top level population. A total of 40,000 cells was analyzed and clustered using the following markers: CD45, CD19, CD11B, CD4, CD8A, CD11C, CD34, CD66B, CD14, CD15, CD3 and CD56. The cells in the ViSNE map are colored according to the median intensity of expression for markers as identified in the top left corner of each figure. **a** Immunophenotyping of CD45+ cells in solid tumor sample. T-cell subsets are identified by expression of CD4 and CD8 markers, B-cells by expression of CD19, NK cell by CD56+, DC cells by CD11C+, Monocytes CD14+, Neutrophils CD15+, and MDSC by CD15+/CD66B+. Checkpoint regulatory receptors are represented by inhibitory (PD-1, BTLA, CTLA-4, TIM-3, and TIGIT) and stimulatory (GITR, CD137, CD27) markers on identified cellular subsets. **b** Immunophenotyping of CD45- cells in solid tumor sample. Specific subsets (Sp) were identified based on these expression patterns; Sp1: CD34^{bright}, CD107a$^+$, HLA-ABC$^+$, HLA-DR^{mid}. Sp2: CCR9$^+$, CD56$^+$, CTLA-4$^+$, PD-L1$^+$, PD-L2$^+$

were greater than 2.0 g in mass. Dissociated cells were used for immediate analysis, and remaining cells were cryopreserved and used in subsequent experiments. 30 to 50 million cells were obtained per tumor sample, allowing for at least four vials containing 2–3 million cells per CM formulation to be frozen. Viability and cell numbers were assessed by Trypan blue exclusion immediately after tumor dissociation and at both recovery time points (Fig. 5a). Decrease in cell viability upon cryopreservation was evident for both RCC and CRC samples (Fig. 5a). The commonly used cryopreservation medium, CM1, containing 90 FBS and 10% tissue grade neat DMSO, was the most effective in preserving cell viability for both tumor types, with approximately 80% of viable cells for both time points. In contrast, samples frozen with 90 FBS and 10% of glycerol (CM3) had viability below 60% at both time points for both tumor types. CM2 formulation contained conditioned media in which the tumors were stored following excision until processing, and the viability for both time points was above 70% at T1 and T2 for both tumor types. Under this condition, the viability measured for the RCC sample was 81.8 and 81.1%, while for the CRC samples the

measured viability was 72.2 and 75.0% at T1 and T2 respectively. Because commercial AQIX media is optimized for preservation of cells and tissue biopsies [63], it is possible that the ability of this media to maintain pH levels at fluctuating temperatures [64], as well as the tissue specific growth factors secreted by cells while in transit, are responsible for preserving cellular viability. CM4, a serum-free, DMSO-free commercial media supplemented with a proprietary cryoprotectant was marked by a decrease in viability for the CRC sample measuring values at T1 of 76.7 and T2 of 66.7%. The viability of the RCC sample as compared to CRC was better with 74.3 viability at T1, and 88.0% at T2.

Although cell viability was best maintained with CM1 media, there still was a significant loss in total cell numbers as observed during both recovery time points. For the RCC sample, close to 90% of cells were lost from T1 to T2 post-freeze thaw time point as compared to other CM formulations. The CRC sample appeared to be more stable during cryopreservation, and cell recovery varied among the different media tested. The greatest decline in cell recovery from first to second thaw was observed with CM4, showing a 94% cell loss (Fig. 5a), while total

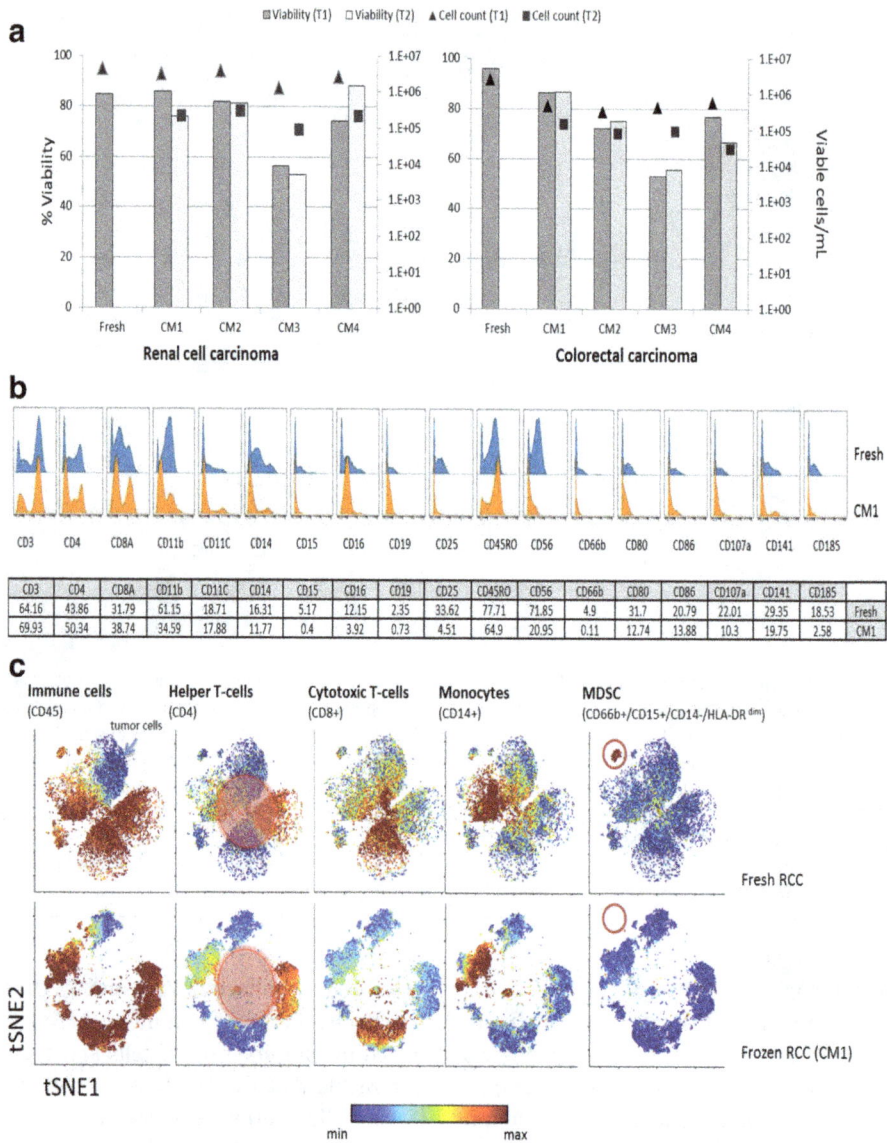

CD3	CD4	CD8A	CD11b	CD11C	CD14	CD15	CD16	CD19	CD25	CD45RO	CD56	CD66b	CD80	CD86	CD107a	CD141	CD185	
64.16	43.86	31.79	61.15	18.71	16.31	5.17	12.15	2.35	33.62	77.71	71.85	4.9	31.7	20.79	22.01	29.35	18.53	Fresh
69.93	50.34	38.74	34.59	17.88	11.77	0.4	3.92	0.73	4.51	64.9	20.95	0.11	12.74	13.88	10.3	19.75	2.58	CM1

Fig. 5 Cryopreservation effects on cellular viability and cell number recovery in renal cell carcinoma and colorectal carcinoma. **a** Viability and cell number determined by Trypan blue exclusion. For each tumor type 2–3 million cells per vial were frozen and samples were recovered in 10 mL complete media. Determinations of viable cells/mL are shown on a log_{10} scale. **b** Cryopreservation effects on surface marker detection and cellular subset identification in primary renal cell carcinoma. Comparison between fresh and CM1-cryo preserved renal cell carcinoma samples is expressed as histogram overlays of surface markers in CD45$^+$ parent population. Percent positive cells as part of CD45+ population associated with selected cell surface markers are summarized in complementary table. **c** ViSNE analysis of fresh and cryopreserved renal cell specimen. The viSNE maps are colored based on median expression of selected cell surface markers, the intensity levels are represented by sliding scale. Equal sampling totaling 25,000 cells for both fresh and frozen specimens was used in this analysis. Singlet-live cells, as determined by cell length and cellular nucleation state, were used as the top level population. Clustering was done using the following markers: CD45, CD19, CD11B, CD4, CD8a, CD11C, CD34, CD66B, CD14, CD15, CD44, CD3, CD56, and CD16. CM1 formulation (T1) was selected for fresh to frozen comparison. Expression of cell surface markers in upper left corner is represented by ViSNE regions colored in gradient of red. Differences in ViSNE scatter plots between fresh and frozen specimens directly highlight differences in expression levels of surface markers used for clustering, and are highlighted by red masking

cell loss measured for other cryomedia formulations was between 65 and 80%.

In addition to cell viability, we examined cryopreservation effects on the expression of common cell surface markers (Fig. 5b). For this analysis, raw median intensities for all surface markers were assessed in the CD45+ cell population. A representation of the different effects of cryopreservation on surface marker expression is depicted as histogram overlays (Fig. 5b). Our data indicates that 24 out of 39 analyzed markers show decreased median intensities upon cryopreservation. The majority of the markers affected by cryopreservation are those used to identify cells of myeloid lineage, such as CD11B, CD14, CD15, CD16, CD66B, CD80, CD86, and CD141. Additionally CD107a and CD25 expression levels are also decreased after cryopreservation. Both of these markers are associated with cellular activation, resulting in functional phenotypes implicated in anti-tumor response [65, 66]. Although most surface markers tested in this study are affected at varying levels, samples preserved in CM1 showed greater median intensities as compared to other cryomedia formulations (Fig. 5b). Expression patterns seen with CM3 had the least agreement with fresh samples. These findings are in alignment with the viability and cell number recovery measurements (Fig. 5a). Considering all aspects of cryopreservation, these data demonstrate that commonly used 90 FBS-10% DMSO formulation, although superior at preserving cellular viability as compared to other CM formulations, still has detrimental effects on expression levels of many surface markers.

To further determine if the observed expression level differences of several cell surface markers between frozen and fresh samples are associated with particular cell subpopulations, we applied a ViSNE analysis using the fresh RCC CM1 frozen sample (Fig. 5c). The resulting scatter plots show differential expression of multiple markers in fresh and frozen samples, thus altering spatial relationships of cells as determined by their phenotypes. While data indicates that Th-cells, Tc-cells and monocytes subpopulations are well identified in frozen cell preparations as compared to fresh samples, it also clearly highlights a specific loss of MDSCs as defined by co-expression of $CD66b^+$ and $CD15^+$, HLA-DR^{dim} and $CD14^-$ phenotype. Similar results have been reported in whole blood sample analysis [62]. Because MDSCs are believed to be involved in regulation of tumor progression [67], preferential decrease in detection of this subpopulation might reduce the value of frozen tumor samples for biomarker research. In addition to common cell surface markers, we have evaluated expression of known immunoregulatory receptors on Th and Tc cell subsets (Additional file 3). Most noticeably, the median intensities of PD-1, its ligands PD-L1 and PD-L2, GITR and Lag-3 are significantly decreased in both T- cell subtypes upon cryopreservation. The observed decrease in median intensity ranged from 2- to 5-fold in all frozen samples, which is in agreement with previous publication using PBMCs [68]. Our results warrant further studies in identifying new cryopreservation media suitable for preserving multiple cellular phenotypes.

Discussion

The ability to quantify effects of therapeutic intervention in heterogeneous cell populations and to correlate these with clinical outcome is of critical importance for the success of drug discovery and development. However, efficacy data from preclinical studies using animal models or immortalized cell lines does not always translate to clinical efficacy [69, 70], nor does it recapitulate the complex interactions responsible for cellular homeostasis. Simultaneous and quantitative measurement of multiple biomarkers that directly reflect cellular functional status in individual, primary patient cells, is, therefore, highly desired, particularly in immuno-oncology, where a deeper understanding of the complex responses of immune cells to tumors can facilitate discovery of new therapeutics and aid in patient stratification strategies. Mass cytometry, although relatively new to the field of single-cell analysis, has attracted significant interest for its ability to simultaneously profile up to 100 phenotypic and functional markers, enabling in-depth understanding of biomarker complexity [71, 72].

While several landmark studies have shown proof-of-concept [25, 43, 73, 74] of the MC analysis, comprehensive comparison to the gold standard of single cell analysis, flow cytometry, as applied to different samples, including tumors, is still limited. The initial analysis of frozen PBMC single donor sample over 9 independent runs enabled us to systematically evaluate precision and accuracy of analytical performance of the MC platform. The results of this study were in agreement with previously published data [73], and demonstrated that the major immune subsets constituting PBMCs are consistently detected using MC, with inter-run variability for all PBMC subpopulations below two-fold difference across nine runs.

Although we observed significant correlation between FC and MC using PBMC samples, the agreement between the two platforms using frozen tumor samples was variable. A number of factors can be considered to explain discrepancy for several tumor samples. Our data indicate that the samples exhibiting substantial discrepancy were marked by significant differences in acquired cell numbers and differences in viability determinations between FC and MC. Additionally the use of multiple panels required for FC, and overall lower sampling efficiencies reported for MC [73] played potential factors which contributed to variability in detected marker frequencies in both platforms. In contrast, tumor samples exhibiting significant correlation between FC and MC analyses had similar detected viability and acquired cell numbers on either platform. These data indicate that both FC and MC platforms are sensitive to quality and quantity of the analyzed samples, specifically evidenced with the commonly used frozen tumor samples.

To assess applicability of the MC platform for biomarker discovery in clinically relevant specimens, a comprehensive phenotyping analysis of fresh renal carcinoma using 39 simultaneous markers, validating detection of immune cell subtypes and various tumor cell subpopulations, was performed. The high multiplexing capability of CyTOF™ enabled identification of major leukocyte populations, as evaluated by the co-expression of various checkpoint regulators, as well as several tumor subtypes. For example, we were able to identify tumor subpopulations marked by presence of CD34[bright] cells, potentially representing cancer stem cells (CSC), implicated in tumor initiation and progression [75]. However given significant heterogeneity reported in CSCs [76], it is impossible to definitively identify these cells as CSC without including additional markers known to be expressed on tumor initiating cells [77] or performing *in-vitro* experiments assessing functional pluripotent responses of these cells [78]. Regardless of the precise cellular identity of this population, the co-expression of CD107a (Lysosome Associated Membrane Protein-1, LAMP1) might suggest a connection to auto-cytolitic activity of NK cells [79]. We identified additional subpopulations marked by expression of CCR9 which potentially represent a subtype of tumor cells in the process of migrating to the small intestine where the CCR9 ligand, CCL25, is expressed [80, 81]. Furthermore, co-expression of inhibitory molecules CTLA-4, PD-L1 and PD-L2 on these tumor subtypes indicates the complex biology of tumor cells [82], suggesting that targeting multiple checkpoints expressed in particular tumors might have an additive therapeutic benefit. The phenotyping results of fresh clinical biospecimens confirm that these samples present a suitable model for understanding cancer pathophysiology.

As the end goal of this study to explore the use of MC analysis for clinical specimens, we further examined effect of cryopreservation on colon and renal cell carcinoma using four commonly used cryomedia formulations. Detrimental effects on both viability and cellular recovery were apparent using all media formulations, however the traditionally used freezing media of 90 FBS and 10% DMSO, was superior as compared to others, possibly due to DMSO's ability to penetrate cells better than glycerol [83]. Extensive publications documenting detrimental effects of cryopreservation on cells and in particular embryonic stem cells [84, 85] could potentially explain the dramatic cell loss observed in this study. Because enzymatic digestion and mechanical dissociation have been implicated as the major contributing factors in inducing cellular apoptosis upon freezing [86, 87], similar effects, as a result of tissue processing and cryopreservation, may cause the observed decrease in DTC cell numbers. Further studies are required to determine if the observed differences in cryopreservation and recovery are organ and specimen specific, or are due to the sample processing methods.

In addition, cryopreservation affected the expression of many myeloid surface markers, possibly explaining the lack of detection of MDSC as previously described in PBMCs [62, 88]. Furthermore the decreased detection of CD107a and CD25 is particularly concerning as both markers are used to asses cellular activation states, as well as identification of CD25+ Treg cells [9], a subset critical for regulating anti-tumor immune response [89]. Our findings are also in agreement with previously published data documenting a damaging cryopreservation effects on PD-1 and PD-L1 detection in PBMCs [68], and further extend these results to tumor samples.

Conclusion
In summary, our data suggests that results generated by MC are comparable to FC for both PBMC and tumor samples. However, MC analysis offers an improved ability for multiplexing of up to 39 markers. The obvious advantage of highly multiplexed MC capabilities is exemplified by the detection of tumor cells expressing markers potentially valuable for diagnosis, prognosis, assessment of treatment efficacy and patient stratification strategies. As the sensitivity and throughput are further improved of this still-developing platform, it is conceivable that MC could become the primary detection method for interrogation of complex interactions between tumor and immune subtypes at real time from clinical biopsies. This can be particularly critical in developing novel immunomodulatory therapies which are aimed at overcoming cancer resistance [90–92]. However, our data also cautions to the quality of frozen specimens used for biomarker discovery. The loss of specific subpopulations, particularly of those implicated in tumor-related biology, presents a challenge for using frozen clinical specimens for immunomodulatory biomarker studies. While additional studies extending to multiple tumors from various organ sources are needed to further corroborate these findings, the present study with renal and colon carcinomas supports further investment in developing more suitable clinical sample handling.

Additional files

Additional file 1: Supplementary Table 1 provides a list of MC antibodies used for immunophenotyping of fresh and frozen RCC and CRC samples. (DOCX 75 kb)

Additional file 2: Supplemental data for Fig. 4 presents expression patterns of immunomodulatory and disease prognostic biomarkers monitored on immune and tumor cell subsets in fresh CRC as delineated by MC analysis. ViSNE analysis of fresh CRC performed using singlet live cells as top level population. A total of 10,902 events were sampled with cellular clustering performed using CD45, CD3, CD4, CD8a, CD20, CD56, CD11B, CD14, CD11C, and CD16 cell surface markers. Median expression levels of the markers listed in upper right corner of each plot is used for identification of cellular subtypes present in this sample. Expression of CD194 and CD183 on CD45⁻ cells are considered as potential clinical biomarkers, correlating with an advanced disease state and associating with significantly poorer prognosis and an increased metastatic potential of colorectal cancers. (DOCX 785 kb)

Additional file 3: Supplemental data for Fig. 5b provides additional information on cryopreservation effects on IMR expression in primary RCC samples. The data is depicted as histogram overlays of median intensities for selected markers as expressed in Th and Tc-cell subtypes. (DOCX 312 kb)

Author details
[1]Department of Pharmacology, Cellular Pharmacology, Merck and Co. Inc, 33 Avenue Louis Pasteur, Boston 02115, MA, USA. [2]Department of Biology-Discovery, Immunooncology, Merck and Co. Inc, Boston, MA, USA. [3]Department of Chemistry, Capabilities Enhancement, Merck and Co. Inc, Boston, MA, USA.

Abbreviations
Ab: Antibody; ACK: Ammonium-chloride-potassium; AML: Acute myeloid leukemia; BSA: Bovine Serum Albumin; BTLA: B-and T-lymphocyte attenuator; CCL25: C-C motif chemokine ligand 25.; CCR9: C-C motif chemokine receptor 9; CM: Cryopreservation medium; CRC: Colorectal carcinoma; CSC: Cancer stem cells; CSM: Cell-staining-medium; CTLA-4: Cytotoxic T-lymphocyte antigen-4; CyTOF: Cytometry by time-of-flight; DC: Dendritic cells; DMSO: Dimethyl sulfoxide; DPBS: Dulbecco's Phosphate-buffered Saline; DTC: Dissociated tumor cells; FBS: Fetal bovine serum; FC: Fluorescent cytometry (flow cytometry); FMM: Flourescent minus multiple; GITR: Glucocorticoid-induced TNFR-related protein; HTS: High-throughput sampler; IMR: Immunoregulatory receptors; Lag-3: Lymphocyte-activation gene 3; LAMP-1: Lysosomal-associated membrane protein 1; MC: Mass cytometry; MDSC: Myeloid derived suppressor cells; MMM: Metal minus multiple; MS: Mass spectrometry; NAT: Normal adjacent tissue; NCAM: Neural cell adhesion molecule; NK-cells: Natural-killer cells; PBMC: Peripheral blood mononuclear cells; PD-1: Programmed cell death-1; PDL-1: Programmed cell death ligand-1; PDL-2: Programmed cell death ligand 2; PPMC: Pearson product moment correlation; RBC: Red blood cells; RCC: Renal cell carcinoma; RPMI medium: Roswell Park Memorial Institute medium; RT: Room temperature; Sp: Subpopulation; T1 and T2: Time point 1 and time point 2; Tc: T-cytotoxic cells; Th: T-helper cells; TIL: Tumor infiltrating lymphocyte; TIL: Tumor infiltrating lymphocyte; Treg: T-regulatory cells

Acknowledgements
Not applicable.

Funding
Not applicable.

Authors' contributions
EK was instrumental in conception, design and carrying out all mass cytometry experiments, including data analysis and elucidation, and was a major contributor to manuscript preparation. RJM performed all flow cytometry experiments, data analysis and interpretation, as well as manuscript editing. YH maintained CyTOF platform, performed QC and calibration experiments, and executed on sample acquisition. AC has been instrumental at the initial stages of setting up CyTOF platform, guiding development of detection methods, and manuscript editing. IK provided scientific guidance to experimental design and data analysis, and was a major contributor to manuscript preparation. All authors read and approved the final manuscript.

Competing interests
The authors declare that they have no competing interests.

References
1. De Visser KE, Eichten A, Coussens LM. Paradoxical roles of the immune system during cancer development. Nat Rev Cancer. 2006;6:24–37.
2. Parish CR. Cancer immunotherapy: the past, the present and the future*. Immunol Cell Biol. 2003;81:106–13.
3. Hamid O, Robert C, Daud A, Hodi FS, Hwu W-J, Kefford R, et al. Safety and tumor responses with lambrolizumab (anti-PD-1) in Melanoma. N Engl J Med. 2013;369:134–44.
4. Sliwkowski MX, Mellman I. Antibody therapeutics in cancer. Science. 2013; 341:1192–8.
5. Prieto PA, Yang JC, Sherry RM, Hughes MS, Kammula US, White DE, et al. CTLA-4 blockade with ipilimumab: long-term follow-up of 177 patients with metastatic melanoma. Clin Cancer Res. 2012;18:2039–47.
6. Robert C, Ribas A, Wolchok JD, Hodi FS, Hamid O, Kefford R, et al. Anti-programmed-death-receptor-1 treatment with pembrolizumab in ipilimumab-refractory advanced melanoma: a randomised dose-comparison cohort of a phase 1 trial. Lancet. 2014;384:1109–17.
7. Smyth MJ, Hayakawa Y, Takeda K, Yagita H. New aspects of natural-killer-cell surveillance and therapy of cancer. Nat Rev Cancer. 2002;2:850–61.
8. Domogala A, Madrigal JA, Saudemont A. Natural killer cell immunotherapy: from bench to bedside. Front Immunol. 2015;6:264.
9. Clarke SL, Betts GJ, Plant A, Wright KL, El-Shanawany TM, Harrop R, et al. CD4 + CD25 + FOXP3+ regulatory T cells suppress anti-tumor immune responses in patients with colorectal cancer. Plos One. 2006;1:e129.
10. Mak IW, Evaniew N, Ghert M. Lost in translation: animal models and clinical trials in cancer treatment. Am J Transl Res. 2014;6:114–8.
11. Peterson JK, Houghton PJ. Integrating pharmacology and in vivo cancer models in preclinical and clinical drug development. Eur J Cancer. 2004;40:837–44.
12. Khleif SN, Doroshow JH, Hait WN. AACR-FDA-NCI cancer biomarkers collaborative consensus report: advancing the use of biomarkers in cancer drug development. Clin Cancer Res. 2010;16:3299–318.
13. Goulart BHL, Clark JW, Pien HH, Roberts TG, Finkelstein SN, Chabner BA. Trends in the use and role of biomarkers in phase I oncology trials. Clin Cancer Res. 2007;13:6719–26.
14. Zips D, Thames HD, Baumann M. New anticancer agents: in vitro and in vivo evaluation. In Vivo. 2005;19:1–7.
15. Hayashi K, Masuda S, Kimura H. Analyzing global trends of biomarker use in drug interventional clinical studies. Drug Discov Ther. 2012;6:102–7.
16. Patel SP, Kurzrock R. PD-L1 expression as a predictive biomarker in cancer immunotherapy. Mol Cancer Ther. 2015;14:847–56.
17. Garon EB, Rizvi NA, Hui R, Leighl N, Balmanoukian AS, Eder JP, et al. Pembrolizumab for the treatment of non-small-cell lung cancer. N Engl J Med. 2015;372:2018–28.
18. Orfao A, Schmitz G, Brando B, Ruiz-Arguelles A, Basso G, Braylan R, et al. Clinically useful information provided by the flow cytometric immunophenotyping of hematological malignancies: current status and future directions. Clin Chem. 1999;45:1708–17.
19. Corver WE, Cornelisse CJ. Flow cytometry of human solid tumours: clinical and research applications. Diagn Pathol. 2002;8:249–67.
20. Williams DM, O'Connor S, Grant JW, Marcus RE, Broadbent V. Rapid diagnosis of malignancy using flow cytometry. Arch Dis Child. 1993;68:393–8.
21. Baumgarth N, Roederer M. A practical approach to multicolor flow cytometry for immunophenotyping. J Immunol Methods. 2000;243:77–97.
22. Perfetto SP, Chattopadhyay PK, Roederer M. Seventeen-colour flow cytometry: unravelling the immune system. Nat Rev Immunol. 2004;4:648–55.
23. Miranda-Lorenzo I, Dorado J, Lonardo E, Alcala S, Serrano AG, Clausell-Tormos J, et al. Intracellular autofluorescence: a biomarker for epithelial cancer stem cells. Nat Method. 2014;11:1161–9.
24. Bandura DR, Baranov VI, Ornatsky OI, Antonov A, Kinach R, Lou X, et al. Mass cytometry: technique for real time single cell multitarget immunoassay

based on inductively coupled plasma time-of-flight mass spectrometry. Anal Chem. 2009;81:6813–22.

25. Di Palma S, Bodenmiller B. Unraveling cell populations in tumors by single-cell mass cytometry. Curr Opin Biotechnol. 2015;31:122–9.

26. Bjornson ZB, Nolan GP, Fantl WJ. Single-cell mass cytometry for analysis of immune system functional states. Curr Opin Immunol. 2013;25:484–94.

27. Ornatsky O, Bandura D, Baranov V, Nitz M, Winnik MA, Tanner S. Highly multiparametric analysis by mass cytometry. J Immunol Methods. 2010;361:1–20.

28. Bodenmiller B, Zunder ER, Finck R, Chen TJ, Savig ES, Bruggner RV, et al. Multiplexed mass cytometry profiling of cellular states perturbed by small-molecule regulators. Nat Biotechnol. 2012;30:858–67.

29. Behbehani GK, Bendall SC, Clutter MR, Fantl WJ, Nolan GP. Single-cell mass cytometry adapted to measurements of the cell cycle. Cytometry. 2012;81A: 552–66.

30. Horowitz A, Strauss-Albee DM, Leipold M, Kubo J, Nemat-Gorgani N, Dogan OC, et al. Genetic and environmental determinants of human NK cell diversity revealed by mass cytometry. Sci Transl Med. 2013;5:208ra145.

31. Han L, Qiu P, Zeng Z, Jorgensen JL, Mak DH, Burks JK, et al. Single-cell mass cytometry reveals intracellular survival/proliferative signaling in FLT3-ITD-mutated AML stem/progenitor cells. Cytometry. 2015;87:346–56.

32. Wang L, Abbasi F, Ornatsky O, Cole KD, Misakian M, Gaigalas AK, et al. Human CD4 + lymphocytes for antigen quantification: characterization using conventional flow cytometry and mass cytometry. Cytometry. 2012;81A:567–75.

33. Nicholas KJ, Greenplate AR, Flaherty DK, Matlock BK, Juan JS, Smith RM, et al. Multiparameter analysis of stimulated human peripheral blood mononuclear cells: a comparison of mass and fluorescence cytometry. Cytometry. 2016;89:271–80.

34. Marina Prilutskaya DS, Pustilnik J, Balukova O, Dyakova N, Fenik L. Quality Bio-specimens for novel biomarker discovery. Transl Med. 2012;S1:2–5.

35. Grizzle WE, Bell WC, Sexton KC. Issues in collecting, processing and storing human tissues and associated information to support biomedical research. Cancer Biomark. 2010;9:531–49.

36. Kushnir MM. Are samples in your freezer still good for biomarker discovery? Am J Clin Pathol. 2013;140:287–8.

37. Guibert EE, Petrenko AY, Balaban CL, Somov AY, Rodriguez JV, Fuller BJ. Organ preservation: current concepts and new strategies for the next decade. Transfus Med Hemtother. 2011;38:125–42.

38. Schroy CB, Todd P. A simple method for freezing and thawing cultured cells. Tissue Culture Assoc Manual. 1976;2:309–10.

39. Leipold MD, Maecker HT. Mass cytometry: protocol for daily tuning and running cell samples on a CyTOF mass cytometer JoVE. J Vis Exp. 2012;4398.

40. Chen TJ, Kotecha N. Cytobank: Providing an Analytics Platform for Community Cytometry Data Analysis and Collaboration. Curr Top Microbiol Immunol. 2014;377:127–57.

41. Zunder ER, Finck R, Behbehani GK, Amir ED, Krishnaswamy S, Gonzalez VD, et al. Palladium-based mass tag cell barcoding with a doublet-filtering scheme and single-cell deconvolution algorithm. Nat Protoc. 2015;10:316–33.

42. Maecker HT, McCoy JP, Nussenblatt R. Standardizing immunophenotyping for the human immunology project. Nat Rev Immunol. 2012;12:191–200.

43. Amir ED, Davis KL, Tadmor MD, Simonds EF, Levine JH, Bendall SC, et al. viSNE enables visualization of high dimensional single-cell data and reveals phenotypic heterogeneity of leukemia. Nat Biotechnol. 2013;31:545–52.

44. van der Maaten L, Hinton G. Visualizing data using t-SNE. J Mach Learn Res. 2008;9:2579–605.

45. Bendall SC, Nolan GP, Roederer M, Chattopadhyay PK. A deep profiler's guide to cytometry. Trend Immunol. 2012;33:323–32.

46. Allan AL, Keeney M. Circulating tumor cell analysis: technical and statistical considerations for application to the clinic. J Oncol. 2010;2010:426218.

47. Majonis D, Ornatsky O, Kinach R, Winnik MA. Curious results with palladium- and platinum-carrying polymers in mass cytometry bioassays and an unexpected application as a dead cell stain. Biomacromolecules. 2011;12:3997–4010.

48. Wersto RP, Chrest FJ, Leary JF, Morris C, Stetler-Stevenson M, Gabrielson E. Doublet discrimination in DNA cell-cycle analysis. Cytometry. 2001;46: 296–306.

49. Perfetto SP, Chattopadhyay PK, Lamoreaux L, Nguyen R, Ambrozak D, Koup RA, et al. Amine-reactive dyes for dead cell discrimination in fixed samples. Curr Protoc Cytom. 2010;9:34. CHAPTER:Unit.

50. Ornatsky OI, Lou X, Nitz M, Sheldrick WS, Baranov VI, Bandura DR, et al. Study of cell antigens and intracellular DNA by identification of element-containing labels and metallointercalators using inductively coupled plasma mass spectrometry. Anal Chem. 2008;80:2539–47.

51. Lorent JH, Quetin-Leclercq J, Mingeot-Leclercq M-P. The amphiphilic nature of saponins and their effects on artificial and biological membranes and potential consequences for red blood and cancer cells. Org Biomol Chem. 2014;12:8803–22.

52. Shenkin M, Babu R, Maiese R. Accurate assessment of cell count and viability with a flow cytometer. Cytometry B Clin Cytom. 2007;72:427–32.

53. Kummrow A, Frankowski M, Bock N, Werner C, Dziekan T, Neukammer J. Quantitative assessment of cell viability based on flow cytometry and microscopy. Cytometry A. 2013;83:197–204.

54. Behbehani GK, Samusik N, Bjornson ZB, Fantl WJ, Medeiros BC, Nolan GP. Mass cytometric functional profiling of acute myeloid leukemia defines cell-cycle and immunophenotypic properties that correlate with known responses to therapy. Canc Discov. 2015;5:988–1003.

55. Atkuri KR, Stevens JC, Neubert H. Mass cytometry: a highly multiplexed single-cell technology for advancing drug development. Drug Metab Dispos. 2015;43:227–33.

56. Le Mercier I, Lines JL, Noelle RJ. Beyond CTLA-4 and PD-1, the generation Z of negative checkpoint regulators. Front Immunol. 2015;6:418.

57. Geissler K, Fornara P, Lautenschläger C, Holzhausen H-J, Seliger B, Riemann D. Immune signature of tumor infiltrating immune cells in renal cancer. Oncoimmunol. 2015;4(1), e985082.

58. Schleypen JS, von Geldern M, Weiß EH, Kotzias N, Rohrmann K, Schendel DJ, et al. Renal cell carcinoma-infiltrating natural killer cells express differential repertoires of activating and inhibitory receptors and are inhibited by specific HLA class I allotypes. Int J Cancer. 2003;106:905–12.

59. Donskov F. Immunomonitoring and prognostic relevance of neutrophils in clinical trials. Sem Cancer Biol. 2013;23:200–7.

60. Lizotte PH, Jones RE, Keogh L, Ivanova E, Liu H, Awad MM, et al. Fine needle aspirate flow cytometric phenotyping characterizes immunosuppressive nature of the mesothelioma microenvironment. Sci Report. 2016;6:31745.

61. Nalin L, Deon BD, Allison RG, Bret CM, Jonathan ML, Justine S, Rondi MK, Jay AW, Akshitkumar MM, Kyle DW, Reid CT, Pierre PM, Mary AH, Mark CK, Lola BC, Rebecca AI, Jonathan MI. Single cell analysis of human tissues and solid tumors with mass cytometry. Cytometry B Clin Cytom. 2017;92: 68–78.

62. Kotsakis A, Harasymczuk M, Schilling B, Georgoulias V, Argiris A, Whiteside TL. Myeloid-derived suppressor cell measurements in fresh and cryopreserved blood samples. J Immunol Methods. 2012;381:14–22.

63. Ozeki T, Kwon MH, Gu J, Collins MJ, Brassil JM, Miller MB, et al. Heart preservation using continuous ex vivo perfusion improves viability and functional recovery. Circ J. 2007;71:153–9.

64. Kay MD, Hosgood SA, Harper SJF, Bagul A, Waller HL, Rees D, et al. Static normothermic preservation of renal allografts using a novel nonphosphate buffered preservation solution. Transpl Int. 2007;20:88–92.

65. Alter G, Malenfant JM, Altfeld M. CD107a as a functional marker for the identification of natural killer cell activity. J Immunol Methods. 2004;294: 15–22.

66. Caruso A, Licenziati S, Corulli M, Canaris AD, De Francesco MA, Fiorentini S, et al. Flow cytometric analysis of activation markers on stimulated T cells and their correlation with cell proliferation. Cytometry. 1997;27:71–6.

67. Gabrilovich DI, Nagaraj S. Myeloid-derived suppressor cells as regulators of the immune system. Nat Rev Immunol. 2009;9:162–74.

68. Campbell DE, Tustin NB, Riedel E, Tustin R, Taylor J, Murray J, et al. Cryopreservation decreases receptor PD-1 and ligand PD-L1 coinhibitory expression on peripheral blood mononuclear cell-derived T cells and monocytes. Clin Vaccine Immunol. 2009;16:1648–53.

69. Crowley Jr WF. Translation of basic research into useful treatments: how often does it occur? Am J Med. 2003;114:503–5.

70. Gillet J-P, Calcagno AM, Varma S, Marino M, Green LJ, Vora MI, et al. Redefining the relevance of established cancer cell lines to the study of mechanisms of clinical anti-cancer drug resistance. Proc Natl Acad Sci U S A. 2011;108:18708–13.

71. Bendall SC, Nolan GP. From single cells to deep phenotypes in cancer. Nat Biotechnol. 2012;30:639–47.

72. Ferrell PB, Diggins KE, Polikowsky HG, Irish JM. Mass cytometry of acute myeloid leukemia captures early therapy response in rare cell subsets. Blood. 2014;124:2381.

73. Yao Y, Liu R, Shin MS, Trentalange M, Allore H, Nassar A, et al. CyTOF supports efficient detection of immune cell subsets from small samples. J Immunol Methods. 2014;415:1–5.

74. Wistuba-Hamprecht K, Martens A, Weide B, Teng KWW, Zelba H, Guffart E, et al. Establishing High Dimensional Immune Signatures from Peripheral Blood via Mass Cytometry in a Discovery Cohort of Stage IV Melanoma Patients. J Immunol. 2017;198:927.

75. Jordan CT, Guzman ML, Noble M. Cancer stem cells. N Engl J Med. 2006; 355:1253–61.

76. Tang DG. Understanding cancer stem cell heterogeneity and plasticity. Cell Res. 2012;22:457–72.

77. Bussolati B, Brossa A, Camussi G, Bussolati B, Brossa A, Camussi G. Resident Stem Cells and Renal Carcinoma, Resident Stem Cells and Renal Carcinoma. Int J Neph. 2011;2011:286985.

78. Lucarelli G, Galleggiante V, Rutigliano M, Vavallo A, Ditonno P, Battaglia M. Isolation and characterization of cancer stem cells in renal cell carcinoma. Urologia. 2015;82:46–53.

79. Cohnen A, Chiang SC, Stojanovic A, Schmidt H, Claus M, Saftig P, et al. Surface CD107a/LAMP-1 protects natural killer cells from degranulation-associated damage. Blood. 2013;122:1411–8.

80. Amersi FF, Terando AM, Goto Y, Scolyer RA, Thompson JF, Tran AN, et al. Activation of CCR9/CCL25 in cutaneous melanoma mediates preferential metastasis to the small intestine. Clin Cancer Res. 2008;14:638–45.

81. Gorski RL, Jalil SA, Razick M, Jalil AA. An obscure cause of gastrointestinal bleeding: renal cell carcinoma metastasis to the small bowel. Int J Sur Case Rep. 2015;15:130–2.

82. Chen L, Flies DB. Molecular mechanisms of T cell co-stimulation and co-inhibition. Nat Rev Immunol. 2013;13:227–42.

83. Farshad A, Khalili B, Fazeli P. The effect of different concentrations of glycerol and DMSO on viability of markhoz goat spermatozoa during different freezing temperatures steps. Pak J Biol Sci. 2009;12:239–45.

84. Bissoyi A, Nayak B, Pramanik K, Sarangi SK. Targeting cryopreservation-induced cell death: a review. Biopreserv Biobank. 2014;12:23–34.

85. Heng BC, Ye CP, Liu H, Toh WS, Rufaihah AJ, Yang Z, et al. Loss of viability during freeze-thaw of intact and adherent human embryonic stem cells with conventional slow-cooling protocols is predominantly due to apoptosis rather than cellular necrosis. J Biomed Sci. 2006;13:433–45.

86. Xu X, Cowley S, Flaim CJ, James W, Seymour L, Cui Z. The roles of apoptotic pathways in the low recovery rate after cryopreservation of dissociated human embryonic stem cells. Biotechnol Prog. 2010;26:827–37.

87. Ohgushi M, Matsumura M, Eiraku M, Murakami K, Aramaki T, Nishiyama A, et al. Molecular pathway and cell state responsible for dissociation-induced apoptosis in human pluripotent stem cells. Cell Stem Cell. 2010;7:225–39.

88. Trellakis S, Bruderek K, Hütte J, Elian M, Hoffmann TK, Lang S, et al. Granulocytic myeloid-derived suppressor cells are cryosensitive and their frequency does not correlate with serum concentrations of colony-stimulating factors in head and neck cancer. I Immunity. 2013;19:328–36.

89. Nishikawa H, Sakaguchi S. Regulatory T cells in tumor immunity. Int J Cancer. 2010;127:759–67.

90. Ishida T, Ueda R. CCR4 as a novel molecular target for immunotherapy of cancer. Cancer Sci. 2006;97:1139–46.

91. Iwai Y, Ishida M, Tanaka Y, Okazaki T, Honjo T, Minato N. Involvement of PD-L1 on tumor cells in the escape from host immune system and tumor immunotherapy by PD-L1 blockade. Proc Natl Acad Sci U S A. 2002;99:12293–7.

92. Van Raemdonck K, Van den Steen PE, Liekens S, Van Damme J, Struyf S. CXCR3 ligands in disease and therapy. Cytokine Growth Factor Rev. 2015;26: 311–27.

2

Cancer immunoprevention: from mice to early clinical trials

Arianna Palladini[1], Lorena Landuzzi[2], Pier-Luigi Lollini[1]*◉ and Patrizia Nanni[1]

Abstract

Cancer immunoprevention is based on the fact that a functioning immune system controls tumor onset and development in humans and animals, thus leading to the idea that the enhancement of immune responses in healthy individuals could effectively reduce cancer risk later in life. Successful primary immunoprevention of tumors caused by hepatitis B and papilloma viruses is already implemented at the population level with specific vaccines. The immunoprevention of human tumors unrelated to infectious agents is an outstanding challenge. Proof-of-principle preclinical studies in genetically-modified or in carcinogen-exposed mice clearly demonstrated that vaccines and other immunological treatments induce host immune responses that effectively control tumor onset and progression, eventually resulting in cancer prevention. While a straightforward translation to healthy humans is currently unfeasible, a number of pioneering clinical trials showed that cancer immunoprevention can be effectively implemented in human cohorts affected by specific cancer risks, such as preneoplastic/early neoplastic lesions. Future developments will see the implementation of cancer immunoprevention in a wider range of conditions at risk of tumor development, such as the exposure to known carcinogens and genetic predispositions.

Keywords: Cancer immunoprevention, Cancer vaccines, Genetically-modified mouse models, HER-2, Oncoantigens

Background

The immune system is a major player in the prevention of diseases. Immunity is best known for the prevention of infectious diseases, however it plays an equally important role in the prevention of tumors. Such a role was first hypothesized half a century ago, but a definitive demonstration came only at the beginning of this century, when it was shown that severely immunodeficient mice invariably develop tumors over time, whereas immunocompetent mice of the same age are tumor-free [1, 2].

While mouse immunologists were struggling to devise appropriate genetically-modified immunodeficient mouse models, human immunologists accumulated evidence on transplant recipients and AIDS patients, showing that, in both cases, human immunodeficiency brought about a strong increase in the risk of virus-related tumors, such as Kaposi sarcoma, caused by human herpesvirus 8, or carcinomas caused by human papilloma viruses [3].

After 50 years of intense research, we have reached general conclusions that apply to humans and mice: any severe, congenital immune deficiency exposes the adult host to a high risk of tumor onset involving all tumor types. Partial or transient immune deficiencies entail a correspondingly reduced tumor risk, possibly limited to specific tumor types, such as highly immunogenic viral tumors [4]. Under non-sterile conditions, severe primary immune deficiencies expose the host to an early septic death, well before the age when the tumor risk would become manifest, hence human cancer risk related to immune deficiency is mostly confined to secondary immune deficiencies and viral tumors [5].

Just as it happens with infectious diseases, the tumor preventive efficacy of the immune system is far from complete and declines with age, thus contributing to the age-related risk of cancer [6]. From a preventive point of view, this leads to the concept of cancer immunoprevention, i.e. the opportunity to further decrease tumor risk through the stimulation of immune defenses [7, 8].

* Correspondence: pierluigi.lollini@unibo.it
[1]Department of Experimental, Diagnostic and Specialty Medicine (DIMES), University of Bologna, Viale Filopanti 22, 40126 Bologna, Italy
Full list of author information is available at the end of the article

Immunoprevention of viral and non-viral tumors

Human cancer immunoprevention is clearly divided in two: on the one hand are tumors related to infectious agents, for which some effective vaccines are already implemented at the population level, even though some difficulties remain, as we shall see. On the other hand are all tumors unrelated to infectious agents (here referred to as noninfectious tumors), which represent the bulk of human tumor burden [9], for which we are beginning to see some early clinical application, after two decades of tantalizing preclinical results in mouse models [10, 11].

One issue that must be clarified in advance is that the notion of cancer prevention, and by extension of cancer immunoprevention, encompasses conceptually different approaches (*see* [12] for a more formal definition of the various types of prevention). *Primary prevention* aims at removing cancer risk factors to reduce tumor incidence. A classic example in the field of chemical carcinogenesis is the avoidance of cigarette smoke, to prevent the onset of lung cancer and many other tobacco-related tumors. Vaccines against oncogenic viruses are a typical example of primary cancer immunoprevention. In the field of primary cancer prevention, the use of drugs that reduce the risk of cancer, for example by preventing exposure to carcinogenic agents, is labeled as chemoprevention. Given that vaccines are drugs, immunoprevention can be also defined as a type of chemoprevention that acts through the immune system [13]. *Secondary prevention* aims at limiting cancer progression toward malignancy, through interventions targeted at early stages of tumor onset. Early diagnosis is the classic human application labeled as secondary prevention, implemented through mass screenings, for example using mammography. However, it must be considered that early diagnosis is only the beginning of secondary prevention, and an early therapeutic intervention is needed to actually avoid progression to malignancy. Thus, immunological treatments applied after an early diagnosis, to prevent tumor progression, are instances of secondary cancer immunoprevention [12].

When one considers that the carcinogenic process is a continuum that goes from a normal tissue to a highly malignant tumor, in some instances it is a matter of definition whether a given intervention should be labeled as primary or secondary prevention. From a practical perspective this can result either in the reduction of incident tumors, through the discovery of lesions labeled as preneoplastic, or in the increase in the number of early neoplastic lesions, eventually producing a higher number of tumor diagnoses. From the point of view of secondary prevention, tumor incidence is not an issue, because what really counts is the decrease in cancer mortality. In this review we will adopt a more conceptual perspective, and we will consider as secondary prevention any intervention taking place after the start of the carcinogenic process, regardless of whether the underlying abnormal tissue is formally labeled as preneoplastic or as early neoplastic.

Prevention of infection-related tumors

Outside of the laboratory, the first successful application of vaccines to the prevention of cancer was in the late 1960s to Marek's disease, an avian leucosis that affected poultry farms, caused by the eponymous herpesvirus MDV [14].

The first human cancer preventive vaccine was against hepatitis B virus (HBV), which in a minority of infected individuals could result in chronic hepatitis, hepatic cirrhosis and eventually hepatocellular carcinoma. The earliest confirmation of the tumor preventive activity of anti-HBV vaccines came from a pediatric Taiwanese cohort, which showed a 70% overall reduction of liver cancer risk, further confirmed in a subsequent long-term re-evaluation [15].

Worldwide implementation of HBV vaccination programs in the 1980s thus represents the first instance of mass cancer immunoprevention. It might be objected that prevention of acute HBV infection is the *raison d'être* of the HBV vaccine, and that cancer prevention is just a nice, but secondary, side effect. The point is well taken, but certainly it does not apply to the second wave of cancer preventive vaccines, directed against human papillomaviruses (HPV), which are essentially oncogenic viruses [16], hence any HPV vaccine is by definition aimed at cancer prevention.

Mass vaccination against HPV begun in the late 2000s, thus long-term results for what concerns cancer prevention at the population level are not yet available, but the results of approval trials, which involved tens of thousands of women worldwide, showed near 100% prevention of neoplastic lesions caused by the viral genotypes included in each vaccine [17]. Furthermore, early analyses of national vaccination programs confirm sizeable reductions in HPV prevalence [18], foreboding corresponding reductions in cancer incidence.

In principle, cervical carcinoma could become the first human cancer eradicated by immunoprevention, much as it happened with smallpox in the late 1970s. However, major obstacles must be overcome before this happens. The major one is that in most countries the proportion of subjects vaccinated each year is low, even down to less than 50% in some US states [19]. The reasons of this phenomenon are beyond the scope of this review, but it is clear that, unless the worldwide level of population compliance rises significantly, the hope to eradicate cervical carcinoma through immunoprevention will remain in the realm of dreams.

We still don't have vaccines approved for two major cancer-related infectious agents, hepatitis C virus (HCV) and *Helicobacter pylori*, however there are highly efficacious drugs that can eradicate both, effectively preventing HCV-related hepatocellular carcinoma and gastric cancer (the efficacy of such drugs also hampers the development of vaccines, but again this is a subject beyond the scope of this review). Altogether, we have in our hands the potential to prevent the vast majority of infection-related cancers, which represent about one sixth of the total human cancer burden [9].

Prevention of non-infectious tumors

Conversely, about 85% of all human tumors are unrelated to infectious agents [9]. What are the perspectives of immunoprevention in such cases?

If one looks at animal models of cancer, the problem is already solved: many researchers, including ourselves, have demonstrated time and again that a variety of immunological treatments, administered to healthy, cancer-prone mice, effectively prevent the onset of tumors later in life [13, 20]. So, what are the obstacles to an immediate translation to humans of the results obtained in mice?

The dirty little trick in all animal studies of cancer immunoprevention is that the researchers know *in advance* which type of tumor will arise in their mice, and when it will appear, whereas humans are exposed to the risk of many different tumor types over several decades of their life. Basically, this means that in the near future we are not going to have a generic "vaccine against cancer" to be administered to all children to reduce their lifetime risk of cancer. However, there are several human cohorts subject to a predictable and measurable risk of a known tumor, who could greatly benefit from the implementation of specific vaccination programs.

In the following sections we will first summarize the results of preclinical studies, then we will examine some examples of the earliest clinical trials of cancer immunoprevention.

Cancer immunoprevention in mice

The two major types of mouse models used to investigate cancer immunoprevention are conventional mice treated with carcinogens and cancer-prone genetically-modified mice [13, 20]. Most studies in the past 20 years used genetically-modified mice, mirroring the generalized success of these model systems in all fields of biomedical research [21]. The standard experiment sees young, tumor-free mice undergoing immunological maneuvers that delay tumor onset later in life, or result in a lower incidence of tumors.

Positive results were obtained against a myriad of cancer types, using either passive approaches, e.g. administration of monoclonal antibodies, or active stimuli, which in turn included antigen-specific vaccines, or non-antigen-specific treatments, such as cytokines or other immunostimulants [2, 13, 20, 22]. It could be concluded that, in mice prone to cancer, immunoprevention is generally doable and is not dependent on model-specific or treatment-specific experimental conditions [13, 20, 23].

The analysis of protective immunological responses revealed some differences with those elicited by vaccines used in cancer immunotherapy, which are mainly focused on cytotoxic T lymphocytes (CTL). Many studies showed a relevant role for helper T cells, B cells and their products, i.e. cytokines and antibodies [24]. A major determinant could be the different time frame of immunoprevention in comparison to immunotherapy. In fact, immunoprevention entails immune responses that must be ideally active during the entire life of the host, and mouse experiments typically last from several months to more than one year. Under these conditions a prolonged CTL response would probably produce relevant toxic side effects, whereas the humoral response can persist indefinitely at protective levels without harm for the host. A similar dichotomy is encountered in viral immunity: in most instances the cure of acute infection requires the CTL response, whereas natural prevention of reinfection and vaccine efficacy are mainly dependent on antibodies [25].

Target antigens

A specific aspect of cancer immunoprevention in relation to cancer immunotherapy is the choice of target antigens [26]. In the field of cancer immunotherapy there is currently much interest for neoantigens, i.e. random alterations of normal molecules resulting from the carcinogenic processes [27]. However the intrinsically unpredictable nature of neoantigens makes them unsuitable as targets in cancer immunoprevention. It has been argued that the best targets for cancer immunoprevention are oncoantigens, i.e. those molecules that are causally involved in the carcinogenic process, because their inhibition in preneoplastic lesions or in early tumors offers the opportunity to block tumor progression and minimizes the emergence of antigen-loss variants [2, 28–30].

The ideal target antigen for cancer immunoprevention would be a molecule expressed only by neoplastic or preneoplastic cells, however only a few molecules fulfill this requirement, such as MUC1, which is differentially glycosylated in normal and neoplastic cells [31, 32], or HPV-encoded molecules in HPV-infected people. In most instances the target antigen would be expressed also by some normal cells. In this case an important issue is the physiological role of the target antigen, because (auto)immune responses directed against targets that play a relevant role in the biology of the healthy adult host are bound to provoke intolerable toxicities. Under this respect, the HER-2 oncogene, which was extensively studied both in mice and in humans, is a good choice, because its most important physiological role appears to be during heart embryogenesis [33], whereas long-term inhibition in adults, as it happens during monoclonal antibody therapy of breast cancer, is well tolerated in the vast majority of patients [34]. Such antigens would traditionally be labeled as oncofetal antigens, but more recently the term "retired antigens" has been proposed in relation to cancer immunoprevention [35].

Early clinical trials

We will examine here some early clinical trials demonstrating that cancer immunoprevention is indeed translatable to appropriate human contexts. A detailed discussion of the countless clinical trials in which vaccines were tested as therapeutic agents against established human tumors goes beyond the scope of this review, in particular because most therapeutic cancer vaccines of the past had limited efficacy against existing human tumors [20, 36]. A renaissance of therapeutic cancer vaccines is currently being fostered by the molecular definition of novel antigens (neoantigens) appearing in individual tumors as a consequence of extensive mutational events in the genome ("mutanome") [37]. New therapeutic vaccines are also being combined with immunomodulatory monoclonal antibodies [37], such as those against CTLA-4, PD-1 and PD-L1 already in clinical use, to remove immunosuppressive mechanisms ("immune checkpoints") that hamper the induction of effective anti-tumor immune responses [38]. We expect that the analysis of current and forthcoming therapeutic trials will reveal which advances in the field of therapeutic vaccines will be applicable to prophylactic vaccines.

Successful proof-of-principle preclinical studies outlined in the previous sections have opened the way to a few pioneering clinical trials which demonstrate that immunoprevention is indeed feasible in a variety of human conditions at risk of cancer development [30, 39]. It must be kept in mind that cancer prevention trials entail specific hurdles in comparison with therapeutic trials: even in populations at risk, tumor onset is relatively rare, hence large number of volunteers need to be recruited, furthermore, when the subjects harbor preneoplastic or early neoplastic lesions, spontaneous regression is common, even in the absence of any treatment, mandating the need for controlled trials.

Dr. Olivera J. Finn and Robert E. Schoen in Pittsburgh are investigating anti-MUC1 vaccines for the prevention of colorectal carcinogenesis. A pilot clinical trial assessed vaccine immunogenicity in patients with intestinal polyps [40, 41], paving the way to a currently ongoing trial (ClinicalTrials.gov identifier NCT01720836) that aims at preventing polyp onset in tumor-free individuals who previously had a polyp removed. Immunological studies of patients enrolled in the pilot trial revealed that vaccination elicited tumor-specific, cytotoxic anti-MUC1 antibodies [41], thus providing a human counterpart of the preventive mechanisms found in mouse studies of primary immunoprevention (see above, Cancer immunoprevention in mice).

The introduction of prophylactic HPV vaccination of girls should not obscure the fact that millions of adult women worldwide harbor a chronic HPV infection that natural immune responses were unable to eradicate, exposing them to a sizeable risk of cervical carcinoma [39]. Prophylactic HPV vaccines, directed against late (L) HPV proteins, lack therapeutic activity against chronic HPV infections [42], thus underlining the need for therapeutic vaccines targeting early (E) HPV proteins [43–45]. One such vaccine, made of electroporated plasmids encoding HPV16/18 oncogenes E6 and E7, increased the occurrence of cervical intraepithelial neoplasia (CIN) regression and of HPV clearance in women harboring HPV-positive CIN 2 or CIN 3 [45].

In mammary carcinogenesis the most obvious target for cancer immunoprevention is HER-2. A neoadjuvant clinical trial conducted in women with HER-2-positive ductal carcinoma in situ (DCIS) undergoing resection within 4–6 weeks showed that the administration of autologous dendritic cells pulsed with HER-2 peptides in vitro elicited anti-HER-2 immune responses in most patients. At surgery, one fourth of all patients had complete tumor regression, the best results was in the ER-negative group, with 38% of complete tumor regressions [46]. Other ongoing vaccination trials are testing an immunodominant HER-2 peptide (nelipepimut-S, also known as E75) in combination with granulocyte-macrophage colony stimulating factor either in a neoadjuvant setting against DCIS (ClinicalTrials.gov NCT02636582) or to prevent the development of metastases after conventional therapy in more advanced, node-positive patients (ClinicalTrials.gov NCT01479244).

A further area in which immunoprevention is already being tested in the clinical arena is that of hematopoietic diseases at risk of progression. After an early clinical trial as single agent [47] a multiepitopic peptide vaccine is being tested in patients with smoldering myeloma in combination with other therapeutic agents to prevent progression to multiple myeloma (ClinicalTrials.gov NCT02886065).

Conclusions and perspectives

The results of countless mouse studies have demonstrated that the risk of cancer development can be significantly reduced by appropriate treatments that enhance immune defenses.

Primary cancer immunoprevention in healthy humans is currently restricted to tumors related to infectious agents, such as HBV and HPV, which cause about one-sixth of the whole tumor burden. Primary prevention of tumors unrelated to infectious agents is presently unfeasible in the general human population, mainly because it would require vaccines completely devoid of significant toxicities that should confer long-term protection against the risk of a wide spectrum of tumors histotypes. Some hope in this direction comes from the possibility to elicit immune responses against the products of some common mutations in cancer genes, such as RAS or dominant negative p53 [48, 49], but proof-of-principle results in humans are still lacking.

A series of pioneering clinical trials have shown that immunoprevention can be successfully applied to selected human groups in which the risk of a specific tumor type is much higher than in the general population.

Future developments of these concepts might lead to a widespread implementation of cancer immunoprevention, because epidemiological, molecular and genetic studies of the past 100 years have uncovered a huge number of human beings with specific cancer risks, including individuals previously exposed to potent carcinogens, such as asbestos workers or tobacco smokers; patients with preneoplastic or early neoplastic conditions at risk of progression; individuals with genetic predispositions, like microsatellite instability or BRCA mutations.

Finally, most lifestyles (e.g. diet, physical activity) and chemopreventive treatments conducive to reductions in cancer risk also seem to have beneficial effects on the immune system [50], leading to the prediction that complex preventive regimes combining behavioral, chemopreventive and immunopreventive components could have additive or synergistic effects.

Abbreviations
AIDS: Acquired immune deficiency syndrome; CIN: Cervical intraepithelial neoplasia; CTL: Cytotoxic T lymphocytes; HBV: Hepatitis B virus; HPV: Human papillomavirus

Acknowledgments
This paper is dedicated to the memory of Giorgio Prodi, thirty years after his untimely demise.

Funding
The research of the authors is funded by the Italian Association for Cancer Research (AIRC), grant IG15324 to PLL, by the University of Bologna (Pallotti Fund) and by the Italian Ministry of Health "Ricerca Finalizzata 2013".

Authors' contributions
PLL drafted the manuscript; AP, LL and PN were involved in research projects covered in this review article and participated in the preparation of the manuscript. All authors read and approved the final manuscript.

Competing interests
The authors declare that they have no competing interests.

Author details
[1]Department of Experimental, Diagnostic and Specialty Medicine (DIMES), University of Bologna, Viale Filopanti 22, 40126 Bologna, Italy. [2]Laboratory of Experimental Oncology, Rizzoli Orthopaedic Institute, Via di Barbiano 1/10, 40136 Bologna, Italy.

References
1. Shankaran V, Ikeda H, Bruce AT, White JM, Swanson PE, Old LJ, Schreiber RD. IFNgamma and lymphocytes prevent primary tumour development and shape tumour immunogenicity. Nature. 2001;410:1107–11. https://doi.org/10.1038/35074122.
2. Roeser JC, Leach SD, McAllister F. Emerging strategies for cancer immunoprevention. Oncogene. 2015;34:6029–39. https://doi.org/10.1038/onc.2015.98 .
3. Vajdic CM, van Leeuwen MT. Cancer incidence and risk factors after solid organ transplantation. Int J Cancer. 2009;125:1747–54. https://doi.org/10.1002/ijc.24439 .
4. Corthay A. Does the immune system naturally protect against cancer? Front Immunol. 2014;5:197. https://doi.org/10.3389/fimmu.2014.00197 .
5. Grulich AE, Vajdic CM. The epidemiology of cancers in human immunodeficiency virus infection and after organ transplantation. Semin Oncol. 2015;42:247–57. https://doi.org/10.1053/j.seminoncol.2014.12.029 .
6. Fulop T, Larbi A, Witkowski JM, Kotb R, Hirokawa K, Pawelec G. Immunosenescence and cancer. Crit Rev Oncog. 2013;18:489–513.
7. Lollini P-L, Nanni P. Immunoprevention. In: Schwab M, editor. Encyclopedia of cancer. 4th ed. Berlin Heidelberg: Springer-Verlag; 2017. p. 2223–8.
8. Umar A. Cancer immunoprevention: a new approach to intercept cancer early. Cancer Prev Res (Phila). 2014;7:1067–71. https://doi.org/10.1158/1940-6207.CAPR-14-0213 .
9. de MC, Ferlay J, Franceschi S, Vignat J, Bray F, Forman D, Plummer M. Global burden of cancers attributable to infections in 2008: a review and synthetic analysis. Lancet Oncol. 2012;13:607–15. https://doi.org/10.1016/S1470-2045(12)70137-7 .
10. Chu NJ, Armstrong TD, Jaffee EM. Nonviral oncogenic antigens and the inflammatory signals driving early cancer development as targets for cancer immunoprevention. Clin Cancer Res. 2015;21:1549–57. https://doi.org/10.1158/1078-0432.CCR-14-1186 .
11. Smit M-AD, Jaffee EM, Lutz ER. Cancer immunoprevention–the next frontier. Cancer Prev Res (Phila). 2014;7:1072–80. https://doi.org/10.1158/1940-6207.CAPR-14-0178 .
12. Lollini P-L, Cavallo F, Nanni P, Quaglino E. The promise of preventive Cancer vaccines. Vaccines (Basel). 2015;3:467–89. https://doi.org/10.3390/vaccines3020467 .
13. Lollini P-L, Nicoletti G, Landuzzi L, Cavallo F, Forni G, De Giovanni C, Nanni P. Vaccines and other immunological approaches for cancer immunoprevention. Curr Drug Targets. 2011;12:1957–73.
14. Schat KA. History of the first-generation Marek's disease vaccines: the science and little-known facts. Avian Dis. 2016;60:715–24. https://doi.org/10.1637/11429-050216-Hist .
15. Chang M-H, You S-L, Chen C-J, Liu C-J, Lee C-M, Lin S-M, et al. Decreased incidence of hepatocellular carcinoma in hepatitis B vaccinees: a 20-year follow-up study. J Natl Cancer Inst. 2009;101:1348–55. https://doi.org/10.1093/jnci/djp288 .
16. Zur Hausen H. Papillomaviruses and cancer: from basic studies to clinical application. Nat Rev Cancer. 2002;2:342–50. https://doi.org/10.1038/nrc798 .
17. Joura EA, Giuliano AR, Iversen O-E, Bouchard C, Mao C, Mehlsen J, et al. A 9-valent HPV vaccine against infection and intraepithelial neoplasia in women. N Engl J Med. 2015;372:711–23. https://doi.org/10.1056/NEJMoa1405044 .
18. Brotherton JML, Fridman M, May CL, Chappell G, Saville AM, Gertig DM. Early effect of the HPV vaccination programme on cervical abnormalities in

Victoria, Australia: an ecological study. Lancet. 2011;377:2085–92. https://doi.org/10.1016/S0140-6736(11)60551-5 .

19. Stokley S, Jeyarajah J, Yankey D, Cano M, Gee J, Roark J, et al. Human papillomavirus vaccination coverage among adolescents, 2007-2013, and postlicensure vaccine safety monitoring, 2006-2014–United States. MMWR Morb Mortal Wkly Rep. 2014;63:620–4.

20. Lollini P-L, Cavallo F, Nanni P, Forni G. Vaccines for tumour prevention. Nat Rev Cancer. 2006;6:204–16. https://doi.org/10.1038/nrc1815 .

21. Fry EA, Taneja P, Inoue K. Clinical applications of mouse models for breast cancer engaging HER2/neu. Integr Cancer Sci Ther. 2016;3:593–603. https://doi.org/10.15761/ICST.1000210 .

22. Finn OJ. Vaccines for cancer prevention: a practical and feasible approach to the cancer epidemic. Cancer Immunol Res. 2014;2:708–13. https://doi.org/10.1158/2326-6066.CIR-14-0110 .

23. Lollini P-L, De Giovanni C, Nanni P. Preclinical HER-2 vaccines: from rodent to human HER-2. Front Oncol. 2013;3:151. https://doi.org/10.3389/fonc.2013.00151 .

24. Nanni P, Landuzzi L, Nicoletti G, De Giovanni C, Rossi I, Croci S, et al. Immunoprevention of mammary carcinoma in HER-2/neu transgenic mice is IFN-gamma and B cell dependent. J Immunol. 2004;173:2288–96.

25. Ada G. Vaccines and vaccination. N Engl J Med. 2001;345:1042–53. https://doi.org/10.1056/NEJMra011223 .

26. Wojtowicz ME, Dunn BK, Umar A. Immunologic approaches to cancer prevention-current status, challenges, and future perspectives. Semin Oncol. 2016;43:161–72. https://doi.org/10.1053/j.seminoncol.2015.11.001 .

27. Schumacher TN, Hacohen N. Neoantigens encoded in the cancer genome. Curr Opin Immunol. 2016;41:98–103. https://doi.org/10.1016/j.coi.2016.07.005 .

28. Lollini P-L, Cavallo F, De Giovanni C, Nanni P. Preclinical vaccines against mammary carcinoma. Expert Rev Vaccines. 2013;12:1449–63. https://doi.org/10.1586/14760584.2013.845530 .

29. Spira A, Disis ML, Schiller JT, Vilar E, Rebbeck TR, Bejar R, et al. Leveraging premalignant biology for immune-based cancer prevention. Proc Natl Acad Sci U S A. 2016;113:10750–8. https://doi.org/10.1073/pnas.1608077113 .

30. Kensler TW, Spira A, Garber JE, Szabo E, Lee JJ, Dong Z, et al. Transforming Cancer prevention through precision medicine and immune-oncology. Cancer Prev Res (Phila). 2016;9:2–10. https://doi.org/10.1158/1940-6207.CAPR-15-0406 .

31. Vlad AM, Kettel JC, Alajez NM, Carlos CA, Finn OJ. MUC1 immunobiology: from discovery to clinical applications. Adv Immunol. 2004;82:249–93. https://doi.org/10.1016/S0065-2776(04)82006-6 .

32. Ryan SO, Gantt KR, Finn OJ. Tumor antigen-based immunotherapy and immunoprevention of cancer. Int Arch Allergy Immunol. 2007;142:179–89. https://doi.org/10.1159/000097020 .

33. Sanchez-Soria P, Camenisch TD. ErbB signaling in cardiac development and disease. Semin Cell Dev Biol. 2010;21:929–35. https://doi.org/10.1016/j.semcdb.2010.09.011 .

34. Farolfi A, Melegari E, Aquilina M, Scarpi E, Ibrahim T, Maltoni R, et al. Trastuzumab-induced cardiotoxicity in early breast cancer patients: a retrospective study of possible risk and protective factors. Heart. 2013;99:634–9. https://doi.org/10.1136/heartjnl-2012-303151 .

35. Tuohy VK. Retired self-proteins as vaccine targets for primary immunoprevention of adult-onset cancers. Expert Rev Vaccines. 2014;13:1447–62. https://doi.org/10.1586/14760584.2014.953063 .

36. Rosenberg SA, Yang JC, Restifo NP. Cancer immunotherapy: moving beyond current vaccines. Nat Med. 2004;10:909–15. https://doi.org/10.1038/nm1100 .

37. Sahin U, Derhovanessian E, Miller M, Kloke B-P, Simon P, Löwer M, et al. Personalized RNA mutanome vaccines mobilize poly-specific therapeutic immunity against cancer. Nature. 2017;547:222–6. https://doi.org/10.1038/nature23003 .

38. Topalian SL, Taube JM, Anders RA, Pardoll DM. Mechanism-driven biomarkers to guide immune checkpoint blockade in cancer therapy. Nat Rev Cancer. 2016;16:275–87. https://doi.org/10.1038/nrc.2016.36 .

39. Finn OJ, Beatty PL. Cancer immunoprevention. Curr Opin Immunol. 2016;39:52–8. https://doi.org/10.1016/j.coi.2016.01.002 .

40. Kimura T, McKolanis JR, Dzubinski LA, Islam K, Potter DM, Salazar AM, et al. MUC1 vaccine for individuals with advanced adenoma of the colon: a cancer immunoprevention feasibility study. Cancer Prev Res (Phila). 2013;6:18–26. https://doi.org/10.1158/1940-6207.CAPR-12-0275 .

41. Lohmueller JJ, Sato S, Popova L, Chu IM, Tucker MA, Barberena R, et al. Antibodies elicited by the first non-viral prophylactic cancer vaccine show tumor-specificity and immunotherapeutic potential. Sci Rep. 2016;6:31740. https://doi.org/10.1038/srep31740 .

42. Hildesheim A, Herrero R, Wacholder S, Rodriguez AC, Solomon D, Bratti MC, et al. Effect of human papillomavirus 16/18 L1 viruslike particle vaccine among young women with preexisting infection: a randomized trial. JAMA. 2007;298:743–53. https://doi.org/10.1001/jama.298.7.743 .

43. de Vos van Steenwijk PJ, Ramwadhdoebe TH, MJG L, van der Minne CE, der Meer DMA B-v, Fathers LM, et al. A placebo-controlled randomized HPV16 synthetic long-peptide vaccination study in women with high-grade cervical squamous intraepithelial lesions. Cancer Immunol Immunother. 2012;61:1485–92. https://doi.org/10.1007/s00262-012-1292-7 .

44. Kenter GG, Welters MJP, Valentijn ARPM, Lowik MJG, Berends-van der Meer DMA, Vloon APG, et al. Vaccination against HPV-16 oncoproteins for vulvar intraepithelial neoplasia. N Engl J Med. 2009;361:1838–47. https://doi.org/10.1056/NEJMoa0810097 .

45. Trimble CL, Morrow MP, Kraynyak KA, Shen X, Dallas M, Yan J, et al. Safety, efficacy, and immunogenicity of VGX-3100, a therapeutic synthetic DNA vaccine targeting human papillomavirus 16 and 18 E6 and E7 proteins for cervical intraepithelial neoplasia 2/3: a randomised, double-blind, placebo-controlled phase 2b trial. Lancet. 2015;386:2078–88. https://doi.org/10.1016/S0140-6736(15)00239-1 .

46. Fracol M, Xu S, Mick R, Fitzpatrick E, Nisenbaum H, Roses R, et al. Response to HER-2 pulsed DC1 vaccines is predicted by both HER-2 and estrogen receptor expression in DCIS. Ann Surg Oncol. 2013;20:3233–9. https://doi.org/10.1245/s10434-013-3119-y .

47. Nooka AK, Wang M, Yee AJ, Thomas SK, O'Donnell EK, Shah JJ, et al. Final results of a phase 1/2a, dose escalation study of Pvx-410 multi-peptide Cancer vaccine in patients with smoldering multiple myeloma (SMM). Blood. 2016;128:2124.

48. Carbone DP, Ciernik IF, Kelley MJ, Smith MC, Nadaf S, Kavanaugh D, et al. Immunization with mutant p53- and K-ras-derived peptides in cancer patients: immune response and clinical outcome. J Clin Oncol. 2005;23:5099–107. https://doi.org/10.1200/JCO.2005.03.158 .

49. Nasti TH, Rudemiller KJ, Cochran JB, Kim HK, Tsuruta Y, Fineberg NS, et al. Immunoprevention of chemical carcinogenesis through early recognition of oncogene mutations. J Immunol. 2015;194:2683–95. https://doi.org/10.4049/jimmunol.1402125 .

50. Singh SK, Dorak MT. Cancer Immunoprevention and public health. Front Public Health. 2017;5:101. https://doi.org/10.3389/fpubh.2017.00101 .

3

Adverse events following immunization with pentavalent vaccine: experiences of newly introduced vaccine

Manoochehr Karami[1,2]* , Pegah Ameri[2], Jalal Bathaei[3], Zeinab Berangi[2], Tahereh Pashaei[4], Ali Zahiri[3], Seyed Mohsen Zahraei[5], Hussein Erfani[3] and Koen Ponnet[6,7]

Abstract

Background: The most important factors that affect the incidence of vaccine-related complications are the constituent biological components of the vaccine, injection site reactions, age and sex. The aim of this study is to determine the incidence rate of adverse events following immunization with pentavalent vaccine (DTPw-Hep B-Hib (PRP-T) vaccine (pentavac) (adsorbed) is manufactured by Serum Institute of India ltd), which was introduced in Iran in November 2014. It is important to monitor vaccine-related adverse events because of the role of vaccine safety in immunization program success.

Methods: This study was a mixed cohort study that included 1119 children less than 1 year of age. In 2015, the children were referred to Hamadan health centers to receive pentavalent vaccine at 2, 4 and 6 months of age. The data were collected from the parents of the children using a questionnaire that was administered either face-to-face or by telephone. The cumulative incidence of side effects and risk ratio was reported with 95% confidence intervals (CI). Chi-squared tests and logistic regressions were used to investigate the association between the variables.

Results: The cumulative incidence rate of pentavalent-related adverse events during 48 h following immunization was estimated to be 15.8% for swelling, 10.9% for redness, 44.2% for pain, 12.6% for mild fever, 0.1% for high fever, 20.0% for drowsiness, 15.0% for loss of appetite, 32.9% for irritability, 4.6% for vomiting and 5.5% for persistent crying. There is no evidence for the occurrence of convulsion and encephalopathy among children who receive pentavalent vaccines.

Conclusion: Further large studies with long time follow up are required to address rare events include convulsions, encephalopathy or persistent crying. However, Findings urge immunization programs to use pentavalent vaccinations and to continue implementing the current immunization program in children under 1 year of age.

Keywords: Immunization, Vaccine, Adverse reactions, Iran

Background

Immunization is a fundamental component of public health policies for controlling infectious diseases. The vaccination program for smallpox effectively eradicated the disease from the world. Moreover, similar vaccination programs successfully led to the regional eradication of other infectious diseases, making vaccination one of the most reliable and cost-effective public health interventions [1]. According to estimations made by the World Health Organization (WHO), approximately two million deaths among children under 5 years of age can be prevented annually through the use of existing vaccines [2]. WHO has recommended the Expanded Program on Immunization (EPI), which integrates *Heamophilus influenza* type b (Hib) vaccine into the routine pediatric immunization program. Hib is a leading cause of life-threatening infectious diseases, including meningitis and pneumonia, that mostly affects children under 5 years of age [3, 4]. Hib is responsible for a significant proportion of the disease burdens of both developed and developing countries. Each year, Hib

* Correspondence: ma.karami@umsha.ac.ir
[1]Social Determinants of Health Research Center, Hamadan University of Medical Sciences, Hamadan, Iran
[2]Department of Epidemiology, School of Public Health, Hamadan University of Medical Sciences, Hamadan, Iran
Full list of author information is available at the end of the article

leads to approximately three million cases of serious illness and 400,000 to 700,000 deaths among children [5].

Some new vaccines, especially multivalent ones, have been added to the immunization program, primarily to add more antigens to vaccines. For example, in most countries, the tetravalent (DTP-Hib or DTP–HepB) or pentavalent (DTP-HepB-Hib) combination vaccines are currently being used instead of the trivalent vaccine (DTP) without the Hib or HepB component [6]. Combination vaccines for pediatric immunization schedules have contributed to a decrease in the number of clinic visits, logistical challenges, operational costs and injections and an increase in parental consent [7, 8]. Moreover, these vaccines improve individual adaptation to the virus and routine vaccination coverage. Therefore, the addition of antigens to existing vaccines with high coverage is considered an effective and appropriate strategy for protecting society from new diseases [9, 10].

Public trust in newly introduced vaccines can be strengthened by monitoring vaccine safety. Surveillance of adverse events following immunization will enable us to monitor the safety of immunization programs and thereby contribute to validating the immunization program. In this way, the undesirable adverse events of the immunization program can be effectively managed, and any inappropriate measures based on reports of adverse effect that may cause concern in society can be prevented [11–13]. As the pentavalent vaccine (DTPw-Hep B-Hib (PRP-T) vaccine (pentavac) (adsorbed) manufactured by Serum Institute of India ltd) has been part of the national pediatric immunization schedule of Iran since 2014, the study of adverse events associated with this vaccine seems to be of paramount importance. After assessing for reactogenicity following immunization with the pentavalent vaccine, we can take effective and useful action toward earning public trust and managing vaccine safety.

The aim of this study is to examine pentavalent vaccine safety and increase the amount of knowledge that might help policy makers in their decisions to continue introducing pentavalent vaccines to immunization programs.

Methods

The sample of the present mixed cohort study was comprised of 1119 children under 1 year of age who were referred to Hamadan health centers to receive pentavalent vaccine at 2, 4 and 6 months of age. More specifically, a sample of approximately 370 children was examined at each point of the three scheduled doses of pentavalent vaccine. Only children under 1 year of age who received the first, second and third dose of pentavalent vaccine were eligible for inclusion in this study.

Urban health centers that are affiliated with the District Health Center in the city of Hamadan were selected using a randomized sampling method, and children under 1 year of age who were referred to these centers to receive pentavalent vaccine at 2, 4 and 6 months of age were recruited consecutively.

The data for the present study were collected through a self-constructed questionnaire from the parents of the children. Ethical approval for the present study was obtained from the Ethics Committee of the Hamadan University of Medical Sciences. Moreover, before the start of the study, parents of all the participants were informed of the study's purpose and the procedure. We obtained verbal consent prior to administering the questionnaires. Because of using non-invasive approach at this study, we did not obtain written consent form. After completing the first part of the questionnaire, which included questions about the socio-demographic characteristics of the children and their parents along with some questions on their history of experiencing adverse events while receiving the last dose of pentavalent vaccine, we gave parents an information sheet that included questions related to the vaccination. After each vaccination (i.e. at 2, 4 and 6 months), they were asked to record any complications they observed in the children within the 48 h following the vaccination. After 48 h, we contacted parent by telephone to complete the second part of questionnaire. In total, we asked about the occurrence of 12 complications: (1) swelling, (2) redness, (3) pain, (4) mild fever, (5) high fever, (6) drowsiness, (7) anorexia, (8) restlessness, (9) vomiting, (10) long-term crying, (11) encephalopathy and (12) convulsion using standard definitions.

If parents reported a suspected occurrence of convulsion in the child, they were asked additional probing questions about all the symptoms they observed in the vaccinated child so that a specialist could make a definite conclusion concerning the occurrence of convulsion afterward. In a similar way, parents could report on other serious complications such as persistent crying and irritability. Parents were asked to report possible adverse events that they remembered in the case of a previous dose pentavalent/DTP vaccine. All children who received the first, second and third doses of the vaccine were followed up on by their parents (who were 98% mothers) 48 h after immunization to determine the incidence of complications.

The cumulative incidence of the outcomes studied (i.e. the adverse events after pentavalent immunization) were calculated with 95% confidence intervals (CI). Moreover, risk ratio (RR) was calculated by dividing the cumulative incidence of adverse events among male children to female children to explore gender differences. Chi-squared tests and logistic regressions were used to investigate the determinants of vaccine-related side effects. RR values have been approximated using logistic regression analysis. All statistical analyses were conducted at a significance level of 0.05 using SPSS software, version 20 (SPSS, Chicago, IL, USA).

Results

In this study, of the children who received pentavalent vaccines in four health centers in Hamadan, 1119 children were included in the study for the final analyses, and all the pertinent data for these children were collected after they received three doses of pentavalent vaccine at 2, 4 and 6 months of age. The numbers of children at the first, second and third doses of vaccine were reported to be 373 (33.3%), 372 (33.2%) and 374 (33.4%), respectively. Moreover, 54.3% of vaccine recipients ($n = 608$) were male, whereas the remaining 45.7% ($n = 511$) were female. The present study demonstrated that the incidence rate of adverse events 48 h after pentavalent immunization in the children under study was estimated to be 15.8% (13.7–18.0) for swelling, 10.9% (9.2–12.9) for redness, 44.2% (41.2–47.2) for pain, 12.6% (10.7–14.6) for mild fever, 0.1% (0.0–0.4) for high fever, 20.0% (17.7–22.5) for drowsiness, 15.0% (12.9–17.2) for loss of appetite, 32.9% (30.2–35.8) for irritability, 4.6% (3.4–6.0) for vomiting and 5.5% (4.2–7.0) for persistent crying. However, there was no evidence for the occurrence of convulsion and encephalopathy among children who received vaccines. Table 1 presents the frequency of reactogenicity following immunization with pentavalent vaccine in the study group based on gender. The only significant gender differences were found with regard to persistent crying: the incidence of this complication in males was higher than in females ($p = 0.01$). We found no other significant gender differences in the incidence of other complications.

With regard to the vaccine dose, the results of statistical analyses indicated that the frequency of adverse events due to pentavalent immunization in our sample were statistically significant for swelling ($p = 0.002$), pain ($p = 0.002$) and mild fever ($p = 0.004$). As shown in Table 2, more fine-grained analyses revealed that the frequency of swelling ($p = 0.003$), pain ($p = 0.001$), mild fever ($p = 0.003$) and redness ($p = 0.02$) were significantly higher after the first dose of vaccination compared to the second dose, but that children were more restless after the second dose than after the first ($p < 0.001$). Furthermore, the symptoms of mild fever were significantly higher in the third dose than in the second dose (($p < 0.001$).

In this study, we further examined the relationship between sex and adverse events following pentavalent vaccination by means of logistic regressions. As shown in Table 1, the results of the analyses indicated that there is no association between sex and adverse events following pentavalent vaccination. Furthermore, we examined the relationship between vaccination dose (i.e. first, second

and third dose) and adverse events following pentavalent vaccination. As shown in Table 3, there is a statistically significant relationship between the vaccination dose and swelling (RR = 0.72 (95% CI: 0.59–0.89)) and pain (RR = 0.85 (95% CI: 0.74–0. 99). These complications decrease with increasing age.

Discussion

The implementation of immunization is meant to protect individuals and society as a whole against vaccine-preventable diseases. Although advances in medicine have made vaccines reliably more effective with minimal adverse events, no vaccine can be found that is free from unwanted adverse events [11]. As the immunization schedule for Hib is similar to that of the DTP vaccine, it can be easily incorporated into the current immunization program [14]. There has been no report of incompatibility between the Hib vaccine and the DTP and hepatitis B vaccines. In general, each new combination vaccine containing the DTP vaccine is acceptable if there is no interference among multiple antigens. Physical and chemical interactions among the components of a combination vaccine and immunological interference may trigger undesirable changes in the immune response to vaccines [15]. Hence, in this study, we attempted to investigate the incidence rate of adverse events following immunization associated with pentavalent vaccine, which has been implemented as a combination vaccine in Iran for the first time. To the best of our knowledge, this is the first study that aims to provide evidence regarding the safety of pentavalent vaccine in Iran.

The results obtained in the present study showed that the most frequently reported reactogenicity associated with pentavalent vaccine was pain, with an incidence rate of 44.23%. This finding is in line with the results obtained by Edna in his meta-analysis, in which some minor reactions such as pain and redness were more prevalent among the children who received the combined vaccine [16]. The results of a study conducted in China revealed that the majority of the adverse events following immunization were reported to be non-serious events; fever and injection site reaction were the most common forms of reactogenicity experienced after immunization [17]. Moreover, in other Iranian studies on the adverse events associated with DTP and pentavalent vaccination, mild fever was found to be the most commonly experienced complication that occurred after vaccination [18–20]. Contrary to the above observation, in our study, the incidence rate of mild fever was a reported 12.2%. The main reason for the difference could be the use of acetaminophen prior to vaccination and a lack of sufficient parental attention to the child's temperature. We observed no significant difference in the incidence rate of complications following vaccination

Table 1 The cumulative incidence rate of adverse events associated with pentavalent vaccination in male and female children and related risk ratios

Adverse events		Incidence (per 100 children) Sex		P-value	Risk ratio (95% CI)[a]
		Male	Female		
Swelling	Yes	103(16.9)	74(14.5)	0.149	1.16 (0.88–1.50)
	No	505(83.1)	437(85.5)		
Redness	Yes	64(10.5)	59(11.5)	0.327	0.91 (0.65–1.27)
	No	544(89.5)	452(88.5)		
Pain	Yes	282(53.6)	213(41.7)	0.065	1.11 (0.97–1.27)
	No	326(53.6)	298(58.3)		
Mild fever	Yes	75(12.3)	66(12.9)	0.420	0.95 (0.70–1.30)
	No	533(87.7)	445(87.1)		
High fever	Yes	0	1(0.2)	0.457	NA
	No	608(100)	510(99.8)		
Drowsiness	Yes	123(20.2)	102(20)	0.486	1.01 (0.80–1.28)
	No	485(79.8)	409(80)		
Anorexia	Yes	91(15)	77(15.1)	0.514	0.99 (0.75–1.31)
	No	517(85)	434(84.9)		
Restlessness	Yes	204(33.6)	165(32.3)	0.351	1.03 (0.87–1.22)
	No	404(66.4)	346(67.7)		
Vomiting	Yes	29(4.8)	23(4.5)	0.474	1.05 (0.62–1.80)
	No	579(95.2)	488(95.5)		
Long-term crying	Yes	43(7.1)	19(3.7)	0.010	1.90 (1.13–3.22)
	No	565(92.9)	492(96.3)		
Encephalopathy	Yes	0	0	1	NA
	No	608(100)	511(100)		
Convulsion	Yes	0	0	1	NA
	No	608(100)	511(100)		
History of convulsion	Yes	3(0.49)	0	0.43	NA
	No	605(99.5)	511(100)		
Family history of convulsion	Yes	10(1.64)	10(1.9)	0.16	0.84 (0.35–2)
	No	598(98.3)	501(98.0)		

NA not applicable
[a]Female gender was considered as reference for RR calculation

between male and female children except for persistent crying, which was significantly more common among males than females.

We have cited some studies that assessing adverse events associated with the pentavalent vaccine with a separate formula or combinations. In a safety study among Indian infants [21], authors have monitored adverse events following a hexavalent vaccine during 1 month after immunization. They found that 37.9% infants experienced at least one injection site reaction. The corresponding value for systemic reaction was 54.6%. Wang YX et al. [22] in a clinical trial to evaluation the safety of a "combined Haemophilus influenzae type b-Neisseria meningitidis serogroup A and C-

tetanus toxoid conjugate vaccine (Hib-MenAC)" found that there is no serious adverse events following immunization with Hib-MenAC. In a retrospective cohort study, Sadoh AE and his/her colleagues [23] have compared the prevalence of adverse events following pentavalent and DTP vaccines in Nigeria. They reported that the rate of pentavalent-related adverse reactions vaccine was higher than DTP one (22.2% vs. 13.5%). Similar studies in Iran have been implemented on different antigen [24].

A comparison of the complication incidence rates of the first and second doses of vaccination with pentavalent showed that all the adverse events were more frequently observed in the first dose of vaccination than the second,

Table 2 Comparison of the cumulative incidence rates of complications in the first, second and third doses of the vaccination in children

Adverse events	Incidence (per 100 children) vaccine dose			P-value (1st and 2nd dose comparison)	P-value (2nd and 3rd dose comparison)
	1st dose (2 months) N = 373	2nd dose (4 months) N = 372	3rd dose (6 months) N = 374		
Swelling	79(0.21)	50(0.13)	48(0.12)	0.003	0.068
Redness	50(0.13)	30(0.08)	43(0.11)	0.026	0.679
Pain	190(0.5)	143(0.38)	62(0.43)	0.001	0.162
Mild fever	45(0.12)	33(0.08)	63(0.16)	0.068	<0.001
High fever	1(0.002)	0(0)	0(0)	0.388	NA
Drowsiness	83(0.22)	72(0.19)	70(0.18)	0.310	0.725
Anorexia	65(0.17)	51(0.13)	52(0.13)	0.126	1
Restlessness	35(0.06)	115(0.3)	119(0.31)	<0.001	0.766
Vomiting	16(0.04)	19(0.05)	17(0.04)	0.510	0.510
Long-term crying	24(0.06)	16(0.04)	22(0.05)	0.210	0.510
Encephalopathy	0(0)	0(0)	0(0)	NA	NA
Convulsion	0(0)	0(0)	0(0)	NA	NA
History of convulsion	0(0)	1(0.002)	2(0.005)	0.387	0.488
Family history of convulsion	0(0)	14(0.037)	6(0.016)	<0.001	0.074

NA not applicable

and this relationship was statistically significant. The only exception was restlessness, which had a higher incidence rate in the second dose of vaccination rather than the first. The meaningful reduction in the incidence rate of these complications with increasing age can be partly accounted for by several factors, including the increase of muscle tissue and deeper intramuscular injections. Moreover, mothers might be more sensitive and worried about the complications their children show after the first dose of vaccination and thus give more detailed reports of the complications their children experience after the first dose of vaccination than after subsequent doses. In addition, due to the experience they have gained after the first dose of the vaccination, some mothers may use acetaminophen prior to subsequent doses. The results of the statistical analyses showed that with the exception of mild fever,

Table 3 Relationship between vaccination dose and the cumulative incidence rate of adverse events associated with pentavalent vaccine in children

Adverse events	Incidence (per 100 children)			RR[a] (95% CI)
	First dose N = 373	Second dose N = 372	Third dose N = 374	
Swelling	79(44.6)	50(28.2)	48(27.1)	0.72(0.59–0.89)
Redness	50(40.7)	30(24.4)	43(35)	0.9(0.72–1.14)
Pain	190(38.4)	143(28.9)	162(32.7)	0.85(0.74–0.99)
Mild fever	45(31.9)	33(23.4)	63(44.7)	1.24(1.00–1.54)
High fever	1(100)	0(0)	0(0)	NA
Drowsiness	83(36.9)	72(32)	70(31.1)	0.89(0.74–1.07)
Anorexia	65(38.7)	51(30.4)	52(31)	0.87(0.71–1.06)
Restlessness	135(36.6)	115(31.2)	119(32.2)	0.9(0.77–1.05)
Vomiting	16(30.8)	19(36.5)	17(32.7)	1.02(0.73–1.44)
Long-term crying	24(38.7)	16(25.8)	22(35.5)	0.94(0.69–1.29)
Encephalopathy	0(0)	0(0)	0(0)	Not applicable
Convulsion	0(0)	0(0)	0(0)	Not applicable
History of convulsion	0(0)	1(0.2)	2(0.5)	3.45(0.5–23.74)
Family history of convulsion	0(0)	14(3.7)	6(1.6)	1.6(0.9–2.83)

NA not applicable

[a]Risk ratios values have been approximated using logistic regression analysis

which was more common in the third dose of vaccination than the second one, there was no significant difference between the incidence rate of all other complications after the second and third doses.

Study limitations

One limitation of the present study is that the limited sample size and the rarity of more serious complications such as convulsion, encephalopathy and persistent crying constrain the generalizability of the study results. Other limitations are the duration of follow up participants and lack of control group. It is evident that some of rare adverse events such as encephalopathy occur after 7–10 days following immunization or later. Therefore, similar studies with long duration follow up, larger sample sizes or the use of surveillance system data associated with adverse events after immunization are recommended. Consider to the above mentioned limitations, findings on mild and moderate reactions after pentavalent vaccine in this study as a field work in the new setting could support licensur studies.

Conclusion

In general, the present findings on usual reactions should move immunization programs to use pentavalent vaccinations and continue implementing the current immunization program in children under 1 year of age. Moreover, the findings of this study show that giving some useful guidelines to parents with children under 1 year of age about avoidable adverse events following vaccination such as pain, redness and swelling is a necessary measure for effectively managing these complications.

Abbreviations

EPI: Expanded Program on Immunization; Hib: Heamophilus influenza type b; WHO: World Health Organization

Acknowledgments

We would like to thank all participants for their participation in this study, as well as the experts without their support this study would not has been possible.

Funding

The present study was approved by the Vice Chancellor for Research and Technology of Hamadan University of Medical Sciences, (Grant No: 9,403,191,394). Hamadan University of Medical Sciences have partially supported this project and does not give the authors of this manuscript any support for publication fee or article processing charge.
The researchers express their gratitude to the participants for sharing their experiences.

Authors' contributions

MK conceived of the idea for the manuscript, conducted the statistical analyses, interpreted the data and drafted the manuscript. MK, PA, JB, ZB, TP, AZ, MZ, and HE conducted the data collection. All authors read, provided feedback, and approved the final submitted version of the manuscript.

Competing interests

The authors declare that they have no competing interests.

Author details

[1]Social Determinants of Health Research Center, Hamadan University of Medical Sciences, Hamadan, Iran. [2]Department of Epidemiology, School of Public Health, Hamadan University of Medical Sciences, Hamadan, Iran. [3]Deputy for Health, Hamadan University of Medical Sciences, Hamadan, Iran. [4]Social Determinants of Health Research Center, Kurdistan University of Medical Sciences, Sanandaj, Iran. [5]Center for Communicable Diseases Control, Ministry of Health, Tehran, Iran. [6]Department of Communication Studies, Ghent University, Ghent, Belgium. [7]Faculty of Social Sciences, University of Antwerp, Antwerp, Belgium.

References

1. Hinman AR, Orenstein WA, Schuchat A, Control CfD, Prevention. Vaccine-preventable diseases, immunizations, and MMWR: 1961–2011. MMWR Surveill Summ. 2011;60(Suppl 4):49–57.
2. Arístegui J, Usonis V, Coovadia H, Riedemann S, Win KM, Gatchalian S, Bock HL. Facilitating the WHO expanded program of immunization: the clinical profile of a combined diphtheria, tetanus, pertussis, hepatitis B and Haemophilus influenzae type b vaccine. Int J Infect Dis. 2003;7(2):143–51.
3. De Serres G, Gay NJ, Farrington CP. Epidemiology of transmissible diseases after elimination. Am J Epidemiol. 2000;151(11):1039–48. discussion 1049–1052
4. Shapiro ED, Ward JI. The epidemiology and prevention of disease caused by Haemophilus influenzae type b. Epidemiol Rev. 1990;13:113–42.
5. WHO Global Programme for Vaccines and Immunization. The WHO position paper on Haemophilus influenzae type b conjugate vaccines. Weekly Epidemiological Record. 1998;73(10):64–68.
6. Gallego V, Berberian G, Lloveras S, Verbanaz S, Chaves TS, Orduna T, Rodriguez-Morales AJ. The 2014 FIFA world cup: communicable disease risks and advice for visitors to Brazil–a review from the Latin American Society for Travel Medicine (SLAMVI). Travel Med Infect Dis. 2014;12(3):208–18.
7. Asturias EJ, Contreras-Roldan IL, Ram M, Garcia-Melgar AJ, Morales-Oquendo V, Hartman K, Rauscher M, Moulton LH, Halsey NA. Post-authorization safety surveillance of a liquid pentavalent vaccine in Guatemalan children. Vaccine. 2013;31(49):5909–14.
8. Happe LE, Lunacsek OE, Marshall GS, Lewis T, Spencer S. Combination vaccine use and vaccination quality in a managed care population. Am J Manag Care. 2007;13(9):506–13.
9. Decker MD. Principles of pediatric combination vaccines and practical issues related to use in clinical practice. Pediatr Infect Dis J. 2001;20(11):S10–8.
10. Kalies H, Grote V, Verstraeten T, Hessel L, Schmitt H-J, von Kries R. The use of combination vaccines has improved timeliness of vaccination in children. Pediatr Infect Dis J. 2006;25(6):507–12.
11. Esteghamati A, Salar Amoli M, Fatemeh A. Guideline for adverse events following immunization. 3th ed. Tehran: Department of Disease Management in Health Ministry; 2005.
12. Crawford NW, Clothier H, Hodgson K, Selvaraj G, Easton ML, Buttery JP. Active surveillance for adverse events following immunization. Expert Rev Vaccines. 2014;13(2):265–76.
13. Tafuri S, Gallone MS, Calabrese G, Germinario C. Adverse events following immunization: is this time for the use of WHO causality assessment? Expert Rev Vaccines. 2015;14(5):625–7.
14. Sharma HJ, Patil VD, Lalwani SK, Manglani MV, Ravichandran L, Kapre SV, Jadhav SS, Parekh SS, Ashtagi G, Malshe N. Assessment of safety and immunogenicity of two different lots of diphtheria, tetanus, pertussis, hepatitis B and Haemophilus influenzae type b vaccine manufactured using small and large scale manufacturing process. Vaccine. 2012;30(3):510–6.
15. Insel RA. Potential alterations in immunogenicity by combining or simultaneously administering vaccine componentsa. Ann N Y Acad Sci. 1995;754(1):35–48.
16. Bar-On ES, Goldberg E, Fraser A, Vidal L, Hellmann S, Leibovici L. Combined DTP-HBV-HIB vaccine versus separately administered DTP-HBV and HIB

vaccines for primary prevention of diphtheria, tetanus, pertussis, hepatitis B
and Haemophilus influenzae B (HIB). *The Cochrane database of systematic
reviews* 2009(3):Cd005530.

17. Hu Y, Li Q, Lin L, Chen E, Chen Y, Qi X. Surveillance for adverse events
     following immunization from 2008 to 2011 in Zhejiang Province, China.
     Clin Vaccine Immunol. 2013;20(2):211–7.

18. Karami M, Holakouie Naieni K, Rahimi A, Fotouhi A, Eftekhar Ardabili H.
     Adverse events following immunization with DTP vaccine in infants and
     children in Kermanshah city: a cohort study. Iran J Epidemiol. 2006;1(3):33–9.

19. Nabavi M, Jandaghi J, Ghorbani R, Khaleghi Hashemian M, Shojaee H,
     Maherbonabi S, Mohammadzade F, Ghadamyari M, Bayat S, Faraji Z. The
     incidence of complications of vaccination in children and infants of
     Semnan, Iran. Koomesh. 2010;11(4):245–54.

20. Sharafi R, Mortazavi J, Heidarzadeh A. Comparison of complications of
     pentavalent and DTP vaccination in infants aged 2–6 months in Anzali, Iran.
     Iran J Neonatology IJN. 2016;7(2):1–6.

21. Chhatwal J, Lalwani S, Vidor E. Immunogenicity and safety of a liquid
     Hexavalent vaccine in Indian infants. Indian Pediatr. 2017;54(1):15–20.

22. Wang YX, Tao H, Hu JL, Li JX, Dai WM, Sun JF, Liu P, Tang J, Liu WY, Zhu FC.
     The immunogenicity and safety of a Hib-MenAC vaccine: a non-inferiority
     randomized, observer-blind trial in infants aged 3–5 months. Expert Rev
     Vaccines. 2017;16(5):515–24.

23. Sadoh AE, Nwaneri DU, Ogboghodo BC, Sadoh WE. Comparison of adverse
     events following pentavalent and diphtheria-tetanus-pertussis vaccines
     among Nigerian children. Pharmacoepidemiol Drug Saf. 2017:1–4.

24. Hashemi A, Taheri Soodejani M, Karami M, Rahimi Pordanjani S. Adverse
     effects of influenza vaccination among healthcare staff in shiraz in 2014,
     Iran. Qom Univ Med Sci J. 2016;10(7):58–64.

4

RNA gene profile variation in peripheral blood mononuclear cells from rhesus macaques immunized with Hib conjugate vaccine, Hib capsular polysaccharide and TT carrier protein

Jing Tang[1,2†], Ying Zhang[1†], Xiaolong Zhang[1], Yun Liao[1], Yongrong Wang[1], Shengjie Ouyang[1], Yanchun Che[1], Miao Xu[2], Jing Pu[1], Qi Shen[2], Zhanlong He[1], Qiang Ye[2] and Qihan Li[1*]

Abstract

Background: The *Haemophilus influenzae* type b (Hib) conjugate vaccine has been widely used in children to prevent invasive Hib disease because of its strong immunogenicity and antibody response induction relative to the capsular polysaccharide (CPS) antigen. The data from vaccine studies suggest that the conjugate vaccine contains carrier proteins that enhance and/or regulate the antigen's immunogenicity, but the mechanism of this enhancement remains unclear.

Methods: To explore the immunological role of the conjugate vaccine, we compared the immune responses and gene profiles of rhesus macaques after immunization with CPS, carrier protein tetanus toxoid (TT) or conjugate vaccine.

Results: A distinct immune response was induced by the Hib conjugate vaccine but not by CPS or carrier protein TT. The genes that were dynamically regulated in conjunction with the macaque immune responses to the conjugate vaccine were investigated.

Conclusions: We propose that these genes are involved in the induction of specific immunity that is characterized by the appearance and maintenance of antibodies against Hib.

Keywords: *Haemophilus influenzae* type b (Hib), Conjugate vaccine, Gene profile

Background

Haemophilus influenzae type b (Hib) is a widely recognized member of the *Haemophilus* genus that directly causes respiratory infectious disease with characteristic manifestations of tympanitis, bronchitis and pneumonia in children of all ages, particularly in infants and 1-year-olds [1–3]. Notably, this pathogen is associated with purulent meningitis in a specific ratio in all Hib-infected patients [1, 4]. Epidemiological studies of this pathogen have primarily been performed in developed countries and have shown that the incidence in children under the age of 5 in areas such as the US, France, and Switzerland is approximately 20–100/100,000 [5–9], but few data have been reported for developing areas. Although no systematic, epidemiological study of Hib has been performed in mainland China, studies of this pathogen in a small number of populations in different regions of China have indicated that the potential incidence of pediatric infections in mainland China is noteworthy [10, 11]. Numerous studies have addressed Hib structure and immunology [12, 13], leading to the licensure of a preventive vaccine against Hib infection in the 1980s [1]. Based on the results of a structural study of the Hib agent that suggested that the bacterium presented a

* Correspondence: liqihan@imbcams.com.cn
†Equal contributors
[1]Yunnan Key Laboratory of Vaccine Research and Development on Severe Infectious Diseases, Institute of Medical Biology, Chinese Academy of Medical Sciences and Peking Union Medical College, No. 935 Jiaoling Road, Kunming, Yunnan 650118, China
Full list of author information is available at the end of the article

capsular polysaccharide (CPS) antigen and thallus anti-gen, the early vaccine was prepared with polyribosylribi-tol phosphate (PRP), which is composed of ribosylribitol phosphate as the basic unit [14, 15]. The CPS antigen is the primary component of the 1st generation Hib vac-cine and has been widely used to vaccinate children. Clinical observation of the use of this vaccine in pediatric populations indicated that it induced a remark-able immune response in children 18 months of age or older but did not provoke a satisfactory response in chil-dren younger than 18 months [16–19]. Subsequent Hib conjugate vaccines were developed based on a CPS antigen-binding protein (i.e., diphtheria toxoid (DT), tetanus toxoid (TT) and the *N. meningitidies* outer membrane protein (OMP) Hib thallus antigen protein) [18, 20]. Previous studies of this conjugate vaccine in mice and macaques have shown that remarkable im-munity is induced by immunization with this vaccine compared to that induced by the CPS vaccine; the im-munity usually presents as an increased antibody re-sponse in serum [21]. The results of additional clinical trials comparing conjugate Hib vaccines produced with various carrier proteins, including DT, TT and OMP, suggested that one or two immunizations induced a lower antibody response in children of various ages than three immunizations [22, 23]. The data indicated that the antibody levels of Hib vaccines conjugated with DT, TT, and OMP were 0.06, 0.05, and 0.83 µg/ml, respect-ively, after the first inoculation and that the levels in-creased to 0.14, 0.26, and 1.22 µg/ml after the second inoculation [23]. However, the levels increased further to 0.28, 3.64, and 1.14 µg/ml after the third inoculation [23]. Based on these data, a routine immunization schedule for the Hib conjugate vaccine has been recom-mended for children worldwide by the WHO [24], and the vaccines have been used extensively in multiple countries, including China [25, 26]. The increased im-munogenicity associated with the Hib conjugate vaccine compared with that of the CPS vaccine suggests that binding of the semi-antigen CPS to the carrier protein would provide an effective antigen for immunization of individuals [27–30].

In previous studies, the immunogenicity of Hib CPS antigen and its protein conjugates were studied in juven-ile and infant rhesus macaques [31, 32], which suggest that the conjugate of CPS and TT, DT and OMP are capable of inducing stronger specific antibody responses than CPS alone in this animal model [31–33]. Although those studies indicated unequal level of antibody in-duced against various conjugate vaccine including Hib-TT, Hib-CT and Hib OMPC and confirmed their im-munogenicity, but also suggested the role of these car-rier protein in the immunogenicity of Hib conjugate vaccine in human should be studied further [33, 34]. To

better understand the immunologic mechanism of this conjugate vaccine, especially the role of carrier protein to enhance immunogenicity of CPS via the immunization schedule of three doses, we conducted a study using rhesus macaques, which are closely genetic-ally related to humans, in which we assessed the mRNA profiles of rhesus macaque peripheral blood mono-nuclear cells (PBMCs) after immunization of the animals with the Hib conjugate vaccine, the Hib polysaccharide antigen or the carrier protein TT. Using comparison and analysis of these mRNA gene profiles, we investigated the molecular mechanism of immunity induced by the Hib conjugate vaccine and identified several genes that are likely to play a role in specific and effective immune responses against Hib in rhesus macaques. These genes might be induced by CPS antigen and carrier protein and might play the roles involved in the enhancement of immunogenicity of Hib conjugate vaccine.

Methods

Animals and ethics

The animal experiments were designed according to the principles of the Guide for the Care and Use of Labora-tory Animals [35] and Guidance for Experimental Ani-mal Welfare and Ethical Treatment [36]. The protocols were reviewed and approved by the Experimental Ani-mal Ethics Committee of the Institute of Medical Biol-ogy, Chinese Academy of Medical Sciences for animal welfare (Approval number: YISHENGLUNZI [2015] 12).

Rhesus monkeys were separately bred in cages and fed according to the guidelines of the Committee on Experimental Animals at the Institute of Medical Biology, Chinese Academy of Medical Sciences. The housing conditions, experimental procedures and ani-mal welfare measures were in accordance with the local laws and guidelines for the use of laboratory non-human primates and were compliant with the recommendations of the Weatherall report [35]. The monkeys were maintained under the care of veterinar-ians. The animals were bred in separate cages in a large room under BSL-2 conditions with sufficient fresh air and natural light; the housing conditions permitted the animals to have visual, olfactory and auditory interactions with other monkeys. The temperature of the room was maintained at approxi-mately 25 °C during the experiments. Food and water were readily available to the animals, and appropriate treats and vitamins were provided. The animals were given access to environmental enrichment, including approved toys, to promote their psychological well-being. None of the animals were sacrificed as part of the experiment. No abnormalities were noted in any of the animals for the 6 months following the study;

during this time, the animals were returned to the colony and remained under the care of a veterinarian.

Antigens used for immunization

The *Haemophilus influenzae* type b conjugate vaccine was purchased from Beijing Zhifei Lvzhu Biopharmaceutical Co., Ltd. (Beijing, China; 10 μg *H. influenza* type b polysaccharide conjugated to 30 μg TT per 0.5 ml). Pure TT and polysaccharide were used as the control antigen (Beijing Zhifei Lvzhu Biopharmaceutical Co., Ltd., Beijing, China).

Vaccination of monkeys

Juvenile rhesus monkeys (Six- to eight-month-old; 1.2 ± 0.5 kg) were randomly immunized in groups of three with the CPS antigen, carrier protein TT or conjugate vaccine via intramuscular injection (i.m.) in the anterolateral thigh on days 0, 30 and 60 using the formulations and immunization doses shown in Additional file 1: Table S1. The monkeys were bled on days 0, 30, 60 and 90. Sera and PBMCs were collected for ELISA analyses and microarray assays, respectively.

ELISA analysis

The anti-PRP antibody concentration in the samples was measured using a standard ELISA protocol [37].Briefly, 96-well plates were coated with Ty-PRP (1:4000; National Institutes for Food and Drug Control, China) overnight. Before adding the sera, the wells were blocked at room temperature (RT). The horseradish peroxidase (HRP)-conjugated goat-anti-monkey IgG/IgA/IgM used as the secondary antibody (Sigma-Aldrich, Inc., St. Louis, MO, USA) was diluted 1:100,000. The substrate (Kinghawk Pharmaceutical Co., Ltd., Beijing, China) was incubated for 30 min at RT, and the reaction was terminated with the stop buffer, followed by absorbance measurements at 450 and 620 nm. With the reason that there was not available of standard anti-serum of macaque, the international standard human serum against Hib obtained from Sanofi-Aventis, was used as reference control. This standard serum was diluted in concentration of antibody in 10, 20, 40, 80, 160, 320 ng/ml and was as the reference for the evaluation of animal serum. The comparison of concentration of human antibody and titer of diluted macaque serum were determined in the light absorbance value in wave length of 450 nm (Additional file 1: Figure S1). The pre-immunization sera of macaques were used as the negative controls for this study. The goat-anti-monkey IgM was used as the secondary antibody (Sigma-Aldrich, Inc., St. Louis, MO, USA) to test the IgM titer induced by the conjugate, polysaccaharide antigen and the TT carrier. The carrier protein-specific IgG was evaluated using ELISA Assay

kit for Tetanus Toxoid IgG (Vida-Bio Co. Ltd., Wuhan, China).

RNA extraction

PBMCs were isolated from the whole blood by density gradient centrifugation over a Lymphoprep (Ficoll-Paque PREMIUM; GE Healthcare, Piscataway, NJ, USA). Total RNA from the PBMCs was isolated using the TRIzol Reagent (Invitrogen, CA, USA) and purified with the RNeasy Mini Kit (QIAGEN, GmBH, Germany). The RNA Integrity Number (RIN) was evaluated to inspect RNA integrity using an Agilent Bioanalyzer 2100 (Agilent, CA, USA). The extracted RNA was frozen in 95% ethanol until further use.

Microarray assay

The Whole Rhesus Monkey Genome Microarray (G2519F-026806, Agilent, CA, USA) was chosen to screen for gene expression in monkey PBMCs. Gene Chip microarray experiments were conducted at the National Engineering Center for Biochip in Shanghai, China, according to the procedures in the Agilent technical manual. Briefly, the mRNA that was purified from total RNA after rRNA removal was amplified and transcribed into fluorescent cRNA using the Low Input Quick Amp Labeling protocol (Agilent).Labeled cRNA was purified using the RNeasy Mini Kit (QIAGEN, GmBH, Germany). Each slide was hybridized with 1.65 μl of Cy3-labeled cRNA using the Gene Expression Hybridization Kit (Agilent) in a hybridization oven (Agilent). After 17 h of hybridization, the slides were washed in staining dishes (Thermo, MA, USA) with the Gene Expression Wash Buffer Kit (Agilent). Slides were scanned using an Agilent Microarray Scanner (Agilent). The raw data were obtained using the Feature Extraction Software 10.7 (Agilent) and normalized using the quantile algorithm with Gene Spring 11.0 (Agilent). The systematic bioinformatic analyses of microarrays were processed by Novel Bioinformatics Co., Ltd. (Shanghai, China). Briefly, the normalization value was set to 1. The differentially expressed genes, with false discovery rate (FDR) values < 0.05 and Log_2 (fold changes) ≥ 1.5, were analyzed compared to the samples collected at day 0. The significant pathway network (Gene-Act-Network) was determined from these differentially expressed genes using the Kyoto Encyclopedia of Genes and Genomes (KEGG) database, according to the relationship among the genes and proteins in the database [17, 38–40]. The raw microarray data were submitted to the Gene Expression Omnibus database and are available under the accession number GSE90481.

Real-time RT-PCR

The gene expression levels were measured by real-time RT-PCR. The primers are listed in Additional file 1: Table S2. Briefly, total RNA was extracted from the PBMCs as described above. For quantification, a single-tube RT-PCR assay was performed using the 1-step RT-PCR Master Mix in a 7500 Fast Real-Time RT-PCR system (Applied Biosystems, Foster City, CA, USA). The following protocol was used for all PCR assays: 5 min at 42 °C and 10 s at 95 °C, followed by 40 cycles at 95 °C for 5 s and 60 °C for 30 s.

Flow cytometry

PBMCs were isolated by density gradient centrifugation with Lymphorprep medium (Ficoll-Paque PREMIUM; GE Healthcare, Piscataway, NJ, USA), and were counted by flow cytometry using anti-monkey CD3$^+$ antibodies (BD Biosciences, San Diego, CA, USA), anti-CD69 antibodies (BD Biosciences) and anti-ITK antibodies (abcam, Cambridge, UK), according with the protocol as previous [41].

T cells proliferation and cytokine production

PBMCs from the rhesus macaques were used to measure T cell proliferation and cytokine secretion. PBMCs were placed in culture with CFSE (1.5 μM/well; BD Biosciences) and the stimulus (10 μg/ml TT) or positive control (LPS, 5 μg/ml) at 2×10^5 cells/ml in RPMI 1640. Then, plates were incubated at 37 °C 5% CO_2. After 36 h, the supernatants (50 μl) were obtained for cytokines analysis and cells were obtained for T cell proliferation by flow cytometry.

— cytokines analysis. The cytokines productions were tested by NHP CBA analysis kit (BD Biosciences) according with the protocol [42].
— T cell proliferation. The newly increased T cells were counted by flow cytometry co-marked with CD3$^+$ antibodies and CSFE (BD Biosciences).

Statistical analysis

The non-parametric Kruskal-Wallis test was applied for comparisons between different groups using the Graph-Pad Prism software (San Diego, CA, USA). A P-value of < 0.05 was considered significant.

Results

A specific immune response was induced in Hib conjugate vaccine-immunized macaques but not in Hib CPS antigen- or carrier protein TT-immunized macaques

Previous Hib conjugate vaccine trials in human subjects demonstrated good immunogenicity in all immunized pediatric groups after three inoculations, including in children of all ages, whereas the Hib polysaccharide

vaccine elicited a lower antibody response in children over 18 months of age [16, 43]. However, a similar study in mice failed to observe age-based variations in immunogenicity [44]. In the present study of rhesus macaques, we selected 6- to 8-month-old animals with physiological features resembling those of 2- to 3-year-old humans [45, 46]. To identify effective immunization outcomes, the conjugate vaccine, the Hib polysaccharide antigen and the TT carrier were used to immunize the macaques according to the routine immunization schedule recommended by the WHO. After three immunizations, the Hib conjugate vaccine elicited an immune response, as shown by higher titer of Hib antibody reached 1:8000, 10,666 and 11,733 in serum after one, two and three immunizations in ELISA assay (Fig. 1a). However, this higher titer was identified being similar the concentration of antibody induced in human pediatric clinical in the comparison with human reference serum (Fig. 1a and Additional file 1: Figure S1). The previous serological analysis suggested that the antibody concentration of 0.15 μg/ml in immunized pediatric population was postulated as the positive conversion, and 1 μg/ml as meaning the immunity of long term [47, 48]. The characteristic of the result observed in macaques and been distinct with that usually observed human is that the conjugate vaccine elicited antibody response after 1st immunization and maintained its increasing after 2nd and 3rd immunization [21, 23], as while Hib polysaccharide antigen did weak work in macaques (Fig. 1a). The specific T cell responses were also remarkably induced by Hib conjugate vaccine (Fig. 1b). In vitro, TT could stimulate proliferation of T cells from the monkeys in Hib vaccine group and cytokines secretion (Fig. 1c and d). This result suggests that the Hib conjugate vaccine is capable of eliciting a distinct immune response in 6- to 8-month-old macaques, similar to the effects observed in children older than 18 months of age, whereas the immune response was weak to the polysaccharide antigen. These results were similar to those reported in previous work of capsular polysaccharide-protein conjugates and suggest that rhesus macaques are suitable to use in comparative analyses of the immunological features of Hib [31, 32]. These data also suggest that this model might be limited to reflect the trend of antibody response elicited in the immunized human individuals by Hib CPS vaccine.

The mRNA gene profile suggested that a synergistic immunologic effect is induced in macaques by the Hib conjugate vaccine compared to CPS and TT

The results of Hib-specific antibody measurements in macaques that were immunized with the Hib conjugate vaccine and Hib capsular antigen or carrier TT protein suggested that the conjugate vaccine, but not the

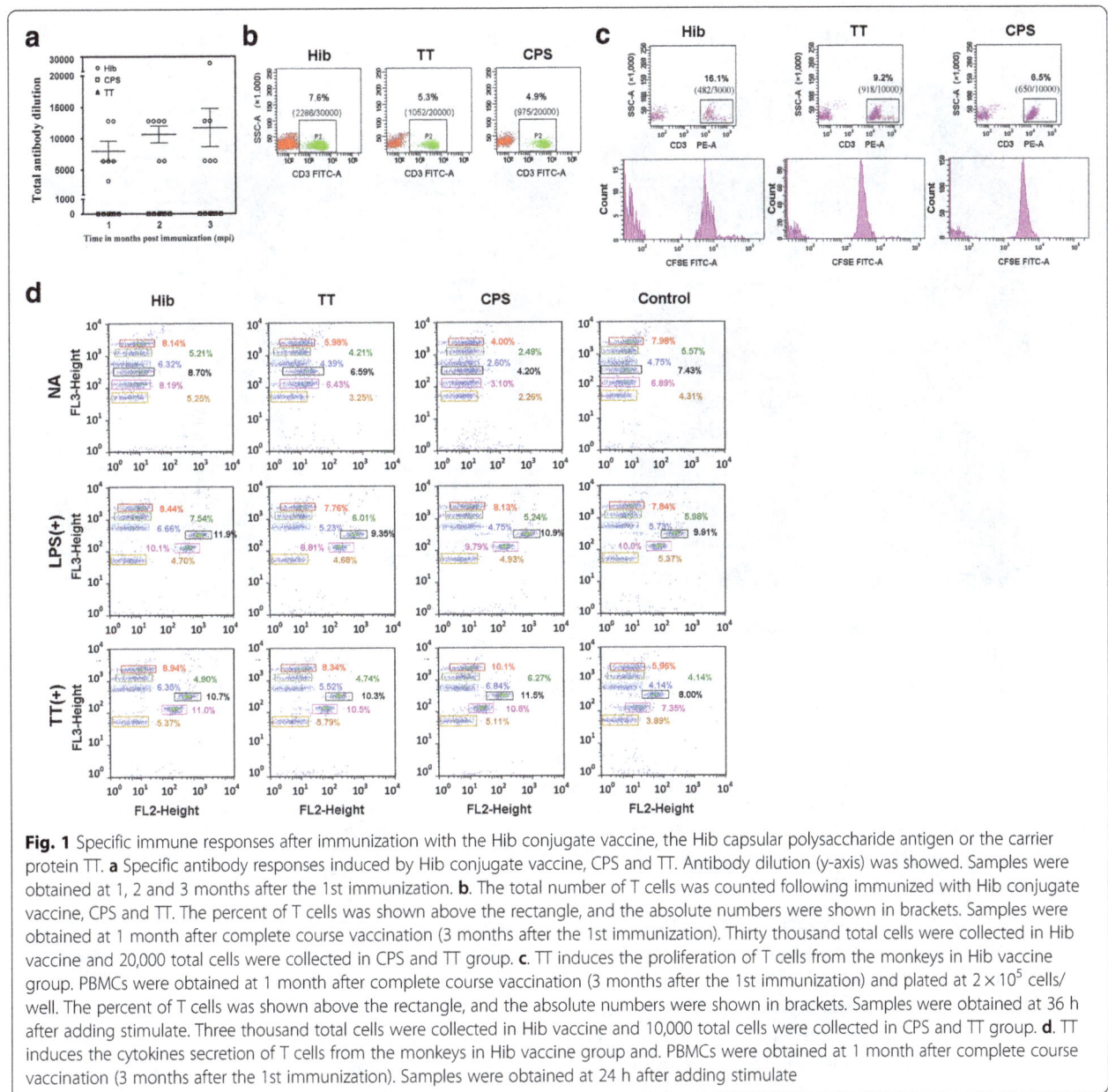

Fig. 1 Specific immune responses after immunization with the Hib conjugate vaccine, the Hib capsular polysaccharide antigen or the carrier protein TT. **a** Specific antibody responses induced by Hib conjugate vaccine, CPS and TT. Antibody dilution (y-axis) was showed. Samples were obtained at 1, 2 and 3 months after the 1st immunization. **b** The total number of T cells was counted following immunized with Hib conjugate vaccine, CPS and TT. The percent of T cells was shown above the rectangle, and the absolute numbers were shown in brackets. Samples were obtained at 1 month after complete course vaccination (3 months after the 1st immunization). Thirty thousand total cells were collected in Hib vaccine and 20,000 total cells were collected in CPS and TT group. **c**. TT induces the proliferation of T cells from the monkeys in Hib vaccine group. PBMCs were obtained at 1 month after complete course vaccination (3 months after the 1st immunization) and plated at 2×10^5 cells/well. The percent of T cells was shown above the rectangle, and the absolute numbers were shown in brackets. Samples were obtained at 36 h after adding stimulate. Three thousand total cells were collected in Hib vaccine and 10,000 total cells were collected in CPS and TT group. **d**. TT induces the cytokines secretion of T cells from the monkeys in Hib vaccine group and. PBMCs were obtained at 1 month after complete course vaccination (3 months after the 1st immunization). Samples were obtained at 24 h after adding stimulate

capsular antigen or TT, effectively activated the immune response. This result implied that a synergistic effect was provided by the carrier TT protein and the CPS antigen during conjugate vaccine stimulation of the immune system. To understand the roles of TT carrier protein and CPS antigen in this immune response, we hypothesized that the immune response elicited by Hib conjugate vaccine is involved in a more complicated event for immune system due to the fact that conjugation of CPS and TT might create a changed antigenic structure, although each of TT or CPS could be capable of stimulating immune system [29]. In this case, two comparisons were performed for their mRNA expression profile. A comparison of PBMCs collected from animals

immunized with the conjugate vaccine or with CPS suggested that the expression of 437 genes varied significantly in the two groups of animals (Fig. 2a). In the comparison of the gene expression profiles of animals immunized with conjugate vaccine and those of animals immunized with TT protein, 596 genes with significantly different levels of expression were identified (Fig. 2b).

To further understand these differentially expressed genes and their relationship to the immune response to Hib, an Ingenuity Pathway Analysis (IPA) of the genes identified in the comparisons between the Hib conjugate vaccine and polysaccharide antigen groups and between the Hib conjugate vaccine and carrier protein TT groups was performed. The results, which are based on the P

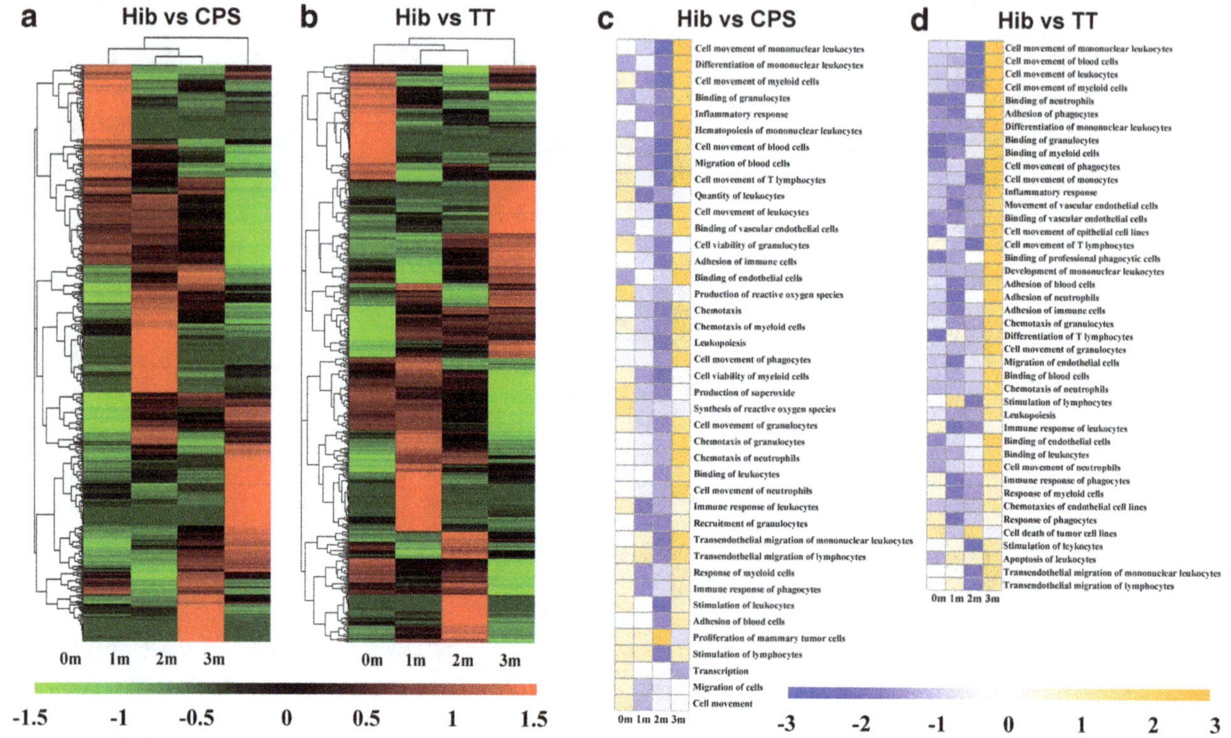

Fig. 2 Comparison of mRNA expression in animals immunized with the Hib conjugate vaccine, Hib CPS antigen or carrier TT protein at various time points and IPA analysis of the genes that showed significant differential expression. **a** Comparison of the expression of 437 genes in macaques immunized with the Hib conjugate vaccine or with CPS antigen at various time points. Each row indicates one gene. The values are expressed as $\log_2$P-values. **b** Comparison of the expression of 596 genes in macaques immunized with the Hib conjugate vaccine or with carrier protein TT at various time points. Each row indicates one gene. The values are expressed as $\log_2$P-values. **c** IPA analysis of the genes that were differentially expressed in macaques immunized with the Hib conjugate vaccine and in macaques immunized with CPS antigen. The values are expressed as $\log_2$P-values. **d** IPA analysis of the genes that were differentially expressed in macaques immunized with the Hib conjugate vaccine and in macaques immunized with carrier protein TT. The values are expressed as $\log_2$P-values

values of the comparisons between the two immunized animal groups (Fig. 2c, d), yielded two findings. First, the genes with the most significant differences in the conjugate vaccine versus CPS antigen groups were associated with inflammatery response, immune cell adhesionand cell movement of immune cells (Fig. 2c). This result suggests that cellular adhesion and cell movement might have been involved in the production of specific immunity against Hib. Second, the genes with the most significant differential expression in the conjugate vaccine versus the carrier TT group were also associated with cellular adhesion, inflammation and cell movement (Fig. 2d). Taken together, the results from the two comparisons suggested that the major events that occurred during the induction of the Hib immune response may have involved molecules with cellular adhesion functions. In addition, more than 19 genes were associated with cellular adhesion (Additional file 1: Table S3). A previous study showed that the bacterial polysaccharides on the thallus surface, which were as the pathogen associated molecular pattern (PAMP) triggering innate immunity, was capable of interacting with the molecules

on human cell surfaces and might play important roles during infection [49], these roles may involve conformational changes in adhesion molecules and subsequent signal transduction and regulation of cellular responses in immune system [50–53]. If these biological processes do occur in immune cells, a functional effect would be involved in the induction of immunity.

Characterization of genes that appear to be involved in the immune response against Hib in conjugate vaccine-immunized macaques

The results of IPA analyses of the comparisons of mRNAs derived from cells of animals that received the conjugate vaccine and from those that were immunized with the CPS antigen or carrier protein TT suggested that most of the genes that are involved in the immune response to Hib encode cellular receptors, transcriptional regulators or inflammatory effectors. Further characterization of the differentially expressed genes identified in animals treated with conjugate vaccine versus CPS antigen and conjugate vaccine versus TT protein was performed in accordance with the biological functions of the gene and the time sequence of immunization. The results indicated two findings. First, 437 and 596 differentially expressed genes from the comparisons of conjugate vaccine verse CPS antigen and conjugate vaccine verse TT protein, respectively, were associated with transcription, signal transduction, immune response, cellular structure and metabolism (Fig. 3a); of these, the percentage of genes related to the immune response was 18% and 16% respectively (Fig. 3a). Second, analysis of the expression of individual genes as a function of time after immunization revealed that the differential expression of 31 genes was maintained in the conjugate vaccine versus CPS antigen comparison at the three time points and that differential expression of 41 genes was maintained in the conjugate vaccine versus carrier protein TT comparison at the three time points (Fig. 3b). Examination of the differentially expressed genes in the two groups at the three time points indicated that 8 genes maintained their variations throughout the immunization period (Fig. 3b). Of these 8 genes, five were directly correlated with the induction of the immune response (Table 1), and the other 3 were indirectly associated with it (Table 1). The genes KLRC1, LGALS13 and VNN2 showed higher expression in the animals that were immunized with the conjugate vaccine than in those that were immunized with CPS antigen or with the carrier protein TT. Although it is not clear whether these 8 genes are involved in the immune response, further analysis showed that although KLRC1

Table 1 The dynamic expressing profile of eight genes associated antibody response in whole immunization period [a]

	Hib vs Capsular			Hib vs Toxoid		
	1mpi	2mpi	3mpi	1mpi	2mpi	3mpi
KLRC1	1.60	6.51	40.85	2.61	14.72	71.36
LGALS13	5.44	4.76	20.84	17.62	29.75	305.67
LTB4DH	1.40	0.82	1.27	1.36	0.59	0.03
NUAK1	1.70	0.77	2.24	2.58	0.82	2.62
VNN2	0.96	35.12	80.82	0.79	47.70	343.50
GALNT3	0.39	0.48	0.58	1.18	1.66	1.01
LOC710050	0.49	0.75	0.65	0.32	0.53	0.57
LOC716305	1.09	0.76	0.03	0.81	0.69	0.24

[a] the fold change indicates the expression levels of the specific gene in the samples from Hib vaccine group compared with the samples from Capsular or Toxoid group. The results were normalized to the level of the same gene in the same group at 0 day

expression increased at all three time points in both the CPS antigen and conjugate vaccine groups, its expression remained lower in the CPS antigen group than in the conjugate vaccine group (Table 2). This resulted in larger differences in the comparisons between the two groups. However, LGALS13 expression increased moderately by 3.7-, 1.19- and 9.17-fold in the conjugate vaccine group at the three time points measured, whereas it maintained its decreasing trend in the CPS antigen and carrier protein TT groups. A similar trend was observed for VNN2. This resulted in large differences between the

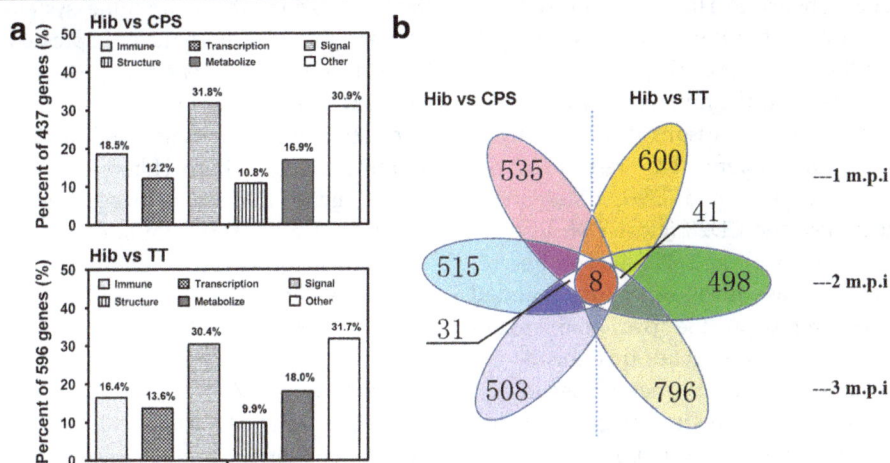

Fig. 3 Analysis of the major genes correlated with the antibody response against Hib. **a** Gene classification. The differentially expressed genes (437 in the Hib conjugate vaccine group versus the CPS group and 596 in the Hib conjugate vaccine group versus the TT group) were classified into groups. The figure shows the percent (y-axis) of each clarification of gene (the intersection) to the differentially expressed genes (437 in the Hib conjugate vaccine group versus the CPS group and 596 in the Hib conjugate vaccine group versus the TT group). Multifunctional genes were put into different classes. The percent of differentially classified genes was showed above the column. **b** Global view of the modulation of gene expression in PBMCs obtained from immunized macaques at 1, 2 and 3 months post-inoculation. The individual sets, which are indicated by different colors, show the numbers of significantly modulated genes at each time point. A total of 39 genes (including a specific set of 8 genes) differed between the Hib vaccine and the CPS antigen groups during the entire immunization period. A total of 49 genes (including the same set of 8 genes) differed between the Hib vaccine and the carrier TT groups during the entire immunization period. Thus, a total of 8 genes (shown in red) differed between the vaccine group (Hib vaccine) and the control groups (CPS and TT) during the whole immunization period

Table 2 Eight different genes in three groups in whole immunization period [a]

	Hib			Capsular			Toxoid		
	1mpi	2mpi	3mpi	1mpi	2mpi	3mpi	1mpi	2mpi	3mpi
KLRC1	1.46	6.77	53.52	0.91	1.04	1.31	0.56	0.46	0.75
LGALS13	3.70	1.19	9.17	0.68	0.25	0.44	0.21	0.04	0.03
LTB4DH	1.50	0.67	0.65	1.07	0.82	0.51	1.10	1.14	22.65
NUAK1	2.14	1.19	4.53	1.26	1.55	2.02	0.83	1.46	1.73
VNN2	0.27	31.96	27.48	0.28	0.91	0.34	0.34	0.67	0.08
GALNT3	5.24	2.97	2.32	13.34	6.16	4.00	4.43	1.79	2.29
LOC710050	0.77	0.82	1.05	1.58	1.09	1.61	2.42	1.56	1.83
LOC716305	0.63	0.41	0.18	0.58	0.54	6.08	0.78	0.59	0.74

[a] the fold change indicates the expression levels of the specific gene in the samples from 1, 2 and 3 m.p.i. compared with the samples from 0 day in the same group

two comparisons (Table 2). These results suggest that there is a logical correlation between the expression of these three genes and the immune response induced by the Hib conjugate vaccine. qRT-PCR analysis of KLRC1, LGALS13, LTB4DH and VNN2 expression in PBMCs of the immunized macaques provided supportive evidence for the results of the other analyses described in this study (Additional file 1: Figure S3).

Analysis of all characterized genes associated with immunity

The divergent immune responses and mRNA gene profiles that were induced by immunization with the conjugate vaccine, the CPS antigen and the TT protein suggested that variation in gene expression related to the specific immune response to Hib in immunized macaques might play a role in the function of the immune system. To address this hypothesis, the direction of our investigation next focused on the differentially expressed genes identified in the two comparisons that are likely to function in the immune system. The results of the characterization of the 437 and 596 differentially expressed genes identified the CD28 (cluster of differentiation 28), IL8 (interleukin 8), and TLR4 (Toll-like receptor 4) genes as well as other genes that showed different and varied trends in the two comparisons (Fig. 4a); the latter genes included genes that encode CD (cluster of differentiation) molecules, chemokines, receptors, transcription factors and cytokines (Fig. 4a). It may be speculated that these genes play important roles in the immune response induced by the conjugate vaccine. Furthermore, the up-regulated expression of CD69, a key marker of T cell activation, was observed in Hib conjugated vaccine group compared to the other two groups based on microarray analysis (Fig. 4a); meanwhile, the expression of CD69 in the PBMCs from monkeys immunized by conjugated Hib vaccine group was increased (Additional file 1: Figure S4). Due to the fact that the conjugate vaccine consisted of CPS and TT, the

differentially expressed genes identified in the comparison of the conjugate vaccine versus the CPS antigen or the TT protein can be presumed to be complementary. Thus, our work compared the differentially expressed genes observed in a comparison of the conjugate vaccine and TT with the differentially expressed genes observed after three immunizations with CPS alone and after three immunizations with TT alone. Sixty-seven genes were found to be differentially expressed in both comparisons (Fig. 4b), whereas 14 and 31 differentially expressed genes, respectively, were distinctive in each comparison (Fig. 4b). If we postulate that the 67 genes that were differentially expressed in both comparisons are involved in the immunity induced by the conjugate vaccine, the 14 genes may be assumed to be related to the stimulation of the immune system by TT protein, whereas the 31 differentially expressed genes are likely to be those that function in the immune response to CPS antigen. Furthermore, there are 2 genes that are associated with immunity and maintained after three immunizations in both Hib-vs-CPS-comparison groups; and 1 gene that is associated with immunity and maintained after three immunizations in both Hib-vs-TT-comparison groups (Additional file 1: Table S4). Further experimental evidence will be required to support this hypothesis.

Discussion

Previous studies of various Hib vaccines have suggested that the conjugate vaccine consisting of the CPS antigen and carrier protein is capable of producing strong immunogenicity in immunized populations, although *Haemophilus influenzae type b* capsular polysaccharide could induce a weak immunogenicity [27, 28, 30]. This success has contributed to the development of several bacterial vaccines based on immunological principles and technical criteria [12, 25]. Millions of clinically infectious pediatric Hib cases worldwide have been controlled through the use of the conjugate vaccine over a

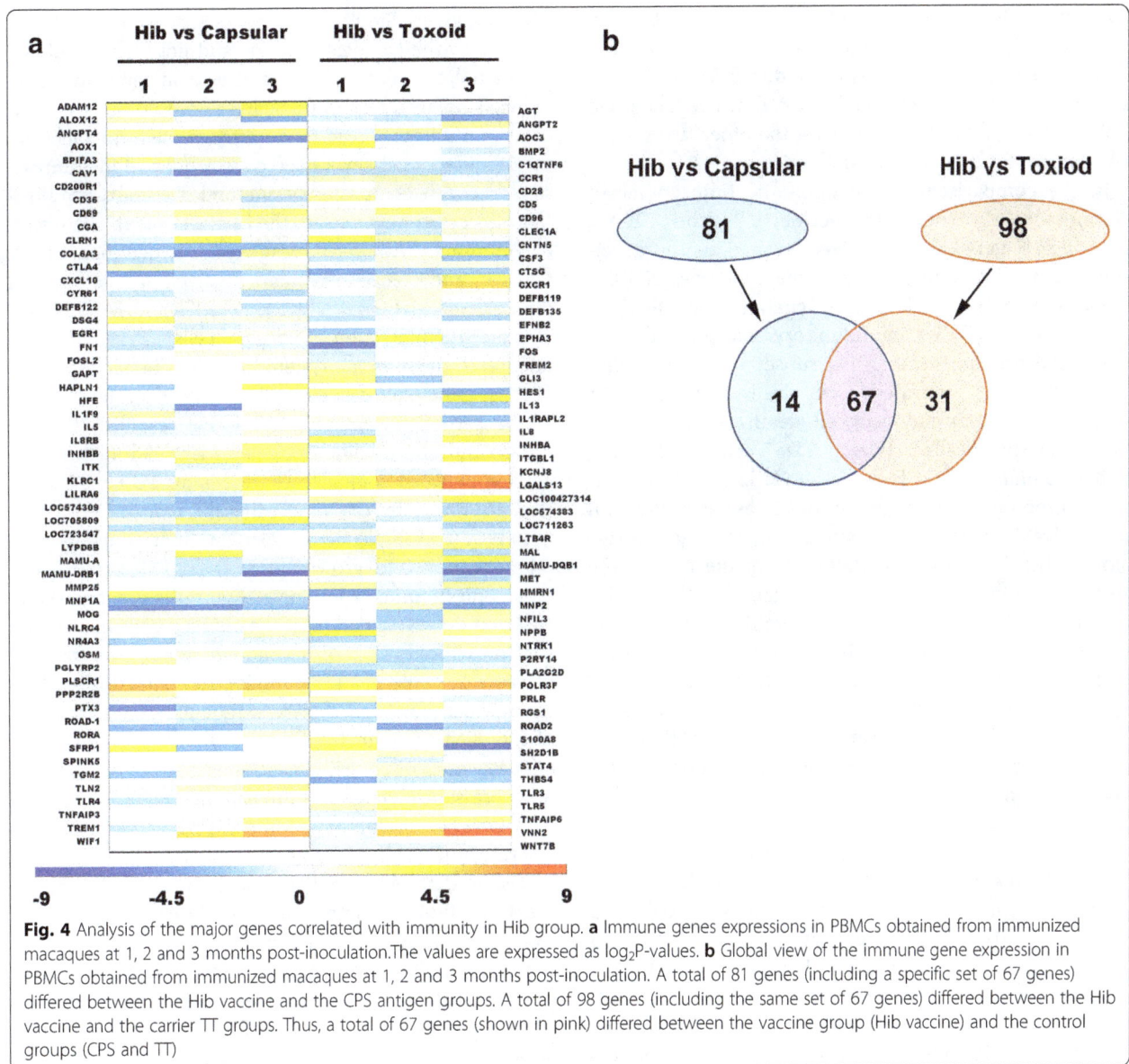

Fig. 4 Analysis of the major genes correlated with immunity in Hib group. **a** Immune genes expressions in PBMCs obtained from immunized macaques at 1, 2 and 3 months post-inoculation. The values are expressed as $\log_2$P-values. **b** Global view of the immune gene expression in PBMCs obtained from immunized macaques at 1, 2 and 3 months post-inoculation. A total of 81 genes (including a specific set of 67 genes) differed between the Hib vaccine and the CPS antigen groups. A total of 98 genes (including the same set of 67 genes) differed between the Hib vaccine and the carrier TT groups. Thus, a total of 67 genes (shown in pink) differed between the vaccine group (Hib vaccine) and the control groups (CPS and TT)

period of several decades, confirming its efficacy [25]. To study the mechanism of this effective Hib conjugate vaccine-induced immunity, our study compared the mRNA gene profiles of macaques that were immunized with the Hib conjugate vaccine, CPS antigen, or the carrier protein TT and identified specific genes that may play major roles in the induction of the immune response against Hib. Knowledge of these genes can improve our understanding of how immunity is developed against Hib. Interestingly, while a higher immune response occurred in conjugate vaccine-immunized macaques than in those immunized by the CPS antigen or carrier protein TT alone, the genes with the greatest differential expression in the comparisons were associated with cellular adhesion, and these genes could be further classified into genes involved in cellular surface

recognition and those involved in interactions between various types of cells in the immune system. This result suggested that the induction of immunity might involve the recognition by immune cells of the conjugated antigen of the polysaccharide and the carrier protein, resulting in subsequent immune cell interactions that activate the adaptive immune response. Several genes whose encoded molecules enabled the induction of the specific immune response and for which dynamic changes in expression were maintained were considered to be significantly correlated with the formation of this immunity. Thus, these genes might play important roles in the immune response. Interesting, the expression of CD69, a key T cell activation marker, was higher in Hib conjugated vaccine group comparing with Capsular and Toxoid groups (Fig. 4a and Additional file 1: Figure S4), supporting that T cells might be activated by Hib vaccine. In addition, unlikely CD69, another gene ITK, which encodes an interleukin 2 induced T cell kinase, was not remarkably changed even down-regulated in Hib vaccine group comparing with the other two groups (Additional file 1: Figure S4 and Fig. 4a).

In the comparisons based upon the time course of response to the conjugate vaccine, CPS and TT, we identified 8 genes that are likely related to the development of immunity; these genes include KLRC1, LGALS13 and VNN2. The encoded product of KLRC1 is NKG2A, an inhibitory receptor that is expressed on the surface of a subset of natural killer (NK) cells and activated CD8$^+$ cells [54]. NKG2A controls activation-induced cell death (ACID), which occurs in specifically activated CD8$^+$ cells, by forming a heterodimer with CD94 [54]. NKG2A/CD94 maintains immune system homeostasis as anti-infection immunity increases. Interestingly, increasing expression of this gene was maintained from the first to the third month after the first immunization with the Hib conjugate vaccine (1.46- to 53.52-fold relative to the background; Table 2), but little variation in its expression was observed in animals immunized with CPS or TT (0.91 to 1.31-fold and 0.56 to 0.75-fold, respectively; Table 2). This observation suggests that this gene may play an important role in the immune response. Conversely, the LGALS13 gene exhibited a small increasing trend (3.7- to 9.17-fold relative to background; Table 2) during the three-month time period, in distinct contrast to the trends observed in animals immunized with CPS or TT (0.68 to 0.44-fold and 0.21 to 0.03-fold, respectively; Table 2). LGALS13 encodes the PP13 protein, which is classified as a member of the galectin family and is involved in multiple biological processes, including signal transduction and cellular adhesion [55–60]. PP13 also induces the secretion of inflammatory agents and chemokines by mononuclear cells [61, 62]. A third gene, VNN2, exhibited conjugate vaccine-induced variation (0.27 to 27.48-fold; Table 2) that was distinctly different from the variations induced by vaccination with CPS or TT alone (0.28 to 0.34-fold and 0.34 to 0.08-fold; Table 2). VNN2 encodes a glycosyl phosphatidylinositol (GPI)-anchored protein that regulates cellular adhesion and promotes neutrophil migration and inflammatory reactivity [63–65].

In addition to the above, we classified the differentially expressed genes identified in various comparisons based upon immunological characterization and tested the hypothesis that the genes whose expression is specifically induced by the conjugate vaccine and not by CPS represent the difference in the integral immunity induced by an intact immunogen and the deficient immunity induced by a hapten antigen. Similarly, the genes that were specifically induced by the conjugate vaccine and not by TT could be postulated to reflect the difference in integral immunity induced by an intact immunogen compared to the deficient immunity induced by a carrier protein. In this case, the 17 differentially expressed genes observed in comparisons between conjugate vaccine and TT and CPS alone (Fig. 4b) could help explain the carrier's role in the resulting immunity. Among these genes, we identified CCR1, CXCL10 and CXCR1, which are involved in inflammation [66], as well as EGR1, NLRC1, NTRK1 and MET, which mediate the interaction of immune cells and signal transduction in the immune system [67–70]. The identification of these genes suggests a possible mechanism for the role of the carrier protein in the immune response. On the other hand, the 67 different genes identified in the comparison between conjugate vaccine and CPS or TT alone (Fig. 4b) may offer clues regarding the role of CPS in immunity; for example, IL5, a cytokine that stimulates the differentiation and growth of B cells [71], showed up-regulation in animals immunized with the conjugate vaccine and down-regulation in the animals immunized with CPS or TT only (Fig. 4b). This finding suggests that IL5 played a key role in the immunity. In contrast, the OSM gene, which has been shown to modulate the expression of IL6, GM-CSF and G-CSF [72, 73] was not induced in animals immunized with the conjugate vaccine, whereas its expression increased in animals that were immunized with CPS or TT only (Fig. 4b). This result also implies a key role of the OSM gene in immunity to Hib.

Despite that we're only allowed to perform the experiments on limited number of animals due to the funding restriction, we still noticed a remarkable immune response in vaccine immunization group. Based on our analyses, we propose that the combination of the Hib polysaccharide antigen and the carrier protein TT produces an antigenic structure that is capable of activating both innate and adaptive immune responses. This Hib conjugate vaccine might achieve this effect through its recognition by the molecules in the surface of some immune cells followed by activation of innate and adaptive immune responses which is characterized by an increase in the level of antibodies against Hib and by the maintenance of that level. The CPS antigen is unable to induce an effective antibody response probably with its lacking the appropriate structure. However, our model will require experimental validation in specific animal models with deficient genes.

Conclusions

Probably as a result of the synergistic effects between the carrier TT and CPS antigen in Hib conjugate vaccine, several special genes associated with specific immunity in the Hib antibody induction and maintenance, were primarily induced.

Additional file

Additional file 1: Table S1. two monkeys in each group were immunized intramuscular injection. Table S2. The primers of eight genes for real-time RT-PCR. Figure S1 ELISA analysis of total antibody titers from immunized rhesus macaques. Figure S2. ELISA analysis of antibody from immunized rhesus macaques. Figure S3. qRT-PCR analysis of mRNA at various time points. Figure S4. qRT-PCR and Flow cytometry analysis of CD69 and ITK expression. Tables S1, S2, S3, S4, Figures S1, S2, S3 and S4. A remarkable immune response induced by Hib conjugate vaccine, in rhesus macaques, because of a result of the synergistic effects between the carrier TT and CPS antigen. (DOCX 1352 kb)

Abbreviations
CD: Cluster of differentiation; CD28: Cluster of differentiation 28; CD69: Cluster of differentiation 69; CPS: Capsular polysaccharide; DT: Diphtheria toxoid; Hib: *Haemophilus influenzae* type b; IL8: Interleukin 8; IPA: Ingenuity Pathway Analysis; ITK: IL2 inducible T cell kinase; OMP: Outer membrane protein; PBMCs: Peripheral blood mononuclear cells; PRP: Polyribosylribitol phosphate; RT: Room temperature; TLR4: Toll-like receptor 4; TT: Tetanus toxoid

Acknowledgments
Many thanks for the help from Dr. Kaili Ma, Dr. Shuaiyao Lu and Ms. Yanyan Li in this study. Special thanks to Dr. Han Zhang for the revision and modification of the manuscript.

Funding
This work was supported by CAMS Initiative for Innovative Medicine (CAMS-I2M-1-019), Medical reserve talents of Yunnan Provincial Health and Family Planning (H-201620), Major science and technology special projects of Yunnan Province (2017ZF020 and 2014HB066) and Central Research Institutes of Basic Research and Public Service Special Operations (2016ZX310180-6).

Authors' contributions
Conceived and designed the experiments: QL, JT and YZ. Performed the experiments: JT, YZ, XZ, YL, SO, JP, ZH, QY. Analyzed the data: QL, JT, YZ, YW. Contributed reagents/materials/analysis tools: MX, QS. Wrote the paper: QL, YC. All authors have approved the manuscript and agree with the submission to BMC Immunology.

Competing interests
All authors have completed the Unified Competing Interest form and declare that they have no competing interests. The sponsors and funders of the present study played no role in the study design, data or sample collection, data processing, or drafting of the manuscript. The corresponding authors had full access to all data generated in the present study and assume full responsibility for the final submission of this manuscript for publication.

Author details
[1]Yunnan Key Laboratory of Vaccine Research and Development on Severe Infectious Diseases, Institute of Medical Biology, Chinese Academy of Medical Sciences and Peking Union Medical College, No. 935 Jiaoling Road, Kunming, Yunnan 650118, China. [2]National Institutes for Food and Drug Control, Beijing, China.

References
1. Zarei AE, Almehdar HA, Redwan EM. Hib vaccines: past, present, and future perspectives. J Immunol Res. 2016;2016:7203587.
2. Briere EC, Jackson M, Shah SG, Cohn AC, Anderson RD, MacNeil JR, et al. Haemophilus influenzae type b disease and vaccine booster dose deferral, United States, 1998-2009. Pediatrics. 2012;130(3):414–20.
3. Bruce MG, Deeks SL, Zulz T, Navarro C, Palacios C, Case C, et al. Epidemiology of Haemophilus influenzae serotype a, north American Arctic, 2000-2005. Emerg Infect Dis. 2008;14(1):48–55.
4. Sell SH, Merrill RE, Doyne EO, Zimsky EP Jr. Long-term sequelae of Hemophilus influenzae meningitis. Pediatrics. 1972;49(2):206–11.
5. Wenger JD. Epidemiology of Haemophilus influenzae type b disease and impact of Haemophilus influenzae type b conjugate vaccines in the United States and Canada. Pediatr Infect Dis J. 1998;17(9 Suppl):S132–6.
6. Gervaix A, Suter S. Epidemiology of invasive Haemophilus influenzae type b infections in Geneva, Switzerland, 1976 to 1989. Pediatr Infect Dis J. 1991; 10(5):370–4.
7. Clements DA, Booy R, Dagan R, Gilbert GL, Moxon ER, Slack MP, et al. Comparison of the epidemiology and cost of Haemophilus influenzae type b disease in five western countries. Pediatr Infect Dis J. 1993;12(5):362–7.
8. Peltola H. Worldwide Haemophilus influenzae type b disease at the beginning of the 21st century: global analysis of the disease burden 25 years after the use of the polysaccharide vaccine and a decade after the advent of conjugates. Clin Microbiol Rev. 2000;13(2):302–17.
9. Reinert P, Liwartowski A, Dabernat H, Guyot C, Boucher J, Carrere C. Epidemiology of Haemophilus influenzae type b disease in France. Vaccine. 1993;11(Suppl 1):S38–42.
10. Yang Y, Shen X, Jiang Z, Liu X, Leng Z, Lu D, et al. Study on Haemophilus influenzae type b diseases in China: the past, present and future. Pediatr Infect Dis J. 1998;17(9 Suppl):S159–65.
11. Zhu H, Wang A, Tong J, Yuan L, Gao W, Shi W, et al. Nasopharyngeal carriage and antimicrobial susceptibility of Haemophilus influenzae among children younger than 5 years of age in Beijing, China. BMC Microbiol. 2015;15:6.
12. Singh B, Su YC, Al-Jubair T, Mukherjee O, Hallstrom T, Morgelin M, et al. A fine-tuned interaction between trimeric autotransporter haemophilus surface fibrils and vitronectin leads to serum resistance and adherence to respiratory epithelial cells. Infect Immun. 2014;82(6):2378–89.
13. Murphy TF, Apicella MA. Nontypable Haemophilus influenzae: a review of clinical aspects, surface antigens, and the human immune response to infection. Rev Infect Dis. 1987;9(1):1–15.
14. Finland M, Sutliff WD. Specific antibody response of human subjects to Intracutaneous injection of Pneumococcus products. J Exp Med. 1932;55(6): 853–65.
15. Hoagland CL, Beeson PB, Goebel WF. The capsular polysaccharide of the type xiv Pneumococcus and its relationship to the specific substances of human blood. Science. 1938;88(2281):261–3.
16. Kayhty H, Karanko V, Peltola H, Makela PH. Serum antibodies after vaccination with Haemophilus influenzae type b capsular polysaccharide and responses to reimmunization: no evidence of immunologic tolerance or memory. Pediatrics. 1984;74(5):857–65.
17. Li C, Li H. Network-constrained regularization and variable selection for analysis of genomic data. Bioinformatics. 2008;24(9):1175–82.
18. Heath PT. Haemophilus influenzae type b conjugate vaccines: a review of efficacy data. Pediatr Infect Dis J. 1998;17(9 Suppl):S117–22.
19. Hoefnagel MH, Vermeulen JP, Scheper RJ, Vandebriel RJ. Response of MUTZ-3 dendritic cells to the different components of the Haemophilus influenzae type B conjugate vaccine: towards an in vitro assay for vaccine immunogenicity. Vaccine. 2011;29(32):5114–21.
20. van den Biggelaar AH, Pomat WS. Immunization of newborns with bacterial conjugate vaccines. Vaccine. 2013;31(21):2525–30.
21. Peeters CC, Evenberg D, Hoogerhout P, Kayhty H, Saarinen L, van Boeckel CA, et al. Synthetic trimer and tetramer of 3-beta-D-ribose-(1-1)-D-ribitol-5-phosphate conjugated to protein induce antibody responses to

21... Haemophilus influenzae type b capsular polysaccharide in mice and monkeys. Infect Immun. 1992;60(5):1826–33.

22. Granoff DM, Anderson EL, Osterholm MT, Holmes SJ, McHugh JE, Belshe RB, et al. Differences in the immunogenicity of three Haemophilus influenzae type b conjugate vaccines in infants. J Pediatr. 1992;121(2):187–94.

23. Decker MD, Edwards KM, Bradley R, Palmer P. Comparative trial in infants of four conjugate Haemophilus influenzae type b vaccines. J Pediatr. 1992;120(2 Pt 1):184–9.

24. Zhao K, Zhang Y, Li H. Haemophilus influenzae vaccine-b type Haemophilus influenzae conjugate vaccine. 2nd ed. medical biological products. Beijing: People's Medical Publishing House; 2007.

25. Morris SK, Moss WJ, Halsey N. Haemophilus influenzae type b conjugate vaccine use and effectiveness. Lancet Infect Dis. 2008;8(7):435–43.

26. Kane MA. Status of hepatitis B immunization programmes in 1998. Vaccine. 1998;16(Suppl):S104–8.

27. Snape MD, Pollard AJ. Meningococcal polysaccharide-protein conjugate vaccines. Lancet Infect Dis. 2005;5(1):21–30.

28. Avery OT, Goebel WF. Chemo-immunological studies on conjugated carbohydrate-proteins: V. The immunological Specifity of an antigen prepared by combining the capsular polysaccharide of type iii Pneumococcus with foreign protein. J Exp Med. 1931;54(3):437–47.

29. Pobre K, Tashani M, Ridda I, Rashid H, Wong M, Booy R. Carrier priming or suppression: understanding carrier priming enhancement of anti-polysaccharide antibody response to conjugate vaccines. Vaccine. 2014;32(13):1423–30.

30. Knuf M, Kowalzik F, Kieninger D. Comparative effects of carrier proteins on vaccine-induced immune response. Vaccine. 2011;29(31):4881–90.

31. Schneerson R, Robbins JB, Chu C, Sutton A, Vann W, Vickers JC, et al. Serum antibody responses of juvenile and infant rhesus monkeys injected with Haemophilus influenzae type b and pneumococcus type 6A capsular polysaccharide-protein conjugates. Infect Immun. 1984;45(3):582–91.

32. Vella PP, Ellis RW. Immunogenicity of Haemophilus influenzae type b conjugate vaccines in infant rhesus monkeys. Pediatr Res. 1991;29(1):10–3.

33. Granoff DM, Rathore MH, Holmes SJ, Granoff PD, Lucas AH. Effect of immunity to the carrier protein on antibody responses to Haemophilus influenzae type b conjugate vaccines. Vaccine. 1993;11(Suppl 1):S46–51.

34. Vella PP, Staub JM, Ellis RW. Biological activity of Hib conjugates. Vaccine. 1991;9(Suppl):S26–9. discussion S42-3

35. Institute for Laboratory Animal Research USA. Guide for the care and use of laboratory animals. 8th ed. Washington, DC: National Academies Press; 2011.

36. Ministry of Science and Technology of the People's Republic of China C. The Guidance to experimental animal welfare and ethical treatment. 2006 [cited 2014 Mar 1]. http://www.most.gov.cn/fggw/zfwj/zfwj2006/200609/t20060930_54389.htm. Accessed 1 Mar 2014.

37. Phipps DC, West J, Eby R, Koster M, Madore DV, Quataert SA. An ELISA employing a Haemophilus influenzae type B oligosaccharide-human serum albumin conjugate correlates with the radioantigen binding assay. J Immunol Methods. 1990;135(1–2):121–8.

38. Jansen R, Greenbaum D, Gerstein M. Relating whole-genome expression data with protein-protein interactions. Genome Res. 2002;12(1):37–46.

39. Wei Z, Li H. A Markov random field model for network-based analysis of genomic data. Bioinformatics. 2007;23(12):1537–44.

40. Spirin V, Mirny LA. Protein complexes and functional modules in molecular networks. Proc Natl Acad Sci U S A. 2003;100(21):12123–8.

41. Wang J, Zhang Y, Zhang X, Hu Y, Dong C, Liu L, et al. Pathologic and immunologic characteristics of coxsackievirus A16 infection in rhesus macaques. Virology. 2017;500:198–208.

42. Wang J, Pu J, Huang H, Zhang Y, Liu L, Yang E, et al. EV71-infected CD14(+) cells modulate the immune activity of T lymphocytes in rhesus monkeys. Emerg Microbes Infect. 2013;2(7):e44.

43. Ward JI, Broome CV, Harrison LH, Shinefield H, Black S. Haemophilus influenzae type b vaccines: lessons for the future. Pediatrics. 1988;81(6):886–93.

44. Granoff DM, Cates KL. Haemophilus influenzae type B polysaccharide vaccines. J Pediatr. 1985;107(3):330–6.

45. Finch CE, Pike MC, Witten M. Slow mortality rate accelerations during aging in some animals approximate that of humans. Science. 1990;249(4971):902–5.

46. Bronikowski AM, Altmann J, Brockman DK, Cords M, Fedigan LM, Pusey A, et al. Aging in the natural world: comparative data reveal similar mortality patterns across primates. Science. 2011;331(6022):1325–8.

47. Kayhty H, Peltola H, Karanko V, Makela PH. The protective level of serum antibodies to the capsular polysaccharide of Haemophilus influenzae type b. J Infect Dis. 1983;147(6):1100.

48. Holmes SJ, Fritzell B, Guito KP, Esbenshade JF, Blatter MM, Reisinger KS, et al. Immunogenicity of Haemophilus influenzae type b polysaccharide-tetanus toxoid conjugate vaccine in infants. Am J Dis Child. 1993;147(8):832–6.

49. Kawai T, Akira S. The role of pattern-recognition receptors in innate immunity: update on toll-like receptors. Nat Immunol. 2010;11(5):373–84.

50. Springer TA. Adhesion receptors of the immune system. Nature. 1990;346(6283):425–34.

51. Gumbiner BM. Cell adhesion: the molecular basis of tissue architecture and morphogenesis. Cell. 1996;84(3):345–57.

52. Aplin AE, Howe AK, Juliano RL. Cell adhesion molecules, signal transduction and cell growth. Curr Opin Cell Biol. 1999;11(6):737–44.

53. Aplin AE, Howe A, Alahari SK, Juliano RL. Signal transduction and signal modulation by cell adhesion receptors: the role of integrins, cadherins, immunoglobulin-cell adhesion molecules, and selectins. Pharmacol Rev. 1998;50(2):197–263.

54. Rapaport AS, Schriewer J, Gilfillan S, Hembrador E, Crump R, Plougastel BF, et al. The inhibitory receptor NKG2A sustains virus-specific CD8(+) T cells in response to a lethal poxvirus infection. Immunity. 2015;43(6):1112–24.

55. Than NG, Pick E, Bellyei S, Szigeti A, Burger O, Berente Z, et al. Functional analyses of placental protein 13/galectin-13. Eur J Biochem. 2004;271(6):1065–78.

56. Than NG, Sumegi B, Than GN, Berente Z, Bohn H. Isolation and sequence analysis of a cDNA encoding human placental tissue protein 13 (PP13), a new lysophospholipase, homologue of human eosinophil Charcot-Leyden crystal protein. Placenta. 1999;20(8):703–10.

57. Burger O, Pick E, Zwickel J, Klayman M, Meiri H, Slotky R, et al. Placental protein 13 (PP-13): effects on cultured trophoblasts, and its detection in human body fluids in normal and pathological pregnancies. Placenta. 2004;25(7):608–22.

58. Sekizawa A, Purwosunu Y, Yoshimura S, Nakamura M, Shimizu H, Okai T, et al. PP13 mRNA expression in trophoblasts from preeclamptic placentas. Reprod Sci. 2009;16(4):408–13.

59. Boronkai A, Bellyei S, Szigeti A, Pozsgai E, Bognar Z, Sumegi B, et al. Potentiation of paclitaxel-induced apoptosis by galectin-13 overexpression via activation of Ask-1-p38-MAP kinase and JNK/SAPK pathways and suppression of Akt and ERK1/2 activation in U-937 human macrophage cells. Eur J Cell Biol. 2009;88(12):753–63.

60. Huppertz B, Meiri H, Gizurarson S, Osol G, Sammar M. Placental protein 13 (PP13): a new biological target shifting individualized risk assessment to personalized drug design combating pre-eclampsia. Hum Reprod Update. 2013;19(4):391–405.

61. Than NG, Balogh A, Romero R, Karpati E, Erez O, Szilagyi A, et al. Placental protein 13 (PP13) - a placental Immunoregulatory galectin protecting pregnancy. Front Immunol. 2014;5:348.

62. Gebhardt S, Bruiners N, Hillermann R. A novel exonic variant (221delT) in the LGALS13 gene encoding placental protein 13 (PP13) is associated with preterm labour in a low risk population. J Reprod Immunol. 2009;82(2):166–73.

63. Yoshitake H, Takeda Y, Nitto T, Sendo F. Cross-linking of GPI-80, a possible regulatory molecule of cell adhesion, induces up-regulation of CD11b/CD18 expression on neutrophil surfaces and shedding of L-selectin. J Leukoc Biol. 2002;71(2):205–11.

64. Yoshitake H, Takeda Y, Nitto T, Sendo F, Araki Y. GPI-80, a beta2 integrin associated glycosylphosphatidylinositol-anchored protein, concentrates on pseudopodia without association with beta2 integrin during neutrophil migration. Immunobiology. 2003;208(4):391–9.

65. Nitto T, Takeda Y, Yoshitake H, Sendo F, Araki Y. Structural divergence of GPI-80 in activated human neutrophils. Biochem Biophys Res Commun. 2007;359(2):227–33.

66. Ubogu EE, Cossoy MB, Ransohoff RM. The expression and function of chemokines involved in CNS inflammation. Trends Pharmacol Sci. 2006;27(1):48–55.

67. McMahon SB, Monroe JG. The role of early growth response gene 1 (egr-1) in regulation of the immune response. J Leukoc Biol. 1996;60(2):159–66.

68. Correa RG, Milutinovic S, Reed JC. Roles of NOD1 (NLRC1) and NOD2 (NLRC2) in innate immunity and inflammatory diseases. Biosci Rep. 2012;32(6):597–608.

69. Pajtler KW, Rebmann V, Lindemann M, Schulte JH, Schulte S, Stauder M, et al. Expression of NTRK1/TrkA affects immunogenicity of neuroblastoma cells. Int J Cancer. 2013;133(4):908–19.

70. Baek JH, Birchmeier C, Zenke M, Hieronymus T. The HGF receptor/met tyrosine kinase is a key regulator of dendritic cell migration in skin immunity. J Immunol. 2012;189(4):1699–707.

71. Harriman GR, Kunimoto DY, Elliott JF, Paetkau V, Strober W. The role of IL-5 in IgA B cell differentiation. J Immunol. 1988;140(9):3033–9.

72. Rose TM, Bruce AG. Oncostatin M is a member of a cytokine family that includes leukemia-inhibitory factor, granulocyte colony-stimulating factor, and interleukin 6. Proc Natl Acad Sci U S A. 1991;88(19):8641–5.

73. Jay PR, Centrella M, Lorenzo J, Bruce AG, Horowitz MC. Oncostatin-M: a new bone active cytokine that activates osteoblasts and inhibits bone resorption. Endocrinology. 1996;137(4):1151–8.

5

Therapeutic cancer vaccine: phase I clinical tolerance study of Hu-rhEGF-rP64k/Mont in patients with newly diagnosed advanced non-small cell lung cancer

Puyuan Xing[1], Hongyu Wang[1], Sheng Yang[1], Xiaohong Han[1,2], Yan Sun[1*] and Yuankai Shi[1*]

Abstract

Background: Hu-rhEGF-rP64k/Mont is a biotechnology product for the treatment of advanced non-small cell lung cancer (NSCLC). The vaccine induces a neutralizing antibody-mediated immune response, against the normal circulating self-protein antigen epidermal growth factor (EGF), which prevents its binding to and activation of the EGF receptor, inhibiting the transduction of the signals that drive cancer cell proliferation, survival and spread. This phase I study aimed to evaluate the safety and the immunological response of Hu-rhEGF-rP64k vaccine in NSCLC patients.

Results: The Hu-rhEGF-rP64k/Mont vaccine showed to be safe and well tolerated, with dizziness, injection-site reactions and tremors being the most commonly reported adverse event. No severe adverse events or death were related to the vaccination. Immune monitoring demonstrated the generation of anti-EGF antibody titers and as a consequence the patients exhibited a decrease in the EGF concentration. In 80% of the vaccinated patients stable disease was achieved.

Conclusion: Hu-rhEGF-rP64k/Mont elicited a valuable immune response, with good safety profile assuring further clinical development of the vaccine in this population to further confirm the potential benefits on survival.

Trial registration: Chinese Clinical Trial Registry, ChiCTR-OID-17014048, date 2017/12/20 (retrospectively registered); Chinese Food and Drug Administration, CFDA 2009 L02105, date 2009/04/03; China Drug Trial, CTR20131039.

Keywords: Cancer vaccine, Lung cancer, Clinical study

Background

Lung cancer is the most common worldwide cancer, with 1.8 million new cases in 2012 (12.9% of the total). It is the most common cancer in men worldwide (1.2 million, 16.7% of the total), reaching rates of 50.4 per 100,000 in Eastern Asia and relatively high rates in women in this geographic region although the tobacco is generally rare in these population. The disease is the leading causes of cancer-related death around the world, responsible for the deaths by cancer in one every five cases of cancer (1.59 million deaths, 19.4% of the total) [1]. Non-small cell histology represents between 75% and 80% of lung tumors. More than 50% of cases are diagnosed in patients with local regional advanced or metastatic disease [2, 3].

The platinum-based doublet chemotherapy has been the standard first-line treatment for non-selected patients with advanced NSCLC [4] and only produce modest survival improve compared with best supportive care. The 1-year survival rate is approximately 35% for patients with wild type tumors whereas 5-year survival rate is still around 5% [5]. There is a great need for novel and more effective treatments for advanced NSCLC.

Hu-rhEGF-rP64k/Mont is a biotechnology product for the treatment of advanced NSCLC. It is a therapeutic vaccine composed by an antigen (recombinant human EGF (rhEGF) chemically conjugated to recombinant P64K (rP64K)) and an adjuvant (Montanide ISA51VG),

* Correspondence: suny@csco.org.cn; syuankai@cicams.ac.cn; syuankaipumc@126.com
[1]Department of Medical Oncology, Beijing Key Laboratory of Clinical Study on Anticancer Molecular Targeted Drugs, National Cancer Center/Cancer Hospital, Chinese Academy of Medical Sciences & Peking Union Medical College, Beijing 100021, China
Full list of author information is available at the end of the article

developed by BIOTECH PHARMA Co., Ltd. and the Center of Molecular Immunology (Havana, Cuba). The antigen is obtained from the chemical conjugation using glutaraldehyde as a linker reagent of drug substance intermediates, the recombinant protein rhEGF, and the recombinant protein rP64K. Hu-rhEGF-rP64k/Mont cancer vaccine can induces a neutralizing antibody-mediated immune response, against the normal circulating self-protein antigen Epidermal Growth Factor (EGF), which is the main ligand of the Epidermal Growth Factor Receptor (EGF-R). This will inhibit the growth of tumor cells and vessels nourishing and lead to the apoptosis of tumor cells. Pre-clinical research results indicated this vaccine is immunogenic, well tolerated and has anti-tumor activity, especially for the NSCLC [6].

The clinical experience in advanced stage (IIIB/IV) NSCLC had demonstrated that the vaccine is very immunogenic, reducing the EGF concentration and increasing the anti-EGF antibody titers and it has been very well tolerated [7–11]. With the purpose of confirming the findings of previous studies, which have been conducted in Western population and considering that the management of NSCLC in China has differences in medical care, drug approval requirements, ethnic variation and clinical behavior we designed this early stage clinical trial in Chinese NSLC patients. In this article, we report the results of a phase I clinical trial approved by the CFDA (2009/04/03, CFDA 2009 L02105), intended to demonstrate the safety, immunogenicity and efficacy of Hu-rhEGF-rP64k/Mont in patients with advanced NSCLC.

Methods
Study design
This monocentric, open label dose-escalation phase I clinical trial enrolled 21 patients with NSCLC, in the National Cancer Center in Beijing, China. All participants were informed about the study and potential risks and required to provide written informed consent prior to undergoing study-related procedures.

A traditional 3 + 3 dose escalation design was implemented [12]. Successive cohorts of patients (3 patients/cohort) were each started on a fixed dose of the vaccine Hu-rhEGF-rP64k/Mont. Patients were assigned sequentially to one of four dose-escalation cohorts. The protocol specified 0.6 mg (group A) of the vaccine on days 4, 18, 32, 46 and 76 (5 vaccine dose), for the first cohort. Successive cohorts were given doses of 1.2 mg (group B), 1.8 mg (group C), 2.4 mg (group D) the same dose intervals. The dose groups were determined on the basis of the vaccine's safety information available from previous clinical studies [8, 13, 14]. Each vaccine dose was administered at 1 injection site, deltoid region (group A), 2 injection sites, deltoids regions (group B),

3 injection sites, deltoids regions and gluteus region (group C) and 4 injection sites, deltoids and gluteus regions (group D).

A DLT was defined as any Grade 3 or 4 adverse event (AE) using the CTCAE 4.03 that was possibly drug-related. CTCAE 4.03 Grade 3 is a severe AE and Grade 4 is a life-threatening or disabling AE. Such events interfere with activities of daily living and include: skin toxicity, diarrhea or antidiarrheal therapy, vomiting at same grade for > 4 days despite aggressive antiemetic therapy, central nervous system, lung or renal toxicity or elevation of liver transaminases or bilirubin lasting more than 1 week. The number of patients who experienced dose-limiting toxicities (DLTs) was assessed at each dose level. If no DLTs were observed for 4 weeks after administration of the last dose of the vaccine, a new cohort of 3 patients was enrolled at the next planned dose level. If DLTs were observed in 1 patient in the cohort, another 3 patients were treated with the same dose level.

The maximum-tolerated dose (MTD) was defined as 1 dose level below the dose in which DLTs were observed in > 33% of the participants. That is, if DLTs were observed in at least 2 of 3 participants, the MTD was determined to be the dose administered to the previous cohort. Similarly, in a cohort of 6 participants, 3 of 6 participants would have to experience DLTs to determine the MTD.

Toxicities were graded using the Common Terminology Criteria for Adverse Events Version 4.03 (CTCAE 4.03) [15]. Health status assessments, including physical exams (vital signs, height, weight, ECOG score, skin of injection site, et al.), complete blood chemistry, electrocardiography was performed at baseline and post vaccination. Chest X-ray, computed tomography (CT) scan, and abdominal ultrasound were conducted at 46 days ±1 week and at 106 days ±1 week to assess clinical response according the Response Evaluation Criteria in Solid Tumors, version 1.1 (RECIST1.1). The objective response rate includes complete response (CR), partial response (PR), stable disease (SD), and progressive disease (PD). Disease control rate (DCR) was defined as CR + PR + SD.

Blood samples were collected at baseline (pre-treatment, day 1) and on days 18, 32, 46, 76 and 106 days post-dose for serum EGF concentration and anti-EGF antibody titers detection. Anti-EGF antibody titers were measured through a validated enzyme linked immunosorbent assay (ELISA), described in previous studies [8, 10] and EGF concentration in serum was measured with a commercial ELISA (Quantikine EGF; R&D Systems Inc., Minneapolis, MN). The detection was conducted by the Beijing Eastern Biotech, Co., Ltd.

The protocol and informed consent documents were reviewed and approved by the hospital human subjects review board and the study was performed in accordance with the Declaration of Helsinki.

Patient eligibility
Inclusion criteria
Adult patients, regardless of gender, aged from 18 to 70 years with histologically or cytologically confirmed NSCLC at stages IIIB or IV and Eastern Cooperative Oncology Group (ECOG) performance status (PS) of 0 to 2 were eligible for the study. All patients received 4 to 6 cycles of platinum-based first-line chemotherapy, from 4 to 8 weeks, and were evaluated as SD or PR after the first line chemotherapy.

Patients were required to have at least 1 measurable lesion (lesions were defined by Response Evaluation Criteria in Solid Tumors (RECIST, 1.1) [16]. If patients have ever received radiotherapy, the disease in the field of radiotherapy cannot be the target lesions and additional requirements were adequate organ function and CBC results and life expectancy of at least 3 months". Women participants should have negative pregnancy test results. All the participants should take contraception measures during the study period. Participants should sign informed consent before the study.

Exclusion criteria
Exclusion criteria included patients receiving immunosuppressant drugs 1 month before study, or receiving other immunotherapy 3 months before the study and patients receiving corticosteroid within 1 month before the research (including oral, intramuscular or intravenous injection). Inhaled corticosteroid for respiratory insufficiency or for local use were not excluded).

Patients with uncontrolled epilepsy seizure; central nervous system dysfunction or cognitive ability lose due to psychosis; CNS metastasis (confirmed or suspicious); chronic alcohol or drug abuse within 6 months before the research; pregnancy or lactation or those who refused to take contraception measures during the study were excluded. Patients with a history of severe allergy or allergic constitution; splenectomy; autoimmune disease or secondary immunodeficiency (such as AIDS, et al.); secondary malignancy within 5 years (except for basal cell carcinoma of the skin or intraepithelial carcinoma of the cervix) were also excluded.

Treatment schedule
The therapeutic cancer vaccine is composed of hu-rhEGF conjugated to the carrier protein, r-P64K, and emulsified with the adjuvant Montanide ISA 51 VG, just prior to administration to patients. Hu-rhEGF-rP64k conjugate injection solution (batch number: 121005, 121006, 121203) and Montanide ISA 51 VG (batch number: 501101, 501201) were mixed in equal parts (0.8 mL of

rhEGF/rP64k conjugate + 0.8 mL of Montanide ISA 51 VG). Hu-rhEGF-rP64k conjugate injection solution and the adjuvant were produced by the Center of Molecular Immunology (Havana, Cuba). CTX (Cyclophosphamide) injection solution (batch number: 04111001) was provided by BIOTECH PHARMA Co., Ltd.

Four to six weeks after finishing first-line chemotherapy, patients were assigned to the group of treatment with the vaccine. All patients received a low-dose of cyclophosphamide intravenously (200 mg/m2) on day 1. The vaccine was administered intramuscular at different dose levels: 0.6 mg (group A), 1.2 mg (group B), 1.8 mg (group C), and 2.4 mg (group D) on days 4, 18, 32, 46 and 76 (5 vaccine doses was administered for each patients. Monthly vaccination was administered according to the best benefits of patients and their wishes, and until the disease progressed or intolerable toxicity occurred.

Study objectives
The primary aims of the study were safety evaluation, to establish the MTD of Hu-rhEGF-rP64k vaccine in NSCLC patients and the immunological response. The secondary outcome was clinical response assessment in NSCLC treated with Hu-rhEGF-rP64k vaccine. Objective Response Rate (CR + PR) and Disease Control Rate (CR + PR + SD) were the standards of assessment.

Results
Patients' disposition
A total of 21 patients were enrolled between April 10, 2012, and May 22, 2013, for four dose levels. The procedure of enrollment, assignment and retention of study participants are carried out according to the CONSORT statement [17] and are described in Fig. 1.

Participants
Participant characteristics are listed in Table 1. Among the included patients, 12 were male while 9 were female, and median age was 54 (37~66). Median height was (167.29 ± 6.91) (158~180) cm. Median weight was (70.64 ± 12.56) (52~98) kg. Median Body Surface Area (BSA) was (1.78 ± 0.17) (1.54~2.10) m2. ECOG score: 5 patients scored 0 (23.81%) and 16 patients scored 1 (76.19%). According the histology, 2 cases were squamous cell carcinoma while 19 cases were adenocarcinoma.

The presence of mutations of the EGFR and KRAS were evaluated preliminary in 5 patients, K-RAS was not mutated and among them 2 patients have EGFR mutations (one has EGFR deletion 19 mutation and the other has EGFR deletion 21 mutation) and in one patient, EGFR mutation was no present. Since EGFR is constitutively activated in tumors with mutations at the intracellular domain, EGF binding will not be required for signal transduction, for this reason the evaluated vaccine would

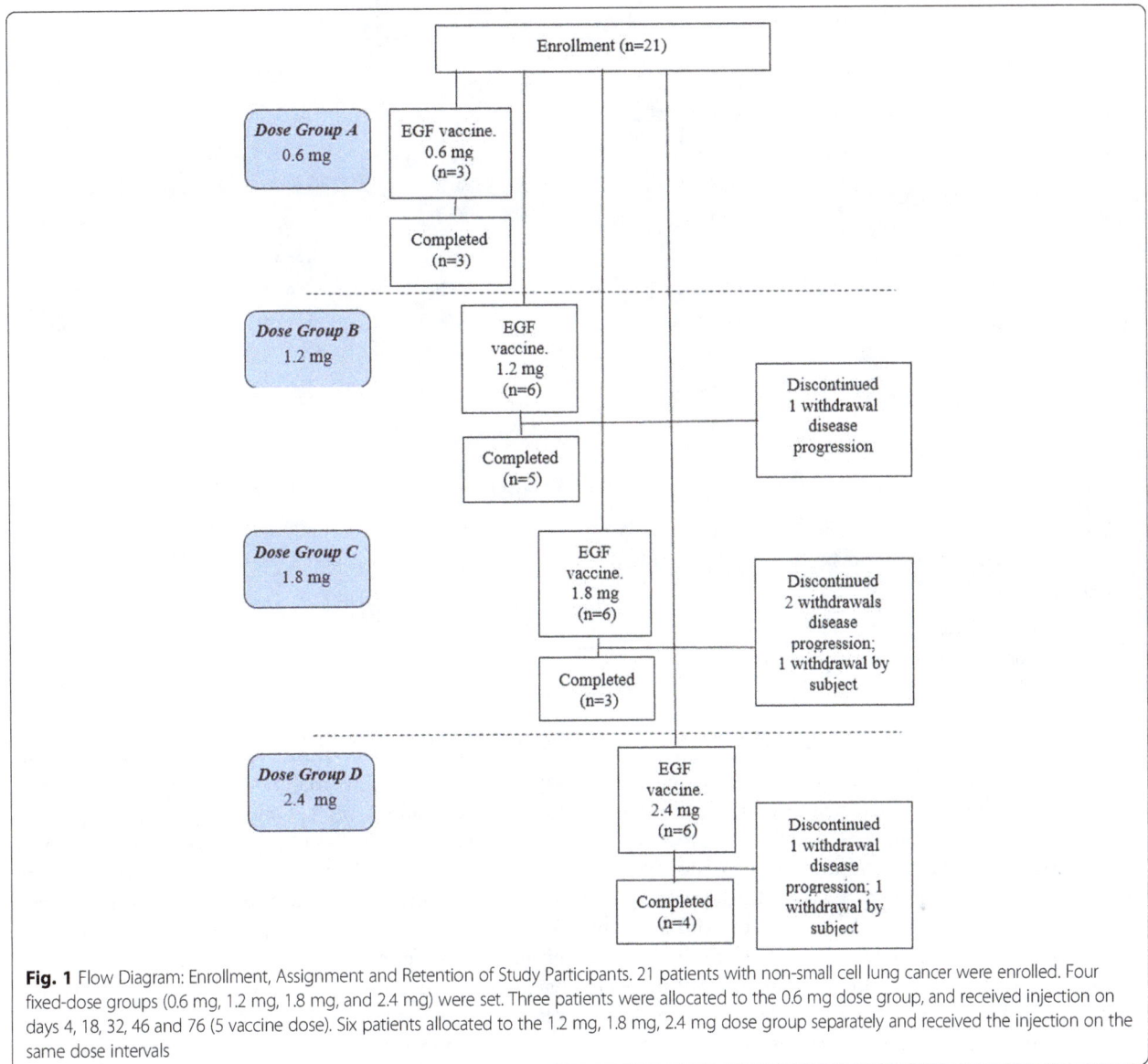

Fig. 1 Flow Diagram: Enrollment, Assignment and Retention of Study Participants. 21 patients with non-small cell lung cancer were enrolled. Four fixed-dose groups (0.6 mg, 1.2 mg, 1.8 mg, and 2.4 mg) were set. Three patients were allocated to the 0.6 mg dose group, and received injection on days 4, 18, 32, 46 and 76 (5 vaccine dose). Six patients allocated to the 1.2 mg, 1.8 mg, 2.4 mg dose group separately and received the injection on the same dose intervals

be effective in patients lacking EGFR mutations. In order to gather more information on the relevance of the individual tumor biology, additional translational studies should be included in the approaching trials, assessing the actual correlation between EGFR mutations and efficacy of the vaccine.

All patients (21) received at least one vaccine dose, 6 subjects (1 patient from group A 0.6 mg, 4 patients from group C 1.8 mg and 1 patient from group D 2.4 mg) received less than 5 doses and the rest 15 patients received 5 or more doses of vaccine. Three patients (2 patients from group A 0.6 mg and 1 patient from group C 1.8 mg) received more than 14 vaccine doses (1-year vaccination), 1 patient from group C 1.8 mg was vaccinated 26 times (2-years vaccination).

Primary endpoints outcomes
Safety profile
In order to determine the primary endpoint, MTD, the number of participants who experienced DLTs was assessed at each dose level. According to the CTCAE 4.03, a DLT was any grade 3 non-hematological toxicity or grade 4 hematological toxicity that was possibly drug-related. CTCAE 4.03 Grade 3 is a severe AE and Grade 4 is a life-threatening or disabling AE. Such events interfere with activities of daily living. The MTD is defined as the dose level below the dose at which > 33% of participants experienced a DLT. The MTD analysis population consisted of all participants who received at least one dose of the vaccine.

No DLTs were observed by patients receiving the 4 doses levels. One patient discontinued the treatment due

Table 1 Baseline demographics and disease characteristic of the patients

Characteristic	Dose groups			
	A (0.6 mg)	B (1.2 mg)	C (1.8 mg)	D (2.4 mg)
Age (years), median	54.00	56.50	46.50	58.00
Gender n (%)				
Female	0(0.00%)	2(33.33%)	4(66.67%)	3(50.00%)
Male	3(100.00%)	4(66.67%)	2(33.33%)	3(50.00%)
Height (cm), Mean (SD)	171.33 (6.35)	167.17 (5.31)	163.67 (6.09)	169.00 (8.99)
Weight (kg), mean (SD)	70.67 (16.92)	72.17 (11.02)	67.67 (16.72)	72.08 (9.97)
BSA (cm2), Mean (SD)	1.82 (0.24)	1.80 (0.14)	1.70 (0.18)	1.82 (0.17)
ECOG[a] PFS n (%)				
0	1(33.33%)	2(33.33%)	1(16.67%)	1(16.67%)
1	2(66.67%)	4(66.67%)	5(83.33%)	5(83.33%)
Histological type n (%)				
Squamous	1(33.33%)	1(16.67%)	0(0.00%)	0(0.00%)
Adenocarcinoma	2(66.67%)	5(83.33%)	6(100.00%)	6(100.00%)
First-line chemotherapy with cisplatin/carboplatin-based combination				
No. of Cycles (SD)	5.33 (0.94)	6.67 (1.15)	4.87 (1.21)	5 (1.53)
Reaction to Chemotherapy, PR/SD[b]	2/1	3/3	1/5	2/4

[a]*ECOG* Eastern Cooperative Oncology Group, *PFS* performance status
[b]*PR/SD* Partial Response/Stable Disease

to disease progression among the three participants receiving 1.2 mg dose, thus three more participants were added to the cohort of which none experienced a DLT. Two patients' withdrawals due to disease progression and 1 patient voluntary withdrawal among the participants receiving 1.8 mg vaccine dose, thus three more participants were added to the cohort of whom none experienced a DLT. One patient withdrawal due to disease progression and 1 patient voluntary withdrawal among the participants receiving 2.4 mg vaccine dose, thus three more participants were added to the cohort of whom none experienced a DLT.

The safety of vaccine was summarized by the number of patients experiencing any adverse event(s), serious and non-serious, which were collected by systematic assessment using terms from the CTCAE 4.03. Adverse events (AE) were reported in 14 cases (66.67%, 48 case-times) among all participants in all 4 cohorts. Ten patients have grade 1 adverse events and three patients have grade 2 adverse events, from them 1 patient in Group A, has WBC decrease; 1 patient in Group B has temporary amaurosis and 1 patient in Group C with erythema, itching and pain at the injection site. Only one patient has grade 3 AE, neutrophil count decreased, which was not related to the vaccine but to the previous chemotherapy. The summary of adverse events is presented in Table 2.

The most frequents adverse event were dizziness (27.1%); injection-site pain (10.4%); tremors (8.3%); headache (6.25%); face flushing (6.25) and injection-site erythema (4.2%). The majority of the adverse events (90%) were grade 1 or 2. Only three cases of grade 3 adverse events, in the 2.4 mg dose level (Group D), were reported, none of them were related to the vaccine. These severe adverse events (SAEs) were: 1 case of grade 3 leukopenia, 1 case of grade 4 neutropenia and 1 case of anal fistula (grade 3), where hospitalization was indicated and the patient was submitted to surgery and recovered from the AE. This last adverse event was reported as non-related SAE. None patients were withdrawn the study due to adverse events.

By the date of submission, 1 case of anemia had been improved, and in 1 case of leukopenia the condition is still ongoing. All other adverse events have been recovered. None patient was dropout of the research due to adverse events. No death cases during the research period.

Immunological response: Serum EGF concentration and anti-EGF antibodies detection

Serum EGF and anti-EGF antibody titers were evaluated in 21 patients before and after vaccination. Blood samples were collected at baseline (pre-treatment, day 1) and on days 18, 32, 46, 76 and 106 days post-vaccination. Anti-EGF antibody titers were measured through an ELISA. EGF concentration in serum was measured with a commercial ELISA (Quantikine; R&D Systems Inc., Minneapolis, MN).

Table 2 Adverse events reported during the study

Adverse events	Group A - 0.6 mg n = 3		Group B - 1.2 mg n = 3		Group C - 1.8 mg n = 3		Group D - 2.4 mg n = 3	
	AEs	Patients	AEs	Patients	AEs	Patients	AEs	Patients
White blood cell decreased	1	1	1	1	1	1	2	1
ALT increased	1	1	0	0	1	1	0	0
Neutrophil count decreased	0	0	0	0	0	0	1	1
AST increased	0	0	0	0	1	1	0	0
Hemoglobin increased	1	1	0	0	0	0	0	0
Headache	0	0	0	0	3	3	0	0
Dizziness	4	2	4	3	5	3	0	0
Temporary amaurosis	0	0	1	1	0	0	0	0
Cough	0	0	0	0	1	1	0	0
Upper respiratory infection	1	1	0	0	0	0	0	0
Hyperhidrosis	0	0	0	0	1	1	0	0
Fever	0	0	1	1	1	1	0	0
Tremors	0	0	2	1	2	1	0	0
Face flushing	3	1	0	0	0	0	0	0
Injection site erythema	0	0	0	0	2	1	0	0
Injection site itching	0	0	0	0	1	1	0	0
injection site pain	3	1	2	2	0	0	0	0
Nausea	0	0	0	0	1	1	0	0
Total	14		11		20		3	

The kinetics of the geometric mean of anti-EGF antibody titers and serum EGF concentration in patients are described in Fig. 2. As showed in the figure, a significant inverse correlation was observed (Spearman rho = − 1.000, $p < 0, 01$) between the anti-EGF antibody titers and serum EGF concentration in patients treated with the vaccine.

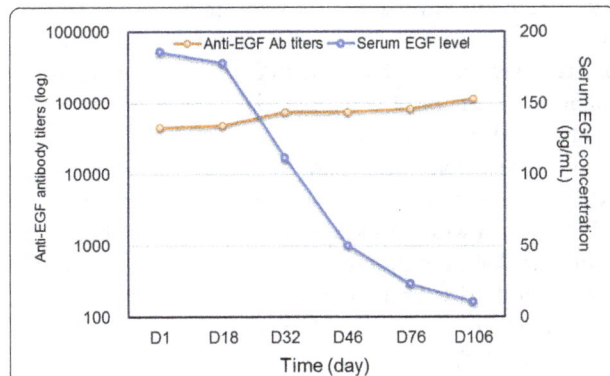

Fig. 2 Kinetics of the anti-EGF antibody titers and serum EGF concentration in patients. A significant inverse correlation was observed (Spearman rho = − 1.000, $p < 0, 01$) between the anti-EGF antibody titers and serum EGF concentration in patients treated with the vaccine

Secondary endpoints
Clinical response evaluation
The first clinical response evaluation was done at 46 days ±1 week and the second evaluation was done at 106 days ±1 week. After the first response assessment ($n = 20$), none patients achieved CR or PR, and 15 patients (75%) were on SD. After the second response evaluation ($n = 15$), no patients had achieved objective response (CR or PR), while 12 (80%) patients had SD and the remaining three (20%) patients had progressive disease. DCR for each dose group were: 100% for 0.6 mg dose group; 60% for 1.2 mg dose group; 66.67% for 1.8 mg dose group and 100% for 2.4 mg dose group. Detailed information is presented on Table 3.

Discussion
Worldwide lung cancer is the main cause of cancer-related death [1]. Among the cases of lung cancer, NSCLC histology prevails, representing between 75 and 80% of lung tumors [2, 3]. Improvements in the treatment of advanced disease with first-line and subsequent therapies are allowing longer survival, disease control and superior quality of life for the patients. Four to six cycles of platinum-based chemotherapy has been the standard first line for the treatment of unselected patients with this cancer subtype. Second-line chemotherapy may include

Table 3 Clinical response to Hu-rhEGF-rP64k vaccine

First evaluation [n (%)] Day 46

Response	Group A–0.6 mg	Group B- 1.2 mg	Group C-1.8 mg	Group D-2.4 mg	Total
	n = 3	n = 6	n = 5	n = 6	n = 20
CR	0(0%)	0(0%)	0(0%)	0(0%)	0(0%)
PR	0(0%)	0(0%)	0(0%)	0(0%)	0(0%)
SD	3(100%)	4(67%)	3(60%)	5(83%)	15(75%)
PD	0(0%)	2(33%)	2(40%)	1(17%)	5(25%)

Second evaluation [n (%)] Day 106

Response	Group A–0.6 mg	Group B- 1.2 mg	Group C-1.8 mg	Group D-2.4 mg	Total
	n = 3	n = 5	n = 3	n = 4	n = 15
CR	0(0%)	0(0%)	0(0%)	0(0%)	0(0%)
PR	0(0%)	0(0%)	0(0%)	0(0%)	0(0%)
SD	3(100%)	3(60%)	2(67%)	4(100%)	12(80%)
PD	0(0%)	2(40%)	1(33%)	0(0%)	3(20%)

pemetrexed in non-squamous cancer and docetaxel or erlotinib (or both) in all types of NSCLC. NSCLC management has positively evolved from the emergence of immunotherapy, currently positioned as second line therapy [18]. Antitumor activity, long lasting response and survival increases in advanced NSCLC patients has been demonstrated with the use of anti-PD-1 passive immunotherapy [19], leading to regulatory approval of an anti-PD-1 drug, nivolumab (Opdivo; Bristol-Myers Squibb) [20] for the treatment of metastatic squamous non–small-cell lung cancer (NSCLC) in patients who have progressed on a platinum-based chemotherapy.

Active cancer immunotherapy is also gaining importance in management of advanced stage. Hu-rhEGF-rP64k vaccine is a therapeutic modality that exerts its anti-cancer activity by targeting the immune system, specifically the self-molecule Epidermal Growth Factor (EGF). The activation of EGF receptor, blocks apoptosis, stimulates cell proliferation, induces malignant transformation, angiogenesis and metastasis [21]. In Hu-rhEGF-rP64k vaccine, the human EGF protein is chemically conjugated to P64K protein, which is a highly immunogenic molecule from Neisseria meningitides, additionally the conjugate is emulsified in the Montanide ISA51 VG adjuvant, enhancing the immunogenicity and promoting the generation of higher titers of anti-EGF antibody titers [22]. The antibodies generated by Hu-rhEGF-rP64k vaccination produced a deprivation of circulating EGF and avoid the activation of the receptor, preventing the initiation of the intracellular signaling cascade. Clinically, the vaccine produces disease stabilization and a prolongation of survival [6, 23].

The preclinical studies found that Hu-rhEGF-rP64k vaccine is immunogenic, well tolerated and has antitumor activity [24–27]. The Phase I to Phase III clinical trials have shown overall survival benefits in addition to an improvement of the quality of life in NSCLC patients [6–9, 11, 22]. It has been demonstrated in NSCLC patients treated with Hu-rhEGF-rP64k vaccine in multiple clinical trials, that high anti-EGF antibodies titers followed by the consequent reduction of serum EGF levels correlates with a significant overall survival benefit for subgroups of patients, especially for those patients with high baseline levels of serum EGF [11]. No serious safety concerns have arisen with the use of Hu-rhEGF-rP64k vaccine and to date the vaccine has shown a mild and very well tolerated adverse event profile.

The primary endpoint in this study was safety. Repeated administration Hu-rhEGF-rP64k vaccine did not result in any dose-limiting toxicities or serious adverse events related to vaccine treatment. The vaccine doses in the four groups (0.6 mg; 1.2 mg; 1.8 mg and 2.4 mg) were well tolerated. MTD was not established in this study. Similar to previous clinical trials [13], the most frequent adverse events were grade 1–2 dizziness, injection-site pain and erythema, tremors and headache. There were no deaths attributed to the vaccine treatment in this clinical trial. The data gathered from this study confirms that under the condition of the study, rhEGF-rP64k vaccine is safe in patients with advanced NSCLC and prolonged vaccination schedule could be administered without inducing severe adverse effects.

Immunological response was also a primary endpoint of this clinical trial. Each dose of Hu-rhEGF-rP64k vaccine was administered from 1 to 4 injections sites, by intramuscular route. The selection of the clinical immunization schedule was based on the previous non-clinical and clinical studies, consisting of an induction phase (to induce maximum antibodies titers) of four bi-weekly immunizations followed by a maintenance phase consisting of monthly re-immunization to maintain the anti-EGF antibodies titers developed during the induction stage [11]. In this phase I trial this dose schedule was effective to induced the production of anti-EGF antibodies that correlated inversely with the EGF concentration. The association between the immunological response and the efficacy parameters was not evaluated in this trial but should be addressed in the subsequent trials since the data of previous studies suggest that a significant survival benefit is achieved mainly in patients having good antibody response after induction period and high EGF concentration after front line chemotherapy [11].

After Hu-rhEGF-rP64k vaccination, 80% of the patients had SD, which confirm that the vaccine after first-line chemotherapy can get high disease control rate. The anti-cancer activity of this novel vaccine target the immune system, inducing an increase in the patient's anti-Epidermal Growth Factor (EGF) antibody titers and reduction of the circulating EGF [13]. The effect of the vaccine on the tumor is not a direct one, it is manifested through the impact on the patient's immune response and may not cause important tumor regression but may significantly slow tumor growth and a final positive impact on survival is achieved.

The data collected from this phase I clinical trial demonstrated that Hu-rhEGF-rP64k vaccination in advanced NSCLC patient is safe and confirm the expected effect on the immune system and on the tumor of the included patients. A new clinical trial to confirm the impact of this vaccine on the survival of patients should be performed.

Conclusion
Hu-rhEGF-rP64k/Mont elicited a valuable immune response, with good safety profile assuring further clinical development of the vaccine in this population to further confirm the potential benefits on survival.

Abbreviations
AE: Adverse event; BSA: Body surface area; CR: Complete response; DCR: Disease control rate; DLT: Dose-limiting toxicity; ECOG: Eastern Cooperative Oncology Group; EGF: Epidermal growth factor; EGF-R: Epidermal growth factor receptor; ELISA: Enzyme linked immunosorbent assay; MTD: Maximum-tolerated dose; NSCLC: Non-small cell lung cancer; PD: Progressive disease; PR: Partial response; PS: Performance status; rhEGF: Recombinant human epidermal growth factor; rP64K: Recombinant P64K; SAE: Severe adverse event; SD: Stable disease

Acknowledgements
We thank M.D. Patricia Piedra Sierra from Center of Molecular Immunology of Cuba for critical review of the manuscript. We also thank Beijing Eastern Biotech, Co., Ltd. for the help with the detection of serum EGF.

Funding
The Chinese Major Project for New Drug Innovation Project (2012ZX09303012-001and2014ZX09102041-006).

Authors' contributions
Conception and design of the trial: YK S, YS and PX Provision of study materials or patients: YK S, YS, PX, HW and SY Collection and assembly of data: YK S, YS, PX, HW, SY and XH Detection of serum EGF, data analysis and interpretation: YK S, PX and XH Manuscript writing: all authors. All authors read and approved the final manuscript.

Competing interests
The authors declare that they have no competing interests.

Author details
[1]Department of Medical Oncology, Beijing Key Laboratory of Clinical Study on Anticancer Molecular Targeted Drugs, National Cancer Center/Cancer Hospital, Chinese Academy of Medical Sciences & Peking Union Medical College, Beijing 100021, China. [2]Department of Clinical Laboratory, National Cancer Center/Cancer Hospital, Chinese Academy of Medical Sciences & Peking Union Medical College, Beijing 100021, China.

References
1. Ferlay J, Soerjomataram I, Dikshit R, Eser S, Mathers C, Rebelo M, Parkin DM, Forman D, Bray F. Cancer incidence and mortality worldwide: sources, methods and major patterns in GLOBOCAN 2012. Int J Cancer. 2015;136: E359–E86.
2. Howlader N, Noone AM, Krapcho M, Miller D, Bishop K, Altekruse SF, Kosary CL, Yu M, Ruhl J, Tatalovich Z, Mariotto A, Lewis DR, Chen HS, Feuer EJ, Cronin KA (eds). SEER Cancer Statistics Review, 1975-2013, Bethesda: National Cancer Institute. https://seer.cancer.gov/csr/1975_2013/, based on November 2015 SEER data submission, posted to the SEER web site, April 2016.
3. Bethesda M. SEER. 2016.
4. Reck M, Popat S, Reinmuth N, De Ruysscher D, Kerr KM, Peters S, Group. EGW. Metastatic non-small-cell lung cancer (NSCLC): ESMO Clinical Practice Guidelines for diagnosis, treatment and follow-up. Ann Oncol. 2014;25:27–39.
5. DeSantis CE, Lin C, Mariotto AB, Siegel RL, Stein KD, Kramer JL, Alteri R, Robbins AS, Jemal A. Cancer treatment and survivorship statistics, 2014. CA Cancer J Clin. 2014;64:252–71.
6. Gisela Gonzalez AL. Cancer vaccines for hormone/growth factor immune deprivation: a feasible approach for cancer treatment. Curr Cancer Drug Targets. 2007:191–201.
7. Gonzalez G, Crombet T, Neninger E, Viada C, Lage A. Therapeutic vaccination with epidermal growth factor (EGF) in advanced lung cancer. Hum Vaccin. 2007;3:8–13.
8. Neninger Vinageras E, de la Torre A, Osorio Rodríguez M, Catalá Ferrer M, Bravo I, Mendoza del Pino M, Abreu Abreu D, Acosta Brooks S, Rives R, del Castillo Carrillo C, González Dueñas M, Viada C, García Verdecia B, Crombet Ramos T, González Marinello G. Phase II randomized controlled trial of an epidermal growth factor vaccine in advanced non-small-cell lung cancer. J Clin Oncol. 2008;26:1452–8.
9. Garcia B, Neninger E, de la Torre A, Leonard I, Martínez R, Viada C, González G, Mazorra Z, Lage A, Crombet T. Effective inhibition of the epidermal growth factor/epidermal growth factor receptor binding by anti-epidermal growth factor antibodies is related to better survival in advanced NSCLC patients treated with the epidermal growth factor cancer vaccine. Clin Cancer Res. 2008;14:840–6.
10. Ramos TC, Vinageras E, Ferrer MC, Verdecia BG, Rupalé IL, Pérez LM, Marinello GG, Rodríguez RP, Dávila AL. Treatment of NSCLC patients with an EGF-based cancer vaccine: report of a phase I trial. Cancer Biol Ther. 2006;5:145–9.
11. Rodriguez PC, Popa X, Martínez O, Mendoza S, Santiesteban E, Crespo T, Amador RM, Fleytas R, Acosta SC, Otero Y, Romero GN, de la Torre A, Cala M, Arzuaga L, Vello L, Reyes D. A phase III clinical trial of the epidermal growth factor vaccine CIMAvax-EGF as switch maintenance therapy in advanced non-small cell lung cancer patients. Clin Cancer Res. 2016;22:3782–90.
12. Le Tourneau C, Lee J, Siu LL. Dose escalation methods in phase I cancer clinical trials. J Natl Cancer Inst. 2009;101:708–20.
13. Rodriguez PC, Rodríguez G, González G, Lage A. Clinical development and

perspectives of CIMAvax EGF, Cuban vaccine for non-small celllung cancer therapy. MEDICC Rev. 2010;12:17–23.

14. Rodriguez PC, Neninger E, García B, Popa X, Lorenzo-Luaces P, Viada C, González G, Lage A, Montero E, Crombet T. Safety, immunogenicity and preliminary efficacy of multiple-site vaccination with an epidermal growth factor (EGF) based cancer vaccine in NSCLC patients. J Immune Based Ther Vaccines. 2011;9:7.

15. Institute NC. 2010. https://evs.nci.nih.gov/ftp1/CTCAE/About.html

16. Eisenhauera EA. New response evaluation criteria in solid tumours: revised RECIST guideline (version 1.1). Eur J Cancer. 2009;45:228–47.

17. Moher D, Hopewell S, Schulz KF, Montori V, Gotzsche PC, Devereaux PJ, et al. CONSORT 2010 explanation and elaboration: updated guidelines for reporting parallel group randomised trials. J Clin Epidemiol. 2010;63:e1–37.

18. Socinski MA, Pennell NA. Best practices in treatment selection for patients. Cancer Control. 2016;23:2–14.

19. Langer CJ. Emerging immunotherapies in the treatment of non-small cell lung cancer (NSCLC): the role of immune checkpoint inhibitors. Am J Clin Oncol. 2015;38:422–30.

20. Ingram I. Cancer network. 2015.

21. Salomon DS, Brandt R, Ciardiello F, Normanno N. Epidermal growth factor-related peptides and their receptors in human malignancies. Crit Rev Oncol Hematol. 1995;19:183–232.

22. Gonzalez G, Crombet T, Torres F, Catala M, Alfonso L, Osorio M, Neninger E, Garcia B, Mulet A, Perez R, Lage A. Epidermal growth factor-based cancer vaccine for non-small-cel llung cancer therapy. Ann Oncol. 2003;14:461–6.

23. Gonzalez G, Crombet T, Catala M, Mirabal V, Hernandez JC, Gonzalez Y, Marinello P, Guilen G, Lage A. A novel cancer vaccine composed of human recombinant epidermal growth factor linked to a carrier protein: report of a pilot clinical trial. Ann Oncol. 1998;9:431–5.

24. Gonzalez G, Sánchez B, Suarez E, Beausouleil I, Perez O, Lastre M, Lage A. Induction of immune recognition of self epidermal growth factor (EGF): effect on EGF biodistribution and tumor growth. Vaccine Res. 1996;5:233–44.

25. Casaco A, Díaz Y, Ledón N, Merino N, Valdés O, Garcia G, Garcia B, González G, Pérez R. Effect of an EGF-cancer vaccine on wound healing and inflammation models. J Surg Res. 2004;122:130–34.

26. Rodriguez PC, Gonzalez I, Gonzalez A, Avellanet J, Lopez A, Perez R, Lage A, Montero E. Priming and boosting determinants on the antibody response to an epidermal growth factor-based cancer vaccine. Vaccine. 2008;26:4647–54.

27. Manceboa A, Casaco A, González B, Ledón N, Sorlozabal J, León A, Gómez D, González Y, Bada AM, González C, Arteaga ME, Ramirez H, Fuentes D. Repeated dose intramuscular injection of the CIMAvax-EGF vaccine in Sprague Dawley rats induces local ánd systemic toxicity. Vaccine. 2012;30: 3329–38.

6

Generation of populations of antigen-specific cytotoxic T cells using DCs transfected with DNA construct encoding HER2/neu tumor antigen epitopes

Maria Kuznetsova[1], Julia Lopatnikova[1], Julia Khantakova[1], Rinat Maksyutov[2], Amir Maksyutov[2,1] and Sergey Sennikov[1*] (iD)

Abstract

Background: Recent fundamental and clinical studies have confirmed the effectiveness of utilizing the potential of the immune system to remove tumor cells disseminated in a patient's body. Cytotoxic T lymphocytes (CTLs) are considered the main effectors in cell-mediated antitumor immunity. Approaches based on antigen presentation to CTLs by dendritic cells (DCs) are currently being intensively studied, because DCs are more efficient in tumor antigen presentation to T cells through their initiation of strong specific antitumor immune responses than other types of antigen-presenting cells. Today, it has become possible to isolate CTLs specific for certain antigenic determinants from heterogeneous populations of mononuclear cells. This enables direct and specific cell-mediated immune responses against cells carrying certain antigens. The aim of the present study was to develop an optimized protocol for generating CTL populations specific for epitopes of tumor-associated antigen HER2/neu, and to assess their cytotoxic effects against the HER2/neu-expressing MCF-7 tumor cell line.

Methods: The developed protocol included sequential stages of obtaining mature DCs from PBMCs from HLA A*02-positive healthy donors, magnet-assisted transfection of mature DCs with the pMax plasmid encoding immunogenic peptides HER2 p369–377 (E75 peptide) and HER2 p689–697 (E88 peptide), coculture of antigen-activated DCs with autologous lymphocytes, magnetic-activated sorting of CTLs specific to HER2 epitopes, and stimulation of isolated CTLs with cytokines (IL-2, IL-7, and IL-15).

Results: The resulting CTL populations were characterized by high contents of CD8+ cells (71.5% in cultures of E88-specific T cells and 90.2% in cultures of E75-specific T cells) and displayed strong cytotoxic effects against the MCF-7 cell line (percentages of damaged tumor cells in samples under investigation were 60.2 and 65.7% for E88- and E75-specific T cells, respectively; level of spontaneous death of target cells was 17.9%).

Conclusions: The developed protocol improves the efficiency of obtaining HER2/neu-specific CTLs and can be further used to obtain cell-based vaccines for eradicating targeted tumor cells to prevent tumor recurrence after the major tumor burden has been eliminated and preventing metastasis in patients with HER2-overexpressing tumors.

Keywords: Cytotoxic T cells, CTLs, Antigen-specific cells, Dendritic cells, HER2/neu, Tumor-associated antigen, Antitumor immune response

* Correspondence: sennikovsv@gmail.com
[1]Federal State Budgetary Scientific Institution "Research Institute of Fundamental and Clinical Immunology", Yadrintsevskaya str., 14, Novosibirsk 630099, Russia
Full list of author information is available at the end of the article

Background

The minimal residual disease remaining after resection of the major tumor burden underlies the existing problems of tumor recurrence and metastasis, which increase the mortality and morbidity rates among cancer patients. In this connection, there is obviously a need for the development of new technologies that can improve the recognition and elimination of single cancer cells remaining in a patient's body after radiation therapy, chemotherapy, or surgical resection.

Currently, cytotoxic T cells are considered the main effectors in cell-mediated antitumor immunity. The presence, number, and adequate function of antitumor cytotoxic T lymphocytes (CTLs) are necessary conditions for the destruction of tumor cells by the immune system [1]. Cytotoxic effects of antigen-specific CTLs against cells of different tumor types have been demonstrated in a number of studies. Back in 2000, it was shown that CTLs specific for HLA-A2-restrictive peptide PR1 could destroy leukemia cells, thus contributing to the elimination of chronic myeloid leukemia [2]. Bernhard et al. demonstrated that CTLs specific for E75 peptide of the HER2/neu tumor antigen could eliminate breast cancer cells in patients after adoptive transfer of HER2-specific CTL populations [3].

Dendritic cells (DCs) are widely used in cancer immunotherapy to stimulate specific antitumor immune responses, because they can effectively recognize and present tumor antigens to T cells both in vitro and in vivo [4–6]. DC vaccines are currently widespread [7]. However, much controversy still surrounds the issue of whether endogenously activated T-cell responses can mediate tumor regression, because tumor progression is often observed even in the presence of high levels of blood-circulating or tumor-infiltrating T cells [8, 9]. Meanwhile, successful ex vivo activation of antitumor cytotoxic T cells (in the absence of immunosuppressive tumor effects) followed by adoptive transfer of activated T cells that eventually retain their ability to eliminate tumor cells in the patient's body has been reported [3]. This advantage of adoptive transfer of autologous T cells activated ex vivo provided grounds to suggest the promising potential of generating an optimal protocol to obtain antigen-specific CTL populations using DCs loaded with a tumor antigen under in vitro conditions, which can be further used to develop effective antitumor cell-based vaccines.

It is currently possible to isolate CTLs specific for certain antigenic determinants from heterogeneous peripheral blood mononuclear cell (PBMC) populations, thus making it possible to target specific cell-mediated immune responses against tumor cells carrying these antigens [7, 10, 11]. A number of procedures employing MHC molecules have been developed to isolate populations of antigen-specific T cells. The principle of these procedures involving MHC molecules is based on use of a T-cell receptor (TCR) ligand, an MHC/antigen peptide complex, as a dye probe via conjugation of the complex to fluorochrome molecules. Recombinant MHC molecules are conjugated to antigen epitopes typical of various types of disease, such as epitopes of tumor antigens. MHC molecules interact with TCR expressed on the T-cell surface. As TCR–MHC interactions are characterized by very weak affinity for one another, monomeric MHC/epitope complexes cannot ensure stable binding. This problem has been solved using multimeric MHC/epitope complexes, which increase the affinity of the binding reaction, and thus facilitate the formation of a stable complex [12]. Thus, MHC multimers can be used to identify and isolate antigen-specific CTLs.

In 2007 the novel Streptamer technology has been developed for the detection and purification of antigen-specific T cells [13]. A distinctive feature of this technology from other MHC multimer-based technologies is the reversibility of staining which allows complete dissociation of all staining reagents from the cell surface after the isolation procedure. Thus, several side effects caused by long-term presence of staining molecules on the surface of labeled cells might be avoided, including T-cell anergy, immune responses directly against the reagents, and loss of the capacity of the transferred T cells to migrate in vivo. Thereby the Streptamer technology significantly improves the quality of the antigen-specific T-cell populations obtained and makes it possible to use the isolated cells in clinical practice for adoptive T-cell transfer [14].

The membrane protein HER2 (human epidermal growth factor receptor 2: HER2/neu) is a tumor-associated antigen whose overexpression is observed in various types of carcinomas, including breast, colon, stomach, pancreatic, and thyroid carcinomas, as well as ovarian cancer [15]. It is known that 20–25% of breast tumors are characterized by HER2 overexpression. Receptor overexpression or HER2 oncogene amplification are associated with the most aggressive phenotype of this type of tumor, shorter relapse-free period after primary therapy, and worse survival rate [16]. HER2 was shown to be a pathological biomarker that can differentiate between tumor and normal mammary gland cells, because HER2 expression on the surface of HER2-overexpressing breast carcinomas can be up to 50 fold higher than its expression on normal cells [17]. The fundamental role of HER2 in triggering the signaling cascade that results in tumor growth determines the trajectory of development of breast cancer therapies toward targeting this antigen.

Hence, the development of optimized protocol for generating populations of antitumor antigen-specific

CTLs using DCs and isolating antigen-specific cells is promising for the most efficient production of T-cell preparations toward adoptive transfer aimed at eliminating the minimal residual disease after removal of the major tumor burden, in the form of tumor cells disseminated in the patient's body.

This study aimed to develop a protocol for obtaining and enriching populations of antitumor cytotoxic T cells specific for tumor-associated protein HER2 and to assess their cytotoxic activity against HER2-expressing MCF-7 tumor cells. The main advantage of the proposed approach is the combination of protocol of generation of an specific cytotoxic antitumor T cell-mediated immune response by dendritic cells transfected with DNA constructs encoding the immunogenic HER2/neu epitopes and the technology of isolation of activated antigen-specific CTLs which allows rapid and complete removal of the staining reagents from the T cells and thus assures the isolation of fully functional T cells with non-affected viability. Combining methods of efficient generation of antigen-specific antitumor T cell populations and subsequent isolation of activated cytotoxic T cells appropriate for clinical use, this approach can be used to generate functionally active antigen-specific T lymphocytes from peripheral blood mononuclear cells of patients with HER2-positive malignancies for adoptive T-cell transfer to eliminate HER2-positive tumor cells, prevent metastasis and relapse.

Methods

Blood samples

Peripheral blood samples from healthy donors carrying the HLA-A02 allele, as shown by genotyping (n = 16), were used in this study. Whole blood samples were obtained from Blood Procurement Station No. 1 of the State-Government-financed Institution of Public Health for the Novosibirsk Region (Novosibirsk Blood Center). Voluntary informed consent was obtained from all the donors. Study design was approved by the local ethics committee of the Research Institute of Clinical Immunology, Siberian Branch of the Russian Academy of Sciences (protocol no. 75 dated April 9, 2013).

DNA constructs and HER2 protein epitopes

To generate strong immune responses, we selected HER2 protein epitopes E75 (HER2 p369–377; KIFG-SLAFL) and E88 (HER2 p689–697; RLLQETELV). These epitopes reported to be most effectively recognized by cytotoxic T cells of HLA-A02-positive donors because of their high affinity for binding to the HLA-A0201 molecule [18–20].

Antigenic activation of mature DCs (mDCs) with HER2 tumor-associated antigens was performed by magnet-assisted transfection with a pMax DNA construct encoding the epitopes E75 and E88 from HER2/neu protein. Proteasomal cleavage and TAP predictions confirmed that flanking sequences are not required for correct processing of selected epitopes. Nevertheless, DNA construct encoding multiple copies of each epitope in different molecular contexts (with or without spacers respectively) was designed for further ensuring a correct antigen presenting and effective stimulation of antigen-specific immune responses by DCs. An ubiquitin was bound to N terminus of prepared DNA construct. The artificial gene encoding poly-CTL epitope immunogen was designed and prepared with an optimization of codon composition for efficient expression in mammalian cells. Next, the artificial gene was cloned into the pmax-Ub vector and resulting DNA construct with N-terminal ubiquitin was prepared. DNA construct was amplified in a preparation form and purified from endotoxins. The nucleotide sequences were verified by sequencing. An additional file shows the resulting amino acid sequences (see Additional file 1).

The construct based on the DNA-vector pDNAVAC-Cultra5 without inserts of immunogenic peptides was used as the control for magnet-assisted transfection of DCs [DNA (p5) construct].

Donor genotyping

DNA for genotyping was isolated from whole blood samples of the donors using the standard phenol–chloroform extraction procedure [21]. HLA-A locus genotyping was carried out by PCR amplification of gene regions using a commercial ALLSET™ GOLD HLA A LOW RES SSP Kit (Invitrogen, USA) according to the manufacturer's protocol. We also used Hot Start Taq DNA polymerase (SibEnzyme, Russia). The amplified DNA fragments were identified by 2% agarose gel electrophoresis. DNA molecular weight markers M16, pUC19/Msp I (SibEnzyme, Russia), and Tris-acetate buffer were used for gel electrophoresis.

Generation of mDCs

RPMI-1640 medium (Biolot, Russia) supplemented with 10% fetal calf serum (Hyclone, USA), 2 mM L-glutamine (Biolot, Russia), 5×10^{-5} mM mercaptoethanol (Sigma, USA), 25 mM HEPES (Sigma, USA), 80 μg/ml gentamicin (KRKA, Slovenia), and 100 μg/ml ampicillin (Sintez, Russia) was used for culture of mononuclear cells (MNCs).

Venous blood samples from healthy donors carrying the HLA-A02 allele were collected into lithium heparin vacuum tubes (Vacuette LH Lithium Heparin; Greiner Bio-One GmbH, Austria). PBMCs were isolated using a conventional density gradient of Ficoll–Urografin [22]. Briefly, 12-ml samples of blood diluted in RPMI-1640 medium to a final volume of 35 ml were layered over 15 ml of Ficoll–Urografin solution (ρ = 1.077 g/L) (Ficoll:

Pharmacia Fine Chemical, Switzerland; Urografin: Scher-ing AG, Germany), centrifuged at 1500 rpm for 40 min, and washed twice with RPMI-1640 medium. Cells with increased adhesion were isolated by incubation for 2 h on plastic Petri dishes (Nunc, Denmark) in 10 ml of cul-ture medium under a humid atmosphere at 37 °C and 5% CO_2. After the incubation, the entire medium containing the fraction of non-adherent PBMCs was transferred into clean centrifuge tubes. Next, 10 ml of RPMI-1640 medium was added to the Petri dishes and the fraction of adherent PBMCs was removed from the bot-tom of the Petri dishes with a scraper (Sigma-Aldrich, USA). The suspensions containing the adherent and non-adherent fractions were centrifuged at 1500 rpm for 10 min. After the centrifugation, the cell pellets were re-suspended in 1 ml of culture medium, and the numbers of cells in both fractions were counted in a Goryaev chamber using acetic acid. The non-adherent cell fraction was then cultured in Petri dishes at a concentration of 2×10^6 cells/ ml in 10 ml of culture medium for 6 days, until the cocul-ture procedure was started.

To stimulate monocyte differentiation of the adherent fraction of PBMCs into immature DCs (iDCs), the ad-herent cell fraction at a concentration of 1×10^6 cells/ml was cultured in culture medium in 48-well plates (Cell-star, USA) under a humid atmosphere at 37 °C and 5% CO_2 in the presence of GM-CSF (50 ng/ml) and IL-4 (100 ng/ml) (Peprotech, USA). After 96 h of culture, the culture medium was replaced and TNFα (25 ng/ml) (State Research Center of Virology and Biotechnology "Vector", Russia) was added to the iDC culture to stimu-late the maturation and generation of mDCs.

Loading of mDCs with tumor antigen

Antigenic activation of mDCs with tumor-associated antigen HER2/neu was performed by magnet-assisted transfection using magnetic nanoparticles (MATra-A Reagent; PromoKine, Germany), a pMax DNA construct encoding two HER2/neu protein epitopes (E75 and E88) and a DNA (p5) construct (without inserts of immuno-genic peptides) as a control. Magnet-assisted transfec-tion was carried out in accordance with the protocol provided by the manufacturer (PromoKine).

To evaluate the effectiveness of transfection into DCs, magnet-assisted transfection of DCs was performed with the pmaxGFP plasmid encoding green fluorescent pro-tein (GFP). The transfection effectiveness was evaluated based on production of the protein encoded by the plas-mid. Specifically, the number of GFP-positive cells was determined in a BD FACS Verse flow cytometry system (Becton Dickinson, USA) at 24 h after the magnet-assisted transfection or nucleofection of DCs. Added propidium iodide (PI) (Sigma, USA) allowed determin-ation of the viability of the cell culture post-transfection.

Phenotyping of DCs and assessment of their functional activity

The phenotype of DCs was assessed by flow cytometry in a BD FACS Aria (Becton Dickinson, USA) using corresponding monoclonal antibodies labeled with fluorochromes (CD3-Pacific Blue, CD14-FITC, HLA-DR-PerCP-Cy5.5, CD11c-PE, CD86-PE-Cy7, and CD83-APC; Becton Dickinson, USA) according to the manufacturer's recommendations. Examples of the used gates are shown in additional files (see Additional file 2).

The criterion for functional activity of DCs was their susceptibility to receptor-mediated endocytosis by FITC-dextran capture (Sigma, USA). Briefly, the cells were in-cubated with FITC-dextran (1 µg/ml) in the complete medium at 4 and 37 °C. Dextran became bound to the surface receptors at 4 °C, and the bound dextran pene-trated into the cells at 37 °C (endocytosis).

Generation of activated HER2-specific T cells

To generate HER2-specific T cells, the monocyte-depleted PBMC culture (non-adherent MNCs, 1×10^6 cells/ml) was cocultured with DCs (1×10^6 cells/ml). The coculture was performed at an MNC:DC ratio of 10:1 in the culture medium (1 ml/well) in 48-well plates (Cellstar, USA) for 4 days.

Streptamer staining and identification of HER2-specific T cells

To identify the population of HER2-specific T cells in the coculture of MNCs and DCs, the cells were stained using MHC I-Strep HLA-A*0201 (plus peptide KIFG-SLAFL of the HER2/neu antigen), Strep-tactin PE, and IS buffer (IBA GmbH, Germany). The stained samples were then analyzed by flow cytometry on the BD FACS Verse system. For staining complex formation, 0.8 µl of MHC and 1 µl of Strep-tactin PE were incubated in the IS buffer solution, at a final volume of 25 µl, for 45 min at 4 °C. After incubation of the cells with the complex, the reaction was stopped by adding 200 µl of IS buffer to the reaction medium. The cells were then washed twice in 200 µl of IS buffer and analyzed using the flow cytometry system. Cells incubated in the presence of 1 µl of Strep-tactin PE only were used as a control for nonspecific binding. All stages of the Streptamer staining were conducted at 4 °C.

Isolation of HER2-specific T cells

HER2-specific T cells were isolated by magnetic-activated cell sorting on MS Columns (Miltenyi Biotec, Germany). HER2-specific T cells were tagged using Strep-Tactin Nano Bead magnetic particles, as well as re-agents MHC I-Strep HLA-A*0201 (plus KIFGSLAFL peptide of the HER2/neu antigen), MHC I-Strep HLA-A*0201 (plus RLLQETELV peptide of the HER-2/neu antigen), IS buffer solution, and D-Biotin (IBA GmbH, Germany). Magnetic-activated cell sorting was carried out in accordance with the manufacturer's protocol with some modifications made by the researchers. To remove magnetic particles from the isolated cells, the eluted fraction of antigen-specific cells were centrifuged at 1400 rpm for 10 min at 4 °C, and the cell pellet was resuspended in 1 ml of 1 mM D-Biotin and incubated for 15 min at 4 °C. Next, the cells were centrifuged at 1400 rpm for 10 min at 4 °C, incubated with 1 mM D-Biotin, and centrifuged again. After resuspension of the cell pellet in 400 μl of culture medium, the cell number and viability were counted in a Goryaev chamber using erythrosine staining. The cells were then transferred into the wells of a 96-well plate (100 μl per well) for further culture.

Stimulation of proliferation of HER2-specific T cells and evaluation of effectiveness of magnetic-activated cell sorting

To effectively culture the isolated HER2-specific T cells required for further experiments, we carried out a preliminary experiment to select the optimal cytokine concentrations for stimulation of T-cell proliferative activity. The cytokine concentrations were titrated with respect to proliferation of $CD8^+$ T cells labeled with CFSE (Molecular Probes, USA) in peripheral blood samples from healthy donors.

To isolate the population of $CD8^+$ T cells, PBMCs from healthy donors were stained with anti-CD8-FITC antibody (eBioscience, USA) by incubation for 30 min at room temperature, and washed by centrifugation at 1500 rpm in 1.5 ml of PBS. $CD8^+$ cells were isolated by flow cytometry in the BD FACS Aria cell sorter (sorting rate, $5–7 \times 10^3$ events per second; sorting effectiveness, 93–95%; purity of sorted cells, 98–99%).

The sorted population of $CD8^+$ cells was labeled with CFSE as follows. Cytotoxic T cells (5×10^6 cells) were resuspended in 0.5 ml of 25 mM PBS containing 0.1% BSA, followed by addition of 2 μM CFSE. The cells were incubated with CFSE at 37 °C for 10 min with occasional shaking. Next, a fivefold volume of cold RPMI-1640 medium supplemented with 10% FCS was added and the mixture was centrifuged at 1500 rpm for 10 min. Following the centrifugation, the supernatant was removed and the cells were washed twice with a fivefold excess of cold RPMI-1640 medium supplemented with 10% FCS. After the final wash, the supernatant was removed and the cell pellet was resuspended in the supplemented RPMI-1640 culture medium to a final concentration of 1×10^6 cells/ml.

The CFSE-labeled $CD8^+$ T cells were cultured for 5 days at 37 °C under 5% CO_2. The proliferative activity was analyzed in the BD FACS Verse flow cytometer. The lymphocyte gate was isolated based on the scatter plot with forward and lateral light scattering. In the CFSE fluorescence histogram, the interval gate of cells that had undergone cell division was isolated.

The optimal combination and concentrations of cytokines were selected based on the results for titration of cytokine concentrations as follows. At the culture stage for the required amount of antigen-specific cytotoxic T cells, the target cell fraction after magnetic-activated cell sorting was cultured in a 96-well plate at a concentration of 1×10^6 cells/ml in the culture medium in the presence of rhIL-7 (50 ng/ml), rhIL-15 (50 ng/ml), and rhIL-2 (50 ng/ml) cytokines (Biozol, Germany) for 10–14 days.

After stimulation of proliferation of the isolated cells, the amount of cells carrying the CD8 surface marker was analyzed by labeling the cells with the anti-CD8-FITC antibodies, followed by analysis in the BD FACS Verse flow cytometer.

Cytotoxicity assay

The human breast adenocarcinoma cell line MCF-7 (cell culture line collection at the Institute of Cytology, Russian Academy of Sciences, St. Petersburg, Russia) was used as the target cells for assessing the direct cytotoxicity of HER2-specific T cells. Frozen MCF-7 cells for the experiment were thawed using a standard procedure, in which the cryoconservation agent was removed by washing. The thawed tumor cells were then cultured in EMEM medium (State Research Center of Virology and Biotechnology "Vector", Russia) supplemented with 10% FCS, 2 mM L-glutamine, 5×10^{-5} mM mercaptoethanol, 10 mM HEPES, 80 μg/ml gentamicin, 100 μg/ml ampicillin, and 10 μg/ml insulin. Prior to use, the tumor cells were subjected to 4–5 passages in culture flasks (Nunc, Denmark) with 5 ml of the culture medium. The cell passages were performed every 3–4 days until a high-density monolayer of tumor cells was obtained. The cells were then detached using trypsin–versene solution, comprising a 1:3 mixture of 0.25% trypsin (Biolot, Russia) and 0.02% versene (Biolot, Russia).

In the cytotoxicity assay, the target cells were tagged with the CFSE label while alive. The tumor cells were detached from the plastic culture flasks using trypsin–versene solution and washed once with EMEM medium, followed by resuspension of the cell pellet in 0.5 ml of 25 mM PBS supplemented with 0.1 BSA. Next, 2 μM CFSE was added to the cell suspension containing ~2–5×10^6 cells, and the mixture was incubated for 10 min in a humid atmosphere at 37 °C in 5% CO_2.

The tagged cells were then washed twice with 5 ml of ice-cold MCF-7 growth medium and cocultured with HER2-specific T cells at a 1:10 ratio in a 96-well plate in 100 μl of RPMI-1640 medium supplemented with 10% FCS, 2 mM L-glutamine, 5×10^{-5} mM mercaptoethanol, 10 mM HEPES, 80 μl/ml gentamicin, and 100 μl/ml ampicillin for 48 h. A coculture of tumor cells and

MNCs, and a culture of MCF-7 cells that were not subjected to coculture with MNCs (control over spontaneous death of target cells) were used as controls.

After incubation for 48 h, the cell cultures were tagged with PI. Briefly, 1 μl of PI (1 μg/ml) was added to 100 μl of cell suspension and the resulting mixture was incubated at room temperature for 10 min. The tagged cells in the control and experimental samples were analyzed by flow cytometry in the BD FACS Verse system.

Statistical analysis

All data were processed using Statistica 7.0 (Dell, Austin, TX, USA). The Wilcoxon test was used to detect statistically significant differences because the statistical samplings exhibited an abnormal distribution. The data are presented as the medians and interquartile ranges. The percentage of proliferating CTLs data are presented as mean and standard error of the mean.

Results

Evaluation of the phenotype and functional activity of the resulting DCs

Phenotyping of adherent MNCs, iDCs, and mDCs using specific antibodies against surface markers described in the literature as DC markers [23–25] was performed to evaluate the effectiveness of the protocol for producing DCs from the adherent fraction of MNCs. DCs were analyzed by flow cytometry in the region of large granular leukocytes. Significant differences in expression of the following markers were demonstrated for the populations of iDCs and mDCs: downregulation of CD14 expression (10.25 and 1.75%, respectively) and upregulation of CD83 expression (24.25 and 37.95%, respectively). In addition, the relative numbers of cells

expressing CD86, HLA-DR, CD11c, and HLA-DR/CD11c markers in cultures of mDCs were shown to be reliably increased compared with cultures of the adherent fraction of MNCs (Fig. 1).

The significant increase in the relative numbers of cells expressing the high-specificity mDC marker CD83 and costimulatory molecule CD86 for cells at the mDC stage compared with those at the iDC stage confirms the effectiveness of the protocol for the generation of mDCs. The reliable increase in the percentages of cells expressing DC markers (HLA-DR, CD11c, HLA-DR/CD11c) in the fraction with mDCs compared with the fraction of adherent cells also attests to the effective differentiation of monocytes to DCs. The decrease in the percentages of cells expressing population markers of other immune cells, such as CD14 (marker of monocytes, macrophages, and neutrophils) and CD3 (T-cell marker) as the degree of maturation increases in the series of fractions under investigation demonstrates that DCs, but not other cell populations carrying cell markers common to those of DCs, predominate in the resulting fractions.

Activity with respect to receptor-mediated endocytosis (via FITC-dextran capture) was evaluated at 4 and 37 °C to examine the antigen-capturing ability of the generated DCs. The degree of FITC-dextran capture by DCs was determined using the formula: index of endocytotic activity = (MFI 37 °C/MFI 4 °C) × 100%, where MFI 37 °C is the fluorescence intensity of labeled cells at 37 °C (specific endocytotic activity) and MFI 4 °C is the fluorescence intensity of labeled cells at 4 °C (nonspecific activity).

Mature DCs were shown to exhibit lower activity for antigen capture compared with iDCs, which were capable of more efficient antigen capture via the mechanism

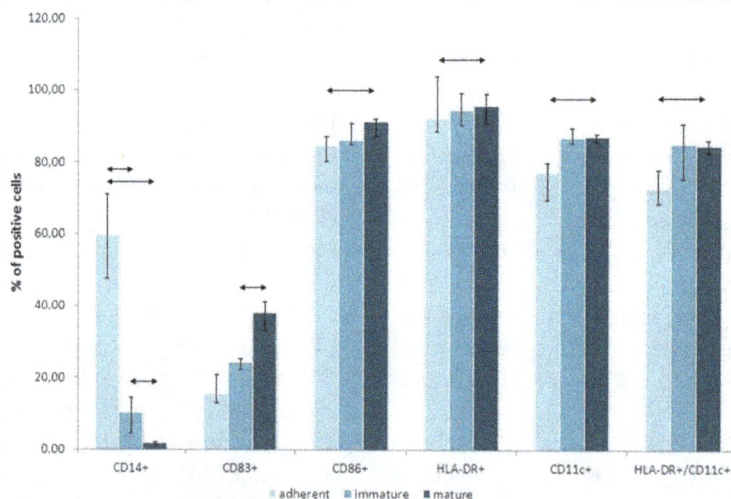

Fig. 1 Relative numbers of cells expressing DC markers. DCs were analyzed by flow cytometry in the region of large granular leukocytes. The data are presented as median and interquartile range. *Arrows* show significant differences ($p < 0.05$; $n = 12$)

of receptor-mediated endocytosis. These findings confirm that myeloid DCs from peripheral blood monocytes undergo directed maturation and differentiation and are consistent with data in the literature [26]. Thus, the protocol used in the present study allows the generation of DCs that have the typical phenotype of the mature stage of antigen-presenting DCs and exhibit proper functional activity.

Loading of mDCs with tumor-associated antigen
The pMaxGFP plasmid, an analogue of the experimental pMax DNA construct that does not encode HER2 epitopes but does encode GFP protein, was used to assess the transfection efficiency with respect to production of the target protein, by analyzing the relative number of cells producing GFP protein using flow cytometry. After magnet-assisted transfection of DCs by the pMaxGFP plasmid, $31,88 \pm 1,93\%$ of the cells were confirmed to express GFP protein [6].

Assessment of the content of HER2-specific T cells
To reveal the population of HER2-specific T cells, MNC/DC cocultures were stained with antigen-specific reagents. The staining protocol was optimized for samples containing 1×10^6 cells. The optimal ratio between the reagents of the staining complex was selected by the results for titration of the MHC concentration: 1 µl of Strep-Tactin-PE and 0.8 µl MHC in a final volume of 25 µl of IS buffer solution. The reagents of the complex were combined and incubated for 45 min at 4 °C. The cells (1×10^6) were incubated in 25 µl of the final complex at 4 °C for 45 min, washed twice with IS buffer, and analyzed in the BD FACS Verse flow cytometer.

Cell populations situated in the lymphocytic region were gated according to the parameters of forward (FSC-A) and side (SSC-A) light scattering for analysis. Cells possessing fluorescence in the PE channel corresponding to the population of HER2-specific T cells stained with PE-conjugated Streptamers were then gated from the lymphocytic region, and the percentage of the subpopulation was measured (Fig. 2).

Cytometric analysis of the stained cells revealed that the relative number of HER2-specific lymphocytes in MNC cultures before coculture with antigen-loaded DCs was not higher than the background fluorescence. An analysis of cocultures of MNCs with DCs transfected with the plasmid DNA encoding HER2 protein epitopes and control cocultures of MNCs with DCs transfected with thr DNA (p5) construct showed that the protocol used allowed the production of MNC cultures containing up to 1.7% T cells specific for the E75 epitope (KIFGSLAFL) of the HER2/neu antigen, while control samples contained only 0.1–0.2% (Fig. 2).

Magnetic-activated sorting of HER2-specific T cells
Magnetic sorting on MS columns was used to isolate the fraction of HER2-specific T cells from cocultures of DCs loaded with tumor antigen and activated MNCs. The manufacturer's protocol for magnetic-activated cell sorting was mastered for isolation of antigen-specific T cells from cocultures of MNCs and DCs consisting of $0.5–1.0 \times 10^7$ cells. The mean number of cells in the sorted fraction of antigen-specific lymphocytes was $0.5–1.0 \times 10^5$ cells, because of the low content of HER2-specific T cells in peripheral blood samples from healthy donors. This was also why their number after stimulation with DCs remained low. Induction of proliferation by cytokines IL-2, IL-7, and IL-15 increased the number of antigen-specific cells by 5–10-fold, up to $0.5–1.0 \times 10^6$ cells.

The effectiveness of the magnetic cell sorting procedure was evaluated by analyzing the content of $CD8^+$ cytotoxic T cells in the cultures of sorted cells, as direct evaluation was not possible using Streptamer cell staining because of the large number of cells required. An analysis of the cells obtained from eight donors showed that the mean content of $CD8^+$ cells was 71.5% in cultures of E88-specific T cells and 90.2% in cultures of E75-specific T cells. Figure 3 shows typical results of the flow cytometry analysis of an experimental sample. Neither monocytic cells (according to the data obtained by forward and side light scattering) nor cells of any morphology other than lymphocytic cells were detected in the experimental sample of antigen-specific cells.

Enrichment of cultures of sorted HER2-specific T cells
Based on the results for titrating the concentrations of cytokines rhIL-2, rhIL-7, and rhIL-15 and the effectiveness of stimulation of $CD8^+$ cell proliferation in cocultures of MNCs in peripheral blood samples from healthy donors, the concentration of 50 ng/ml was selected for each stimulant (Fig. 4). An analysis was carried out using CFSE-labeled cell cultures, in which the numbers of cells that had undergone several divisions were assessed.

Cytotoxicity assay
Experimental assessment of the cytotoxic effectiveness of the resulting cultures against cells carrying the target antigens on their surface was performed after culture for 10–14 days in the presence of rhIL-2, rhIL-7, and rhIL-15 stimulants.

Specifically, after the antigen-specific cells and target cells were cocultured, the cytotoxic activity of T cells was assessed by flow cytometry according to the percentage of PI-positive tumor cells (MCF-7 cells with damaged membranes) in the samples. Based on the results for titration of cell concentrations, the optimal number of cells per probe was selected: 1×10^5 effector

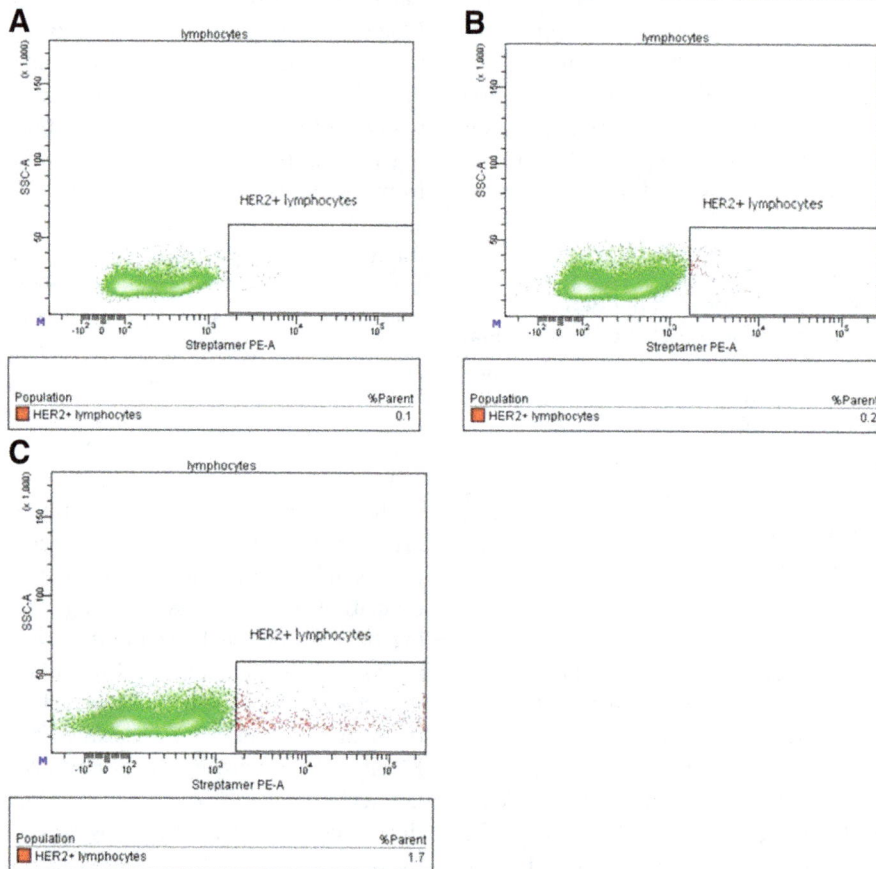

Fig. 2 Relative content of HER2-specific lymphocytes in MNC/DC cocultures. **a** Scatter plot showing the distribution of events from lymphocytic region in the nonspecific binding control sample (unstained cells, incubated only in the presence of Strep-tactin PE) is identified. **b** Scatter plot showing the events from the lymphocytic region in the DC-transfection control sample (Streptamer-stained cells of MNC/DC coculture containing DCs transfected with the control DNA (p5) construct without inserts of immunogenic peptides). **c** Scatter plot showing the events from the lymphocytic region in an experimental sample (Streptamer-stained cells of MNC/DC coculture containing DCs transfected with the pMax DNA construct encoding the HER2 protein epitopes)

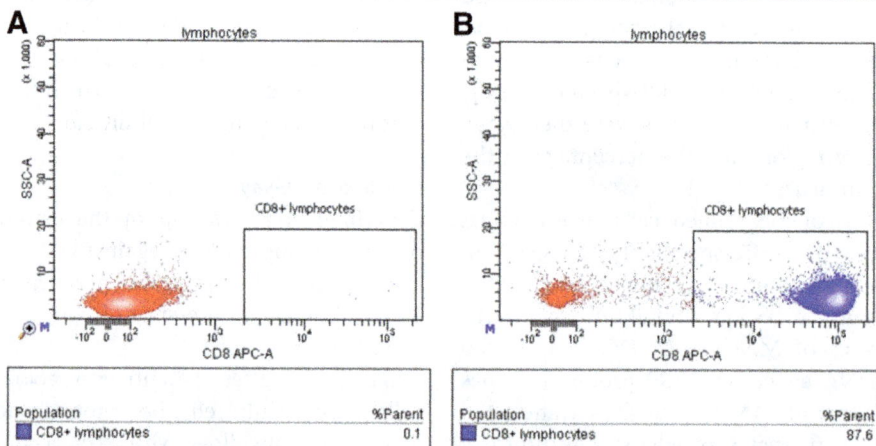

Fig. 3 Relative content of CD8[+] cells in the isolated cultures of HER2-specific T cells (E75-specific cells). The content of CD8+ cytotoxic T cells in isolated fraction was analyzed after culture for 10–14 days in the presence of rhIL-2, rhIL-7, and rhIL-15 stimulants. **a** The scatter plot shows the events from the lymphocytic region in control sample (unlabeled cells). **b** Scatter plot showing the events from the lymphocytic region in an experimental sample (anti-CD8-FITC-labeled cells)

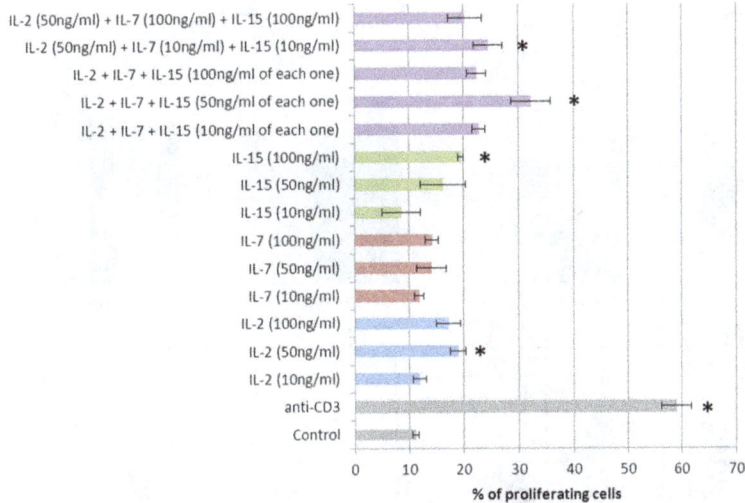

Fig. 4 Proliferation of CD8$^+$ lymphocytes in the presence of different stimulants ($n = 6$). *$p < 0.05$, significant difference compared with the control group. Data are presented as mean and standard error of the mean. The column labels show the set and concentrations of stimulants were used. Control – spontaneous CD8+ cell culture. Anti-CD3 – positive control of proliferation (4 μg/ml)

cells and 1×10^4 target cells at a final cell concentration of 1×10^6 cells/ml.

The gating scheme involved gating of cells exhibiting fluorescence in the FITC channel, corresponding to the emission parameters of the CFSE label. Next, events corresponding to MCF-7 cells in terms of their phenotypic parameters (forward and side light scattering) were gated among the events in this region. An additional file shows the gating scheme in details (see Additional file 3). An analysis of cell fluorescence from MCF-7 region in the PE channel showed cells with damaged membranes stained with PI (Fig. 5, b – d).

The mean relative number of damaged tumor cells in the test samples consisting of HER2-specific T cells and MCF-7 cells was 60.2% for E88-specific T cells and 65.7% for E75-specific T cells, while the control value characterizing the level of spontaneous death of the target cells was 17.9% (Fig. 5, a).

Discussion

Cell transfection with plasmid DNA as a means to effectively deliver antigens into DCs is a modern approach to the design of immune therapeutic vaccines in cancer treatment [6, 27]. Currently research groups worldwide are using many different methods for loading of DCs with tumor antigens [6, 28, 29]. In a number of studies, DCs have been loaded by passive capture of soluble immunogenic proteins, or synthetic or eluted peptides [3], coculture of DCs with tumor lysates [28] and delivery of DNA and RNA constructs encoding tumor antigens into DCs [30]. In addition, antigen loading of DCs can be performed using recombinant viral vectors [31], exosomes [32], and apoptotic bodies [33].

We decided to use magnet-assisted transfection of DNA cells with a construct encoding HER2/neu protein epitopes. The use of DNA constructs allows targeted modulation of the immune response against tumor cells expressing a certain antigen, and several genes encoding different antigenic epitopes can be inserted into the DNA plasmid. Different sequences encoding the most immunogenic epitopes can be inserted into the DNA construct, while immunosuppressive fragments of the tumor antigen can be excluded. Moreover, antigenic activation of mDCs generated with a DNA construct encoding immunogenic peptide fragments ensures strong and long-lasting interactions between MHC molecules and the presented antigenic epitopes, thus making it possible to improve antigen presentation to T cells by DCs. In turn, this increases the effectiveness of in vitro generation of antigen-specific T cells.

Sorting of cells carrying TCRs specific for the selected antigenic peptides (epitopes E75 and E88 of the HER2/ neu protein) was required to obtain a pure fraction of antigen-specific cells. As the protocol for generating antigen-specific CTLs under development was intended for further use toward designing cell-based drugs for adoptive transfer to cancer patients, we needed to use a technology for sorting antigen-specific cells that would enable the production of target cells that did not carry any staining molecules or magnetic beads on their surface, as their presence is not permitted in a patient's body. According to data in the literature, the Streptamer technology [13] is currently the optimal method, because it allows complete dissociation of staining reagents from the cell surface. A number of studies have confirmed that TCRs return into their inactivated state, while the

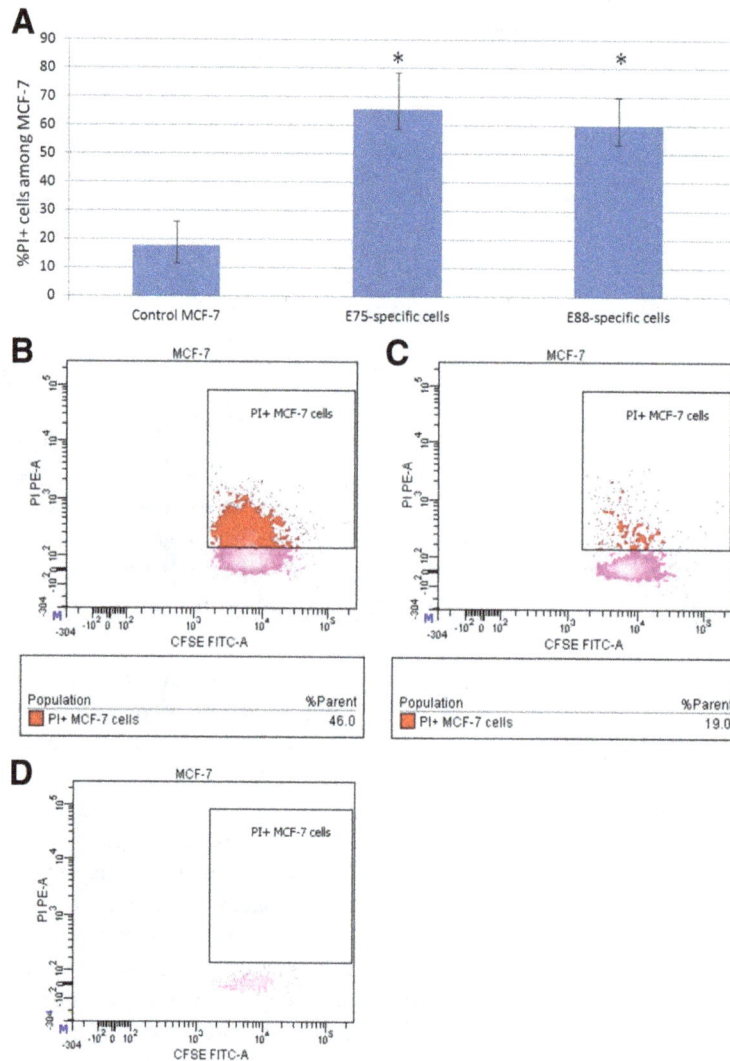

Fig. 5 Results of the cytotoxicity assay. **a** Cytotoxic activity of cultures of HER2-specific T cells against the MCF-7 cell line ($n = 6$). Control MCF-7 – Control over spontaneous death of the target cells. E75-specific cells – Cell culture after magnetic-activated cell sorting at HER2/neu epitope E75 (KIFGSLAFL). E88-specific cells – Cell culture after magnetic-activated cell sorting at HER2/neu epitope E88 (RLLQETELV). *$p < 0.05$, significant difference compared with the control. Data are presented as median and interquartile range. **b** Scatter plot of the experimental sample (PI-labeled coculture of MCF-7 cells and HER2-specific cells). **c** Scatter plot of the control over spontaneous death of target cells (PI-labeled MCF-7 cells). **d** Scatter plot showing the distribution of events from MCF-7 region in control sample contained MCF-7 cells labeled with FITC but not labeled with PI

viability and functions of the isolated cells are retained after the staining and isolation procedure [14, 34–36].

Sorting of antigen-specific cells using Streptamer reagents can be performed by flow cytometry or magnetic cell sorting. A high sorting speed is one of the benefits of using flow cytometry compared with magnetic cell sorting. However, as HER2-specific CTLs comprise a rare and rather small cell population in PBMC cultures from healthy donors, the flow-through sorting procedure would be associated with higher damage to the target cells caused by high pressure resulting from the high sorting speed. Meanwhile, the magnetic sorting

procedure has no noticeable negative effect on the viability of the target cells, because the cellular suspension being sorted passes through a column by gravity acting on the fluid drops, without any additional pressure applied in the system. We took these features into account and selected magnetic sorting as the method for isolating our target cells.

The obtained high percentage of isolated cells carrying the CD8 marker is indirectly indicative of the effectiveness of the magnetic-activated cell sorting procedure. The findings that neither monocytic cells nor cells of any morphology other than lymphocytic cells were detected in the experimental sample of antigen-specific cells also attest to the purity of the resulting population. Furthermore, the magnetic sorting procedure was based on the interactions between magnetic beads conjugated to class I MHC molecules carrying the target epitopes and antigen-specific TCRs. Hence, all of these findings provide grounds for stating that the isolated population was indeed composed of CD8$^+$ HER-specific T cells.

The experimental findings demonstrated that resulting antigen-specific CTL populations displayed strong cytotoxic effects against the MCF-7 cell line We argue that the death of MCF-7 cells was mediated by the cytotoxic action of T cells, because the samples under investigation contained only tumor cells and the fraction of antigen-specific T cells, thereby ruling out possible roles of other factors and taking into account the control samples for spontaneous death of the target cells. In this study, we have demonstrated that the generated T-cell fractions possessed cytotoxic properties against MCF-7 cells. Cells of this line are morphologically large and significantly different from tumor cells that develop in vivo. Hence, a hypothesis can be put forward that the cytotoxic effect on autologous tumor cells will be more pronounced.

Conclusions

A method for generating antitumor cytotoxic T cells specific for the epitopes of the HER2/neu tumor-associated antigen is proposed in this study. The method includes stages of generation and magnet-assisted transfection of mDCs by a DNA construct encoding two immunogenic epitopes of the HER2/neu tumor-associated protein, coculture of antigen-loaded DCs with autologous MNCs, identification and isolation of populations of HER2-specific CTLs from MNC/DC cocultures using reversible Streptamer staining, and enrichment of the isolated cells. The present findings provide grounds for claiming that the designed protocol allows the generation of antigen-specific CTLs that have a pronounced cytotoxic effect with respect to tumor cells expressing the HER2/neu marker.

Additional files

Additional file 1: The amino acid sequences of pMax DNA construct with N-terminal ubiquitin. N-terminal ubiquitin is underlined; C-terminal G replaced by V in ubiquitin for the protease cleavage site elimination. (DOCX 140 kb)

Additional file 2: Typical scatter plots of gates used in DCs phenotyping analysis. DCs were analyzed by flow cytometry in the region of large granular leukocytes. A – Events corresponding to large granular leukocytes in terms of their phenotypic parameters (forward and side light scattering) are gated. B – Events corresponding CD14-FITC-labeled cells are gated. C – Events corresponding CD83-APC-labeled cells are gated. D – Events corresponding CD86-PE-Cy7-labeled cells are gated. E – Events corresponding double-positive HLA-DR-PerCP-Cy5 and CD11c-PE-labeled cells are gated. (DOCX 785 kb)

Additional file 3: Typical scatter plots of the experimental sample showing the gating scheme. The experimental sample is the propidium iodide (PI)-labeled coculture of MCF-7 cells and HER2-specific cells. A – Scatter plot showing the distribution of all events corresponding to the emission parameters of the CFSE label in the FITC channel. Events corresponding CFSE-labeled cells are gated. B – Scatter plot showing the distribution of events from region of CFSE-labeled cells. Events corresponding to MCF-7 cells in terms of their phenotypic parameters (forward and side light scattering) are gated. C – Scatter plot showing the distribution of all events in the experimental sample with respect to parameters of forward and side light scattering. D – Scatter plot of the experimental sample (PI-labeled co-culture of MCF-7 cells and HER2-specific cells). E – Scatter plot of the control over spontaneous death of target cells (PI-labeled MCF-7 cells). (DOCX 160 kb)

Abbreviations

CTLs: Cytotoxic T lymphocytes; DCs: Dendritic cells; HER2: Human Epidermal growth factor Receptor 2, HER2/neu; iDCs: Immature dendritic cells; mDCs: Mature dendritic cells; MNCs: Mononuclear cells (meaning monocyte-depleted non-adherent fraction of peripheral blood mononuclear cells); PBMCs: Peripheral blood mononuclear cells; PI: Propidium iodide

Acknowledgments

The authors are grateful to the staff of the Laboratory of Molecular Immunology, Federal State Budgetary Scientific Institution "Research Institute of Fundamental and Clinical Immunology" for assistance and State Research Center of Virology and Biotechnology "VECTOR" for provided technical help. We also want to thank all the members of Blood Banking Station No. 1 of "Novosibirsk Blood Center" for providing the human blood samples. No writing assistance was utilized in the production of this manuscript.

Funding

This work was supported by the Federal Special-purpose Program "Research and Development in Priority Areas of the Russian Scientific and Technological Complex Development for 2014-2020" (Agreement no. 14.607.21.0043. Unique identifier, RFMEFI60714X0043).

Authors' contributions

MK: design, experimental work and optimization of each experimental stage, analysis and interpretation of data, drafting of the manuscript. LJ: conception, design and interpretation of data. KJ: contributions in experimental work (phenotyping of DCs) and interpretation of data. MR + MA: contributions in experimental work (preparation of DNA construct) and revising of the manuscript. SS: conception, design, final approvement of the manuscript. All authors read and approved the final manuscript.

Competing interests

The authors declare that they have no competing interests.

Author details

[1]Federal State Budgetary Scientific Institution "Research Institute of Fundamental and Clinical Immunology", Yadrintsevskaya str., 14, Novosibirsk 630099, Russia. [2]State Research Center of Virology and Biotechnology "VECTOR", Koltsovo, Novosibirsk Region 630559, Russia.

References

1. Aerts JG, Hegmans JP. Tumor-specific cytotoxic T cells are crucial for efficacy of immunomodulatory antibodies in patients with lung cancer. Cancer Res. 2013;73:2381–8. doi:10.1158/0008-5472.CAN-12-3932.
2. Molldrem JJ, Lee PP, Wang C, Felio K, Kantarjian HM, Champlin RE, Davis MM. Evidence that specific T lymphocytes may participate in the elimination of chronic myelogenous leukemia. Nat Med. 2000;6:1018–23. doi:10.1038/79526.
3. Bernhard H, Neudorfer J, Gebhard K, Conrad H, Hermann C, Nährig J, Fend F, Weber W, Busch DH, Peschel C. Adoptive transfer of autologous, HER2-specific, cytotoxic T lymphocytes for the treatment of HER2-overexpressing breast cancer. Cancer Immunol Immunother. 2008;57:271–80. doi:10.1007/s00262-007-0355-7.
4. Boudreau JE, Bonehill A, Thielemans K, Wan Y. Engineering dendritic cells to enhance cancer immunotherapy. Mol Ther. 2011;19:841–53. doi:10.1038/mt.2011.57.
5. Jeras M, Bergant M, Repnik U. In vitro preparation and functional assessment of human monocyte-derived dendritic cells-potential antigen-specific modulators of in vivo immune responses. Transpl Immunol. 2005;14:231–44. doi:10.1016/j.trim.2005.03.012.
6. Sennikov SV, Shevchenko JA, Kurilin VV, Khantakova JN, Lopatnikova JA, Gavrilova EV, Maksyutov RA, Bakulina AY, Sidorov SV, Khristin AA, Maksyutov AZ. Induction of an antitumor response using dendritic cells transfected with DNA constructs encoding the HLA-A*02:01-restricted epitopes of tumor-associated antigens in culture of mononuclear cells of breast cancer patients. Immunol Res. 2016;64:171–80. doi:10.1007/s12026-015-8735-0.
7. Gelao L, Criscitiello C, Esposito A, De Laurentiis M, Fumagalli L, Locatelli MA, Minchella I, Santangelo M, De Placido S, Goldhirsch A, Curigliano G. Dendritic cell-based vaccines: clinical applications in breast cancer. Immunotherapy. 2014;6:349–60. doi:10.2217/imt.13.169.
8. Qin Z, Blankenstein T. A cancer immunosurveillance controversy. Nat Immunol. 2004;5:3–5. doi:10.1038/ni0104-3.
9. Willimsky G, Blankenstein T. Sporadic immunogenic tumours avoid destruction by inducing T-cell tolerance. Nature. 2005;437:141–6. doi:10.1038/nature03954.
10. Frankenberger B, Schendel DJ. Third generation dendritic cell vaccines for tumor immunotherapy. Eur J Cell Biol. 2012;91:53–8. doi:10.1016/j.ejcb.2011.01.012.
11. Schürch CM, Riether C, Ochsenbein AF. Dendritic cell-based immunotherapy for myeloid leukemias. Front Immunol. 2013;4:1–16. doi:10.3389/fimmu.2013.00496.
12. Knabel M, Franz TJ, Schiemann M, Wulf A, Villmow B, Schmidt B, Bernhard H, Wagner H, Busch DH. Reversible MHC multimer staining for functional isolation of T-cell populations and effective adoptive transfer. Nat Med. 2002;8:631–7. doi:10.1038/nm0602-631.
13. Neudorfer J, Schmidt B, Huster KM, Anderl F, Schiemann M, Holzapfel G, Schmidt T, Germeroth L, Wagner H, Peschel C, Busch DH, Bernhard H. Reversible HLA multimers (Streptamers) for the isolation of human cytotoxic T lymphocytes functionally active against tumor- and virus-derived antigens. J Immunol Methods. 2007;320:119–31. doi:10.1016/j.jim.2007.01.001.
14. Schmitt A, Tonn T, Busch DH, Grigoleit GU, Einsele H, Odendahl M, Germeroth L, Ringhoffer M, Ringhoffer S, Wiesneth M, Greiner J, Michel D, Mertens T, Rojewski M, Marx M, von Harsdorf S, Döhner H, Seifried E, Bunjes D, Schmitt M. Adoptive transfer and selective reconstitution of streptamer-selected cytomegalovirus-specific CD8+ T cells leads to virus clearance in patients after allogeneic peripheral blood stem cell transplantation. Transfusion. 2011;51:591–9. doi:10.1111/j.1537-2995.2010.02940.x.
15. Goebel SU, Iwamoto M, Raffeld M, Gibril F, Hou W, Serrano J, Jensen RT. HER-2/neu expression and gene amplification in gastrinomas: Correlations with tumor biology, growth, and aggressiveness. Cancer Res. 2002;62:3702–10.
16. Subbiah IM, Gonzalez-Angulo AM. Advances and Future Directions in the Targeting of HER2-positive Breast Cancer: Implications for the Future. Curr Treat Options Oncol. 2014;15:41–54. doi:10.1007/s11864-013-0262-4.
17. Dev K, Mandal AK, Husain E. Immunohistochemical expression of Her-2/neu and its correlation with histological grades and age in IDC of breast. Int J adv Sci Tech Res. 2013;3:230–47.
18. Baleeiro RB, Rietscher R, Diedrich A, Czaplewska JA, Lehr C-M, Scherließ R, Hanefeld A, Gottschaldt M, Walden P. Spatial separation of the processing and MHC class I loading compartments for cross-presentation of the tumor-associated antigen HER2/neu by human dendritic cells. Oncoimmunology. 2015;4:e1047585. doi:10.1080/2162402X.2015.1047585.
19. Baxevanis CN, Sotiriadou NN, Gritzapis AD, Sotiropoulou PA, Perez SA, Cacoullos NT, Papamichail M. Immunogenic HER-2/neu peptides as tumor vaccines. Cancer Immunol Immunother. 2006;55:85–95. doi:10.1007/s00262-005-0692-3.
20. Rongcun Y, Salazar-Onfray F, Charo J, Malmberg KJ, Evrin K, Maes H, Kono K, Hising C, Petersson M, Larsson O, Lan L, Appella E, Sette A, Celis E, Kiessling R. Identification of new HER2/neu-derived peptide epitopes that can elicit specific CTL against autologous and allogeneic carcinomas and melanomas. J Immunol. 1999;163:1037–44.
21. Maniatis T, Frich E, Sambrook J. Methods of Gene Engineering. Molecular Cloning [Russian translation]. Moscow: Mir; 1984.
22. Boyum A. Separation of leukocytes from blood and bone marrow. Scand J Clin Lab Invest. 1968;21:97.
23. Jarnjak-Jankovic S, Hammerstad H, Saebøe-Larssen S, Kvalheim G, Gaudernack G. A full scale comparative study of methods for generation of functional Dendritic cells for use as cancer vaccines. BMC Cancer. 2007;7:119. doi:10.1186/1471-2407-7-119.
24. Obermaier B, Dauer M, Herten J, Schad K, Endres S, Eigler A. Development of a new protocol for 2-day generation of mature dendritic cells from human monocytes. Biol Proc Online. 2003;5:197–203.
25. Tanaka F, Yamaguchi H, Haraguchi N, Mashino K, Ohta M, Inoue H, Mori M. Efficient induction of specific cytotoxic T lymphocytes to tumor rejection peptide using functional matured 2 day-cultured dendritic cells derived from human monocytes. Int J Oncol. 2006;29:1263–8.
26. Kato M, Neil TK, Fearnley DB, McLellan AD, Vuckovic S, Hart DN. Expression of multilectin receptors and comparative FITC-dextran uptake by human dendritic cells. Int Immunol. 2000;12:1511–9. doi:10.1093/intimm/12.11.1511.
27. Kulikova EV, Kurilin VV, Shevchenko JA, Obleukhova IA, Khrapov EA, Boyarskikh UA, Filipenko ML, Shorokhov RV, Yakushenko VK, Sokolov AV, Sennikov SV. Dendritic Cells Transfected with a DNA Construct Encoding Tumour-associated Antigen Epitopes Induce a Cytotoxic Immune Response Against Autologous Tumour Cells in a Culture of Mononuclear Cells from Colorectal Cancer Patients. Scand J Immunol. 2015;82:110–7. doi:10.1111/sji.12311.
28. Ruben JM, van den Ancker W, Bontkes HJ, Westers TM, Hooijberg E, Ossenkoppele GJ, de Gruijl TD, van de Loosdrecht AA. Apoptotic blebs from leukemic cells as a preferred source of tumor-associated antigen for dendritic cell-based vaccines. Cancer Immunol Immunother. 2014;63(4):335–45. doi:10.1007/s00262-013-1515-6.
29. Sabado RL, Bhardwaj N. Dendritic cell immunotherapy. Ann N Y Acad Sci. 2013;1284:31–45. doi:10.1111/nyas.12125.
30. Aarntzen EH, Schreibelt G, Bol K, Lesterhuis WJ, Croockewit AJ, de Wilt JH, van Rossum MM, Blokx WA, Jacobs JF, Duiveman-de Boer T, Schuurhuis DH, Mus R, Thielemans K, de Vries IJ, Figdor CG, Punt CJ, Adema GJ. Vaccination with mRNA-electroporated dendritic cells induces robust tumor antigen-specific CD4+ and CD8+ T cells responses in stage III and IV melanoma patients. Clin Cancer Res. 2012;18:5460–70. doi:10.1158/1078-0432.CCR-11-3368.
31. You H, Liu Y, Cong M, Ping W, You C, Zhang D, Mehta JL, Hermonat PL. HBV genes induce cytotoxic T-lymphocyte response upon adeno-associated virus (AAV) vector delivery into dendritic cells. J Viral Hepat. 2006;13:605–12. doi:10.1111/j.1365-2893.2006.00734.
32. Schnitzer JK, Berzel S, Fajardo-Moser M, Remer K a, Moll H. Fragments of antigen-loaded dendritic cells (DC) and DC-derived exosomes induce protective immunity against Leishmania major. Vaccine. 2010;28:5785–93. doi:10.1016/j.vaccine.2010.06.077.
33. Frisoni L, Mcphie L, Colonna L, Monestier M, Gallucci S, Sriram U, Caricchio R. Nuclear Autoantigen Translocation and Autoantibody Opsonization Lead to Increased Dendritic Cell Phagocytosis and Presentation of Nuclear Antigens: A Novel Pathogenic Pathway for Autoimmunity? J Immunol. 2005;175:2692–701.
34. Bouquié R, Bonnin A, Bernardeau K, Khammari A, Dréno B, Jotereau F, Labarrière N, Lang F. A fast and efficient HLA multimer-based sorting procedure that induces little apoptosis to isolate clinical grade human tumor

specific T lymphocytes. Cancer Immunol Immunother. 2009;58:553–66. doi:10. 1007/s00262-008-0578-2.

35. van Loenen MM, de Boer R, van Liempt E, Meij P, Jedema I, Frederik Falkenburg JH, Heemskerk MHM. A Good Manufacturing Practice procedure to engineer donor virus-specific T cells into potent anti-leukemic effector cells. Haematologica. 2014;99:759–68. doi:10.3324/haematol.2013.093690.

36. Wang Z, Li P, Xu Q, Xu J, Li X, Zhang X, Ma Q, Wu Z. Potent Antitumor Activity Generated by a Novel Tumor Specific Cytotoxic T Cell. PLoS ONE. 2013;8:e66659. doi:10.1371/journal.pone.0066659.

7

Analysis of differences between total IgG and sum of the IgG subclasses in children with suspected immunodeficiency –indication of determinants

Gerard Pasternak[1,2]* iD, Aleksandra Lewandowicz-Uszyńska[1,2] and Katarzyna Pentoś[3]

Abstract

Background: Deficits in disorders of humoral immunity associated with a deficit of antibodies are the most common primary immunodeficiency. Total IgG and IgG subclasses measurements are used to diagnose, differentiate and control in patients with primary and secondary immunodeficiencies.

Methods: The purpose of the study was to analyze the structure patients group according to difference between total IgG and sum of the IgG subclasses and to determine factors affecting the level of this difference. This study was based on data collected from 670 children referred to the Department of Clinical Immunology and Pediatrics in order to diagnose the immune disorders. For all children the level of the total of immunoglobulins IgG and of the IgG subclasses (IgG1, IgG2, IgG3, IgG4) were determined. The group of children was divided into subgroups according to gender, age (under 6 years of age, 6.5–12 years, and 12–18 years), and IgG abnormality (below the normal range, normal and above the normal range). In the patients group, the total IgG values were on average higher than sum of the IgG subclasses.

Results: Statistical analysis shown the all parameters under study (age, gender and IgG abnormality) influence statistically significant on the discrepancy between the sum of the IgG subclasses and total IgG. Assessment of IgG and IgG subclasses levels is based on different methods what causes the discrepancy between the sum of the IgG subclasses and total IgG.

Conclusions: Standardization in that regard is crucial. In addition, we have shown the reliability of the results obtained. Despite the determination in two different laboratories and on different analyzers, as well as the freezing process does not affect the test results.

Background

Primary Immunodeficiencies (PID) are a heterogeneous group of diseases. These are rare diseases, but not as rare as one might expect. According to Lim and Elenitoba-Johnson (2004), approximately 400 new PID cases are diagnosed annually in the United States [1]. The course of these diseases can be extremely severe and the high risk other of infections can lead to life-threatening conditions. Delays in making the right diagnosis often results in extremely severe clinical conditions and numerous complications. The speed and accuracy of diagnosis, as well as the implementation of appropriate treatment, will lead to significant benefits for the health and life of the patient.

Most common among PIDs are disorders of the humoral response associated with deficiency of antibodies, a heterogeneous group of proteins present in the body fluids of all vertebrates and characterized by a common pattern of construction. The most important element of the humoral response in the human body are immunoglobulins and the most important of these are

---

* Correspondence: gerard.pasternak@umed.wroc.pl

[1]3rd Department and Clinic of Paediatrics, Immunology and Rheumatology of Developmental Age, Wroclaw Medical University, L. Pasteura 1, Wroclaw 50-367, Poland

[2]Department of Immunology and Paediatrics, Provincial Hospital J. Gromkowski, Koszarowa 5, Wroclaw 51-149, Poland

Full list of author information is available at the end of the article

immunoglobulins of the IgG class which account for about 75% of all immunoglobulins contained in serums. Within the variable parts of immunoglobulins, there are subtle structural differences that determine antigenic properties and affect effector functions associated with, among other things, complement activation and binding to one or more Fc antibody receptors present among others present on phagocytic cells. Because of the molecular structure, 4 subclasses of this immunoglobulin – IgG1,2,3 and 4 are distinguished. Irregularities in the concentrations of particular IgG subclasses may condition various disease states. The most common IgG1 deficiency is the result of a generalized deficiency of antibodies [2]. IgG2 deficiency is associated with recurrent viral and bacterial infections [3]. IgG3 deficiency is observed in viral infections of the urinary tract; IgG2 and IgG3 deficiency predisposes to recurrent respiratory tract infections [4]. IgG4 deficiency is diagnosed in chronic bronchial and lung diseases [5].

For the correct interpretation of the concentrations of immunoglobulins IgG and IgG subclasses in serums, it is important to know the reference ranges of concentrations of immunoglobulins, depending on the age of the patient. The production of immunoglobulins changes during the natural maturation of the immune system in healthy populations. Immunoglobulin production begins during fetal stage. Up to 6 months of age, the baby's blood circulates immunoglobulins obtained through the placenta from the mother. During this period, their own immunoglobulin production gradually increases in response to stimulation with food antigens and microorganisms. From 6 months of age, intensive individual antibody production begins. Causes of deficiency in the production of immunoglobulins, the so-called hypogammaglobulinemia, include primary and secondary immunodeficiency.

The essence of carrying out a reliable diagnosis of PID is largely dependent on an accurate medical history. The data obtained from an interview will determine the direction of further investigation, mainly laboratory based testing. In our department, we routinely evaluate IgG in every patient with suspected PID. In specific cases, we evaluate the IgG subclasses. Samples are usually taken one day apart (total IgG and IgG subclasses).

To the best of the authors' knowledge, there is a lack of analysis concerning differences between total IgG and sum of the IgG subclasses in children (by age group and sex) with suspected immunodeficiency, according to the difference of IgGsum and IgG [5–8].This study aimed to assess frequency and degree of such discrepancies in routine samples. Data was collected retrospectively from 670 children (aged 2 months to 18 years) referred to the Department of Clinical Immunology and Paediatrics for the purpose of diagnosis of immune disorders. All children were screened, among other things, for the total of immunoglobulins IgG and of the IgG subclasses (IgG1, IgG2, IgG3, IgG4). The group of patients was divided into subgroups according to age (under 6 years of age, in the age range between 6 and 12 years, and in the age range between 12 and 18 years), gender, and IgG abnormality (below the normal range, normal and above the normal range).

Methods

Each year in the Department of Immunology and Paediatrics, we treat about 1300 children (aged 6 months to 18 years). These are patients referred to us for diagnostic purposes of primary immunodeficiencies. Most of them are children aged 0–6 years and the majority of these are children with recurrent respiratory tract infections. In our geographic area (Central and Eastern Europe), 6–8 fever infections per year we treat as a norm. All children were screened routinely, for among other things, the total of the IgG in serum. Using our own experience as well as Jeffrey Modell Foundation criteria, in some cases we mark IgG subclasses (IgG1, IgG2, IgG3, IgG4) depending on the individual indications for the patient. Mostly, economic conditions cause us to freeze samples and send them to another lab. The most common sample for IgG subclasses is taken the next day from the sample of total IgG.

The ARTITECT cSystem by immunoturbidimetric method is used for total IgG determination. In contrast, IgG subclass levels are measured by the nephelometric method with the use of a BN ProSpec Siemens analyzer. Both analyzers use a set of reagents provided by the manufacturers.

Statistical analysis was based on the t-test, Kruskal–Wallis test and Mann-Whitney U test, with a significance level of 5% ($p \leq 0.05$). The data analyses were carried out using Statistica version 10 software.

All procedures performed in studies involving human participants were 'in accordance' with the ethical standards in compliance with the Helsinki Declaration. Bioethical committee of Wroclaw Medical University approval number 638/2017.

Results and Discussion

Data from medical tests of 670 children aged between 2 months and 18 years were used in this research. The median age of patients was 4.2 years with 421 males (62,8%) and 249 females (37,2%). The summary statistics for each analysis is detailed in Table 1.

For each patient, parameter D proposed by authors (discrepancy between IgGsum and IgG expressed as a percentage of IgGsum) was calculated as follows:

Table 1 Mean, median, and standard deviation for IgG, IgGsum, and IgG subclasses

Subclasses	Median [g/l]	Mean [g/l]	Standard deviation [g/l]
IgG	7,33	7,79	3,38
IgGsum	6,96	7,36	3,12
IgG1	4,76	5,05	2,16
IgG2	1,34	1,57	1,02
IgG3	0,26	0,31	0,23
IgG4	0,17	0,42	0,69

$$D = \frac{IgGsum - IgG}{IgGsum} \cdot 100\%$$

where IgGsum is the sum of subclasses (IgG1+ IgG2+ IgG3+ IgG4), IgG is the total of the IgG in serum.

In the group of 670 children, there were 22 patients with D parameter exceeding 40% who were excluded from further analysis.In the course of the investigation, it was demonstrated that these were samples (IgG total and IgG subclasses) obtained at intervals greater than one day.

In the group of 648 children considered for further analysis, 245 (37.8%) were female and 403 (62.2%) were male; 428 were under 6 years of age, 151 were in the age range between 6 and 12 years and 69 were in the age range between 12 and 18 years (66.0, 23.3 and 10.7%, respectively); for 80 patients IgG was below the normal range, for 496 patients IgG was normal, and for 73 patients IgG was above the normal range (12.3, 76.5 and 11.2%, respectively).The group of 80 patients with Total IgG deficiency can be divided according to the medical history into three clinical subgroups: recurrent respiratory tract infections (RRT), primary immunodeficiency (PID) and transient hypogammaglobulinemia of infancy (THI).

In this group 55 patients had RRT, 20 PIDs and 5 THI. In PIDs group was: 1 patient with Netherton syndrome, 1 patient with complement deficiency, 1 patient with Nijmegen breakage syndrome, 1 patient with ELANE-related neutropenia, 1 patient with common variable immunodeficiency (CVID), 1 patient with IgA deficiency, 3 patients with ataxia-telangiectasia syndrome, 11 patients with phagocytic disorders.

Significant correlation was observed between IgG and IgGsum as shown in Fig. 1.

Similar results were presented by McLean-Tooke et al. (2013) for 571 patients aged 0.5–83.6 years [9].

The D parameter was used for dividing the population into subgroups: D < 5% (0–5%); D < 10% (0–10%); D < 15% (0–15%); D > 15% (15–40%). Results of IgG were on average 5.8% higher than IgGsum. The results of statistical analysis (t-test) show that there is a statistically significant difference ($p < 0.05$) between total IgG and IgGsum. Of 648 samples, 102 (15.7%) had D value > 15%. In this group, 95 (93%) had an IgG above IgGsum. In the case of the other 546 patients, 416 (64.2% of the whole population) had a difference of IgGsum from IgG < 10% and 238 (36.7% of the whole population) had this difference < 5%. In the group with D value < 10%, 272 (65.4%) had an IgG above IgGsum. In the case of the group with D value < 5%, 137 patients (57,5%) had an IgG higher than IgGsum. Comparing these results with those presented by McLean-Tooke et al. (2013) (IgGsum were on average 3.9% higher than IgG) can lead to the conclusion that the child population is different from adults according to the discrepancy between IgG and IgGsum.

Statistical analysis based on Pearson Correlation Coefficientshowed no statistically significant correlation ($p < 0.05$) between D value and IgG1 ($r = 0.016$), IgG2 ($r = -0,049$), IgG3 ($r = -0,035$) or IgG4 ($r = 0,002$).Based on

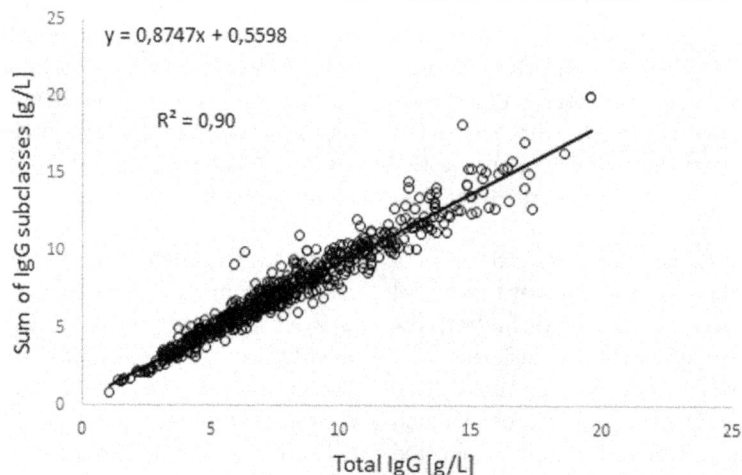

Fig. 1 Scatter plot of IgG versus sum of IgG subclasses

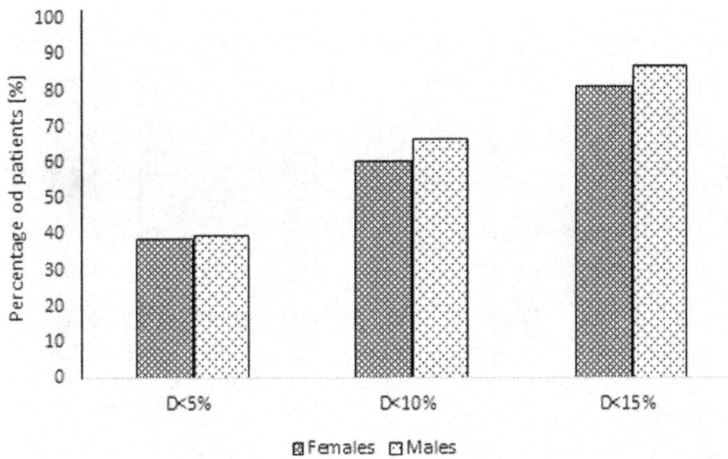

Fig. 2 Percentage of males and females according to the difference of IgGsum and IgG for the whole patient population

the Kruskal–Wallis test results, statistically significant differences were identified between the D value affected by age ($p = 0.022$), gender ($p = 0.003$), and IgG abnormality ($p = 0.000$).

Taking into account gender groups, among 245 females patients 198 (80.8%) with D value < 15%, 148 (60.4%) with D value < 10% and 94 (38.4%) with D value < 5% wereobserved. The proportion of subjects with IgG above IgGsum was 74.7, 70.3 and 64.9%, respectively. In the male population, there were 348 (86.4%) patients with D value < 15%, 268 (66.5%) with D value < 10% and 159 (39.5%) with D value < 5%. The proportion of males with IgG higher than IgGsum was 67.5, 62.7 and 54.7%, respectively. In Fig. 2, the percentage of males and females according to D value is presented. The Fig. 3

shows the total concentration of IgG, IgGsum, and IgG subclasses among males and females.

When considering age groups, among 428 patients aged under 6 years, 360 (84.1%) had D value < 15%, 275 (64.3%) had D value < 10% and 158 (36.9%) had D value < 5%. The proportion of children with IgG greater than IgGsum was 70.6, 65.5 and 58.9%, respectively. In the population of 151 patients aged between 6 and 12 years, there were 130 (86.1%) with D value < 15%, 98 (64.9%) with D value < 10% and 56 (37.1%) with D value < 5%. The proportion of children with IgG higher than IgGsum in this group was 73.1, 69.4 and 58.9%, respectively. Among 69 patients in the age range between 12 and 18 years, 56 (81.2%) with D value < 15%, 43 (62.3%) with D value < 10% and 24 (34.8%) with D value < 5%

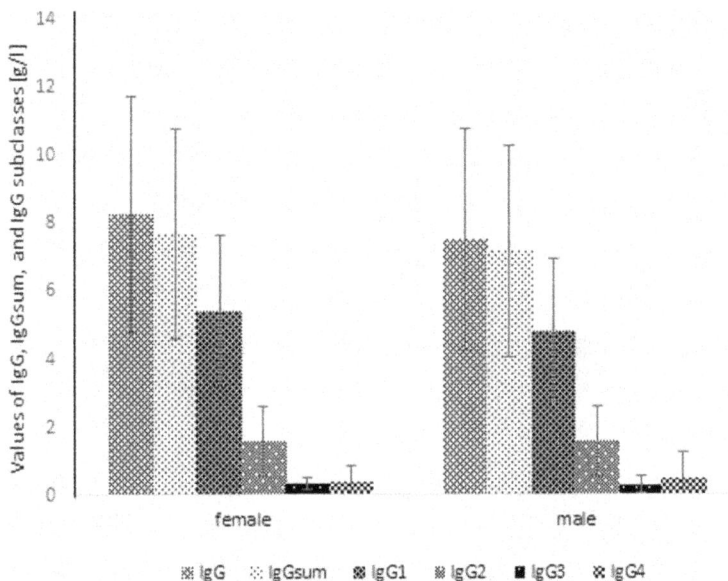

Fig. 3 Mean and standard deviation of IgG, IgGsum, and IgG subclasses by gender

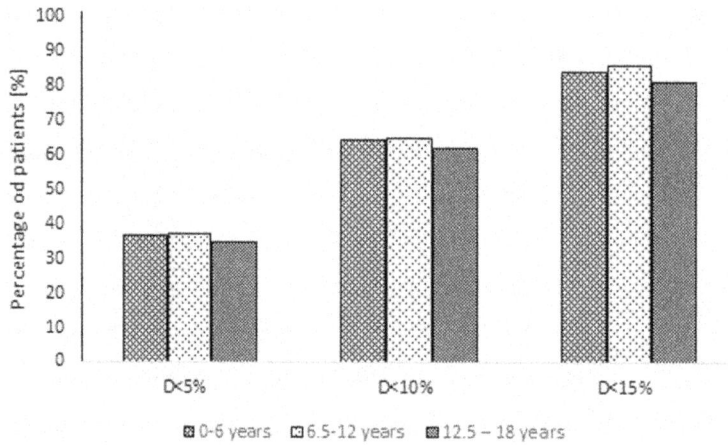

Fig. 4 Percentage of patients belonging to a certain age group according to the difference of IgGsum and IgG for the whole patient population

were observed. The percentage of patients having IgG greater than IgGsum was 60.7, 55.8 and 45.8%, respectively. In Fig. 4, the percentage of patients belonging to a certain age group according to D value is presented. The Fig. 5 shows the total concentration of IgG, IgGsum, and IgG subclasses in certain age group.

When analyzing groups according to IgG measured versus a normal IgG range, of80patients with IgG below the normal range, 68 (85.0%) had D value < 15%, 51 (63.8%) had D value < 10% and 23 (28.8%) had D value < 5%. The proportion of patients with IgG greater than IgGsum was 58.8, 54.9 and 56.5%, respectively. Among 496 patients with IgG normal, there were 423 (85.3%) with D value < 15%, 333 (67.1%) with D value < 10% and 193 (38.9%) with D value < 5%. The percentage of children having IgG greater than IgGsum was 70.7, 66.7 and

59.6%, respectively. In the population of 73 patients having IgG above the normal range, 55 (75.3%) with D value < 15%, 33 (45.2%) with D value < 10% and 22 (30.1%) with D value < 5% were observed. The proportion of children with IgG higher than IgGsum in this group was 81.8, 66.7 and 54.5%, respectively. In Fig. 6, the percentage of patients having IgG normal, below or above normal range according to D value is shown. The Fig. 7 shows the total concentration of IgG, IgGsum, and IgG subclasses for patients with immunodeficiency and those with IgG normal and above normal range.

The figure below (Fig. 8) shows the results of IgG, IgGsum, and IgG subclasses of patients with total IgG deficiency divided into 3 clinical groups: recurrent respiratory tract infections (RRT), primary immunodeficiency (PID) i transient hypogammaglobulinemia of

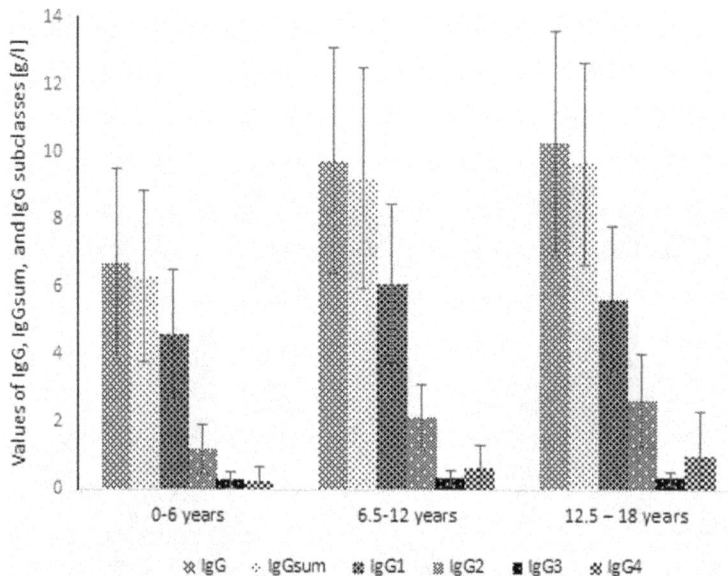

Fig. 5 Mean and standard deviation of IgG, IgGsum, and IgG subclasses by age

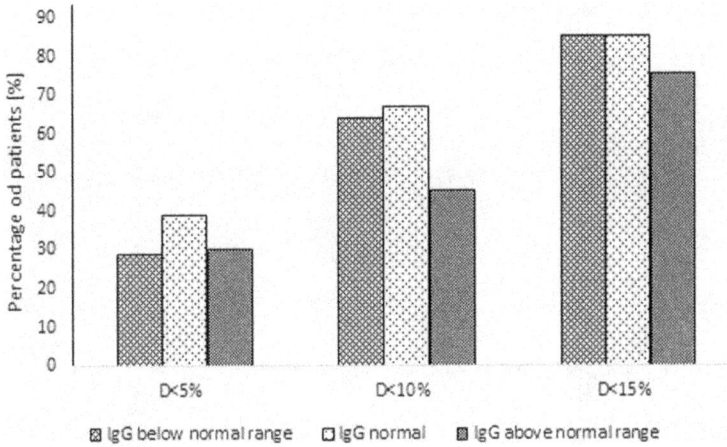

Fig. 6 Percentage of patients with certain IgG abnormality according to the difference of IgGsum and IgG for the whole patient population

infancy (THI). The Mann-Whitney U test indicated that there are no significant differences in IgG, IgGsum, and IgG subclasses between clinical diagnosis.In addition, a whole group of patients (670) was analyzed for clinical diagnosis and shortages in subclasses as presented in Table 2.

Considering gender, a higher percentage of patients with D value > 15% and a higher percentage of patients with IgG greater than IgGsum is observed in the female group than in the male group. The average value of discrepancy between IgG and IgGsum was recognized more in the female group (9.4%) than in the male group (8.5%). In the case of age groups, a significantly lower percentage of patients with D value > 15% is observed for children aged between 12 and 18 years. The percentage of patients with IgG greater than IgGsum decreases as age increases. The average D value is highest for the group aged between 12 and 18 years (9.3%). Comparable values were recognized for other groups – 8.8% for children aged under 6 years and 8.6% for children aged between 6 and 12 years. Analyzing IgG abnormality groups, it can be concluded that for the population with IgG greater than IgGsum, there is a lower proportion of patients with IgG below normal range than with IgG normal or above normal range. The average values of discrepancy between IgG and IgGsum were: 9.1% for children with IgG below normal range, 8.5% for children with IgG normal and 10.7% for children with IgG above normal range.

Summary

The study analyzed the effects of three parameters: age, sex, and IgG deviation from normal to the value

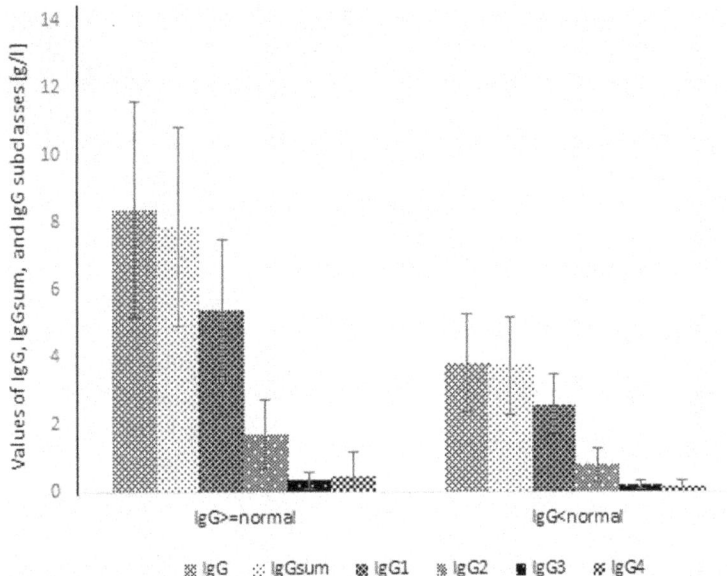

Fig. 7 Mean and standard deviation of IgG, IgGsum, and IgG subclasses by IgG abnormality

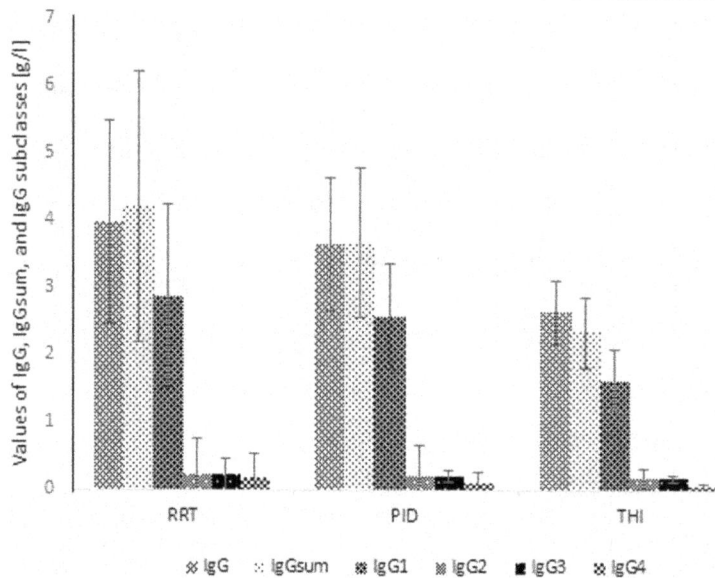

Fig. 8 Mean and standard deviation of IgG, IgGsum, and IgG subclasses by clinical diagnosis

of the difference between IgG and the sum of IgG of each subclass (IgGsum = IgG1 + IgG2 + IgG3 + IgG4). Patients were divided into groups according to these parameters:

1. women and men
2. age up to 6 years, between 6 and 12 years, and between 12 and 18 years
3. IgG below norm, IgG norm and IgG above norm.

The main purpose of the analysis was to determine whether the values of the aforementioned parameters significantly affects the difference between IgG and IgGsum.

Patients' total IgG values were on average higher than IgGsum and there is a statistically significant difference ($p < 0.05$) between total IgG and IgGsum. In the results published by McLean-Tooke et al., for a group of adult patients, the tendency was opposite. This shows that there is a difference between children and adults in this respect.

Statistical analysis (Kruskal-Wallis test) indicates that all three parameters: age, sex, and IgG deviation from the norm, have statistically significant effects on the amount of difference between IgG and IgGsum.

Table 2 The percentage of patients with a deficiency of IgG subclasses division for clinical diagnosis

IgG subclasses	RRT [%]	PID [%]	THI [%]
IgG1	81	15	4
IgG2	76	24	–
IgG3	79	21	–
IgG4	84	16	–

In the case of sex, the greater mean difference between IgG and IgGsum was observed in women. In the group of women, we observed a greater proportion of patients with IgG and the difference between IgGsum exceeding 15% of patients, and for which IgG is greater than IgGsum.

In the case of age, the oldest children had significantly fewer patients with a percentage of the difference between the total IgG and IgGsum exceeding 15% than in the other two child age groups. Increase in patient age results in an increase in the difference between IgG and IgGsum and a decrease in the number of patients for whom IgG is greater than IgGsum.

Analyzing the deviation of the total IgG from the norm, we found that the average value difference between IgG and IgGsum is the smallest in patients with normal IgG. Deviation from the normal range (up or down) results in an increase in the mean difference between total IgG and IgGsum.

Conclusion

Determination of serum immunoglobulin levels is an increasingly available and relatively inexpensive laboratory test performed not only in specialized departments but also in primary care. Assessment of IgG levels as well as IgA and IgM is one of the fundamental studies on the function of the immune system. The indications for their markings are very different and primarily include diagnostics for primary and secondary immunodeficiencies.

In addition, we have shown the reliability of the results obtained. Their determination in two different laboratories and on different analyzers, as well as the freezing process, does not adversely affect the test results.

Abbreviations
CVID: Common variable immunodeficiency; PID: Primary Immunodeficiency; RRT: Recurrent respiratory tract infections; THI: Transient hypogammaglobulinemia of infancy

Authors' contributions
This study was designed by GP. Data collection and analysis was performed by GP. KP participated in statistical analysis. ALU assisted in revised the manuscript. GP prepared the final manuscript which was approved by all authors.

Competing interests
The authors declare that they have no competing interests.

Author details
[1]3rd Department and Clinic of Paediatrics, Immunology and Rheumatology of Developmental Age, Wroclaw Medical University, L. Pasteura 1, Wroclaw 50-367, Poland. [2]Department of Immunology and Paediatrics, Provincial Hospital J. Gromkowski, Koszarowa 5, Wroclaw 51-149, Poland. [3]Institute of Agricultural Engineering, Wroclaw University of Environmental and Life Sciences, J. Chełmońskiego 37/41, Wroclaw 51-630, Poland.

References
1. Lim MS, Elenitoba-Johnson KS. The molecular pathology of primary Immunodeficiencies. J Mol Diagn. 2004;6(2):59–83.
2. Jefferis R, Kumararatne DS. Selective IgG subclass deficiency: quantification and clinical relevance. Clin Exp Immunol. 1990;81(3):357–67.
3. Kuijpers TW, Weening RS, Out TA. IgG subclass deficiencies and recurrent pyogenic infections, unresponsiveness against bacterial polysaccharide antigens. Allergol Immunopathol. 1992;20(1):28–34.
4. Vidarsson G, Dekkers G, Rispens T. IgG subclasses and allotypes: from structure to effector functions. Front Immunol. 2014;5:520. https://doi.org/10.3389/fimmu.2014.00520.
5. de MoraesLui C, Oliveira LC, Diogo CL, Kirschfink M, Grumach AS. Immunoglobulin G subclass concentrations and infections in children and adolescents with severe asthma. Pediatr Allergy Immunol. 2002; 13(3):195–202.
6. Schauer U, Stemberg F, Rieger CH, Borte M, Schubert S, Riedel F, Herz U, Renz H, Wick M, Carr-Smith HD, et al. Clin Chem. 2003;49(11):1924–9.
7. Ludwig-Kraus B, and Kraus FB. Similar but not consistent: Revisiting the pitfalls of measuring IgG subclasses with different assays. J Clin Lab Anal. 2017;31:e22146. https://doi.org/10.1002/jcla.22146.
8. Bossuyt X, Marien G, Meyts I, Proesmans M, De Boeck K. Determination of IgG subclasses: a need for standardization. J Allergy ClinImmunol. 2005;115:872–4.
9. McLean-Tooke A, O'Sullivan M, Easter T, Loh R. Differences between total IgG and sum of the IgG subclasses in clinical samples. Pathology. 2013;45:675–7.

8

Utility of dominant epitopes derived from cell-wall protein LppZ for immunodiagnostic of pulmonary tuberculosis

Jinjing Tan[1†], Xiaoguang Wu[2†], Suting Chen[3], Meng Gu[1], Hairong Huang[3*] and Wentao Yue[1,4*]

Abstract

Background: Serological antibodies tests for tuberculosis (TB) are widely used in developing countries. They appear to have some advantages- faster, simple and could be used for extrapulmonary TB. However, most of current commercial TB serological tests are failed to provide sufficient sensitivity and specificity. Improved serological biomarkers were essential. In this study, we present an approach using peptide array to discover new immunodiagnostic biomarkers based on immunodominant epitopes of TB antigens.

Results: The Probable conserved lipoprotein LppZ, which is difficult to express and purify in vivo was selected as the model antigen. We use two-step screening for dominant epitope selection. Based on peptide array data from 170 TB patients and 41 control samples, two dominant epitopes were identified to have diagnostic value for TB patients. Truncation assay was used to identify the core reactive sequence. Peptide- based ELISA was used to evaluate the diagnostic ability of pep-LppZ-1 and pep-LppZ-13. Pep-LppZ-1 has a sensitivity of 49.2% and a specificity of 83.3% in TB diagnose. Pep-LppZ-13 has a sensitivity of 43.3% and a specificity of 88.5% in TB diagnose.

Conclusions: Our result demonstrated that peptide array screening would be an advantage strategy of screening TB diagnostic peptides.

Keywords: Tuberculosis peptide arrays, LppZ, Serologic test

Background

Tuberculosis (TB) ranks as the second major cause of death among infectious diseases around the world. In 2014, 9.6 million people around the world became sick with TB disease. There were 1.5 million TB-related deaths worldwide. Only 66% of the TB-cases worldwide are correctly diagnosed [1]. China is one of the 22 high TB burden countries in the world, second only to India [2]. About 550 million people was infected with *Mycobacterium*

tuberculosis (*Mtb*). Early diagnosis of TB is especially important for improving early treatment. The gold standard in TB diagnosis remains to be the bacteria culture from sputum or body fluid specimens, which is time-consuming and low efficiency.

Serological tests that rely on the detection of TB-specific antigens or antibodies against TB-specific antigens possess several advantages: simple, inexpensive and feasible for the diagnosis of TB compared with traditional bacteria culturing. Moreover, it could be used to diagnose extrapulmonary TB. Many TB-specific antigens have been evaluated and applied to develop serological assays [3–5]. However, based on meta-analysis of commercial TB serological test from 1990 to 2010, current TB serological assays were failed to provide sufficient sensitivity and specificity [6]. In China, the diagnosis accuracy of these serological tests was major limited by reduced specificity. The low specificity

* Correspondence: Huanghairong@tb123.org; yuewt@ccmu.edu.cn
[†]Equal contributors
[3]National Clinical Laboratory on Tuberculosis, Beijing Key laboratory on Drug-resistant Tuberculosis Research, Beijing Chest Hospital, Capital Medical University/Beijing Tuberculosis and Thoracic Tumor Institute, Beijing 101149, China
[1]Department of Cellular and Molecular Biology, Beijing Chest Hospital, Capital Medical University/Beijing Tuberculosis and Thoracic Tumor Research Institute, Beijing 101149, China
Full list of author information is available at the end of the article

can be attributed to cross-reactivity with other mycobacteria involving environment *Mtb* exposure. World Health Organization (WHO) warned against the use of current inaccurate serological test for TB clinic diagnose [7]. The WHO expert group strongly encouraged further study on identifying improved serological tests.

From the previous proteomic studies, many *Mtb* proteins can be detected by serum antibodies [8]. However, due to complicated post-translational modification, most *Mtb* proteins were difficult to express and purify [9]. For the matter of fact, epitopes of *Mtb* proteins are essential for the antibody reaction to reach the diagnostic accuracy. Protein array research revealed that several protein fragments from bacteria culture filtrate or protein lysate were immunoreactive with serum antibodies [10, 11]. Therefore, instead of expressing recombinant antigens, using epitope peptides is an alternative approach to develop novel biomarkers of serodiagnosis [12]. Recent studies demonstrated that peptide epitopes may even improve the detection efficiency in diagnostic assays for TB [13]. High-throughput proteomic study could help to screen diagnostic antigens in form of peptides or protein fragments that contain immunodominant epitopes. In this context, combinatorial phage display has emerged as a direct method for discovering novel antigens [14–16]. Since high quality peptides are easy to access through chemical synthesis, peptide arrays become an advanced technology. Without translating DNA to protein, designed libraries of peptides display on solid surface usually a cellulose membrane or a glass chip [17]. Systematically screening immunoreactive peptides for serodiagnosis of TB provided large data of specific TB epitopes [18]. These data also indicated that the segregation between TB and healthy individuals does not cluster into specific proteins, but into specific peptide epitope 'hotspots' at different location of the same protein [19]. Therefore, there needs large clinical specimens to validate the candidate peptides, which were screened out by peptide arrays.

Antigen array performed on TB protein fractionations revealed several TB lipoprotein fractionations including LppZ could be recognized by serum antibodies from TB patients [11]. LppZ(Rv3006) is a cell-wall lipoprotein that contains a post-translational modification involved in glycosylation. Expressing recombinant LppZ antigen is time-consuming and challenged by the need for correct folding and modification. An alternative approach of constructing a high-content peptide array, which displays the LppZ antigen in the form of linear peptide could be used to obtain anti-peptide antibodies in sera. These peptides contained dominant epitope sequence that could recognize by serum IgG.

Therefore, we utilize cell-wall protein LppZ as an example, through two-step screening on peptide array to characterize the immunogenicity of LppZ and identify novel antigens as potential candidates for serological diagnosis of tuberculosis. Here, the entire LppZ protein sequence were dissembled and synthesized on cellulose membrane for IgG reactive epitope mapping. Reactive epitopes ware evaluated by ELISA assay and truncation assay.

Results
LppZ epitope mapping using peptide array
To identify the serum IgG-binding epitope, a set of 121 different 15-mer peptides generated from LppZ epitope mapping library was synthesized on cellulose membranes for the first round screening. Each peptide was shift 3 amino acids from its neighboring peptide. We used serum pools, which contained equivalence mixture of 10 serum samples from TB patients for immunoblotting (Additional file 1: Figure S1). A total 16 immunoreactive spots were obtained after first round screening.

Second round of screening for dominant epitopes
Then those 16 selected IgG-bond epitopes were integrated on a small array for the second round of screening of dominated epitope. A large-scale of individual serum samples of TB patients and health control were used in immunoblotting (Fig. 1a). The clinical character of TB patients was sorted in Additional file 1: Table S1. In order to normalize between arrays, we spotted FLAG-tag peptide as a positive reference probe on the array membrane. Data of each array was generated by image analysis software including spot gray value and background gray value. The signal value was created after normalization transformation including background correction and baseline conversion. The signal values of 16 spots immunoblotting with 170 TB patients and 41 health controls were summarized in Fig. 1b. The sequence and statistic characteristics of each spot were summarized in Additional file 1 Table S2 & S3.

The criteria for selecting peptides with diagnostic potential included a) high ability to react with TB serum sample; b) low ability to react with health control serum sample; c) statistically significant difference between reactivity with TB serum and health controls. AUC (area under the curve) of ROC (Receiver operator characteristic curve) curve of each spot was also under consideration. Based on these criteria, pep-LppZ-1 and pep-LppZ-13 were selected as dominated epitopes for further studies. The positive reactivity rate of pep-LppZ-1 and pep-LppZ-13 among the TB patients were 20.6% (35/170) and 15.3% (26/170) respectively. Both pep-LppZ-1 and pep-LppZ-13 were negative reactivity among health controls. Both AUC of pep-LppZ-1 and pep-LppZ-13 were above 0.7, which indicated a reliable discriminatory ability between TB and health group on chip.

Core sequence identification
Truncation peptide libraries of selected peptides were constructed to identify the shortest amino acid essential for antigen-antibody interactions. To narrow down the

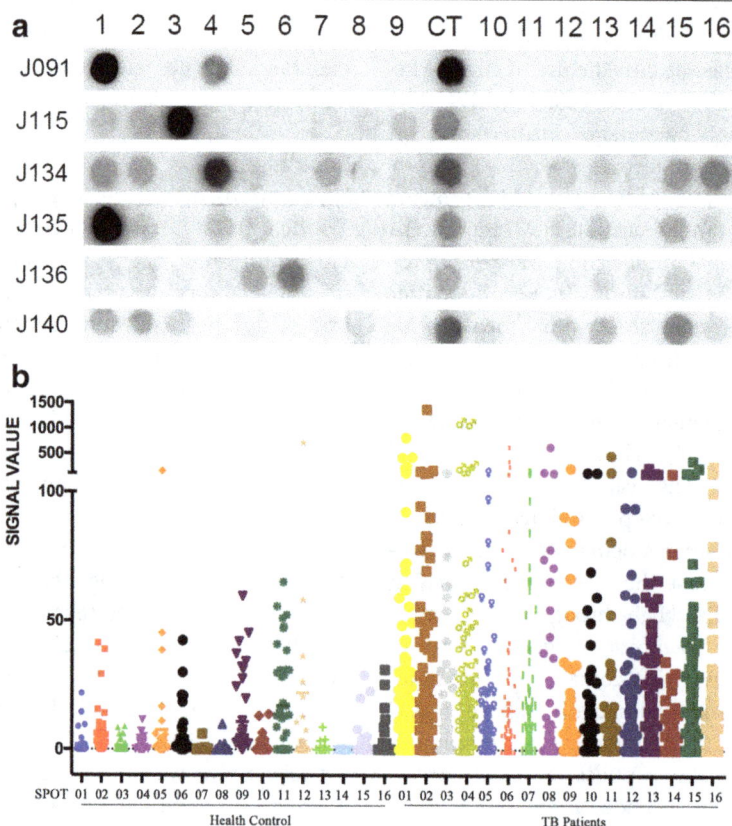

Fig. 1 Screening for LppZ dominated epitopes. **a** Second round peptide array screen of 16 candidate epitope peptides selected from first round screening. J091 to J140 stands for serum sample name; CT represents positive control. **b** Scattergram of peptide arrays signals. Data were normalized by CT signal on each array. Full-length blots are presented in Additional file 1: Figure S1

core activity sequence, the library is constructed by systemically removing the flanking residues of the original peptide. While the essential amino acid was truncated, the peptide was failed to interact with the antibody.

For two of the dominant peptides identified from the screening array, the key interaction residues were located at N terminus of pep-LppZ-1 and middle of pep-LppZ-13. When cutting the first amino acid from the N terminal of pep-LppZ-1, the peptide failed to react with the serum antibodies. The reactivity ability was not affected until the eighth amino acid of pep-LppZ-1 was removed from C terminal. The pep-LppZ-13 failed to interact with serum antibodies when either removes the fifth amino acid from N terminal or the fourth amino acid from C terminal (Fig. 2). As the result showed the core sequence of pep-LppZ-1 and pep-LppZ-13 were A-R-F-N-D-A-Q-S-Q and A-W-A-L-R-M-S-P-D, respectively.

Validation and evaluation by ELISA

The reactivity of dominated epitopes was validated by ELISA assay. KLH-peptide conjugates on microtiter plates were tested with 170 TB serum samples and 78 health controls. An equivalence mixed serum pool was served as

standards using gradient dilution methods. The IgG levels of serum sample were calculated according to the standard curve as relative concentration to serum pool, which was 10. The statistic characteristics of relative concentration of peptide detected IgG are illustrated in Table 1. In accordance with the peptide array result, the IgG reactivity against peptide pep-LppZ-1 and pep-LppZ-13 was significantly higher in the TB patients group when compared to the health control group. The difference between TB patients and health controls was statistically significant ($p < 0.001$) for both of the peptides (Fig. 3a).

The diagnostic value of dominant epitope

ROC curves for these peptides for TB patients with the control group as reference were plotted (Fig. 3b & c). The AUC for pep-LppZ-1 and prp-LppZ-13 were 0.738 and 0.757 respectively, indicating their discriminatory ability for TB infection detection from test group. When cut-off value for pep-LppZ-1 is > 13.5, the overall sensitivity and specificity of the ELISA test are 49.2% and 83.3%. When cut-off value for pep-LppZ-13 is > 16.3, the overall sensitivity and specificity of the ELISA test are 43.4% and 88.5% (Table 1). Combinative use of two

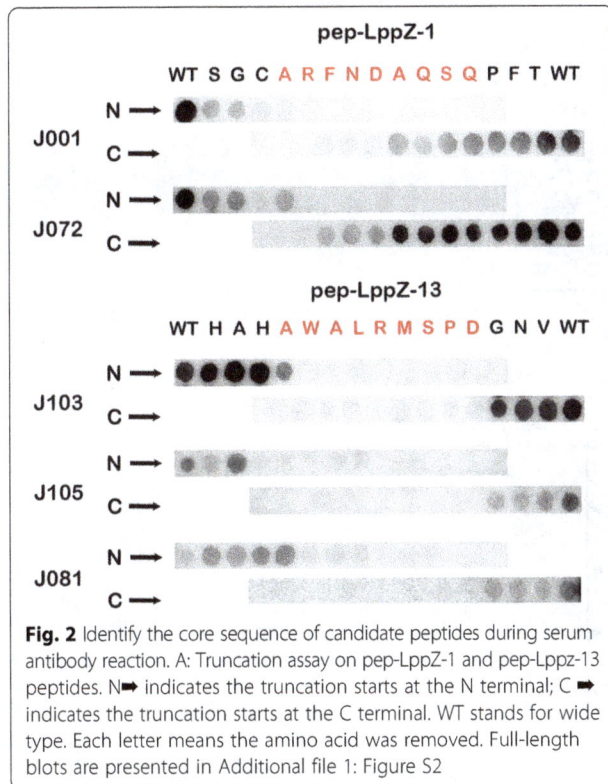

Fig. 2 Identify the core sequence of candidate peptides during serum antibody reaction. A: Truncation assay on pep-LppZ-1 and pep-Lppz-13 peptides. N➡ indicates the truncation starts at the N terminal; C ➡ indicates the truncation starts at the C terminal. WT stands for wide type. Each letter means the amino acid was removed. Full-length blots are presented in Additional file 1: Figure S2

peptides could improve specificity to 90.0% with sensitivity of 39.9%.

Since BCG vaccination is considered as the main interference factor in TB serological diagnose, we compared the diagnose rate of pep-LppZ peptides in BCG vaccination positive and negative groups. The diagnostic sensitive showed not much difference between BCG vaccination positive and negative groups (Table 2). The result suggested that the peptide diagnose value would not be disturbed by individual BCG vaccination condition.

We then analyze the diagnostic consistency of peptide based ELISA and traditional methods including AFB stain (Acid Fast Bacilli stain) and IGRA test (T-SPOT) (Interferon Gamma Release Assay) (Table 3). In TB diagnose, the judgment of peptide ELISA has 60.8% overlap with IGRA test, 44.6–46.4% overlap with sputum smear and 50.5–51.5% overlap with bacteria culture. When comparing the sensitive of peptide ELISA in TB diagnose between smear/ culture/ IGRA positive group and smear/

culture /IGRA negative group, it hardly showed bias, which revealed that the mechanism of peptide diagnoses differ from that of traditional methods (Table 4). Hence, using peptide ELISA as a complement would greatly improve the detection rate of TB (Table 5).

Discussion

This study was focused on the use of peptide array screening to discover novel serological biomarkers for TB diagnose. The cell-wall protein LppZ was utilized as an example for proving the possibility of synthetic peptides to improve the early diagnosis of patients infected with TB. Even though there will be post-translation modifications of LppZ protein such as amidation, glycosylation, and phosphorylation or other modifications, previously studies have shown that all the isoforms of LppZ protein fragments were serologically reactive, suggesting that the epitopes recognized by serum antibodies are on the peptide backbone of the core protein and not on probable modification sites [10]. Therefore, overlap mapping was performed on LppZ protein basic sequence regardless of post-translation modification.

In the process of screening, we designed two-step approach for higher probability of success. At the first round of screening, we performed epitope mapping based on the entire LppZ sequence to obtain serum IgG-bound epitopes. The second round of screening was performed by large group of individual serum samples. Based on the peptide array's result, the diagnostic capability of each candidate epitope was given out at certain diagnostic value (Additional file 1: Table S3). After two rounds of screening, two dominant epitopes, pep-LppZ-1 and pep-LppZ-13, were selected according to our selection criteria. Truncation assay revealed that the core reaction sequence was narrow down to 8 mer amino acids for each peptide. However, when the last unnecessary amino acid was deleted, the binding affinity has been reduced (Fig. 2). Therefore, protective amino acids were needed for immunoreaction.

Then we used traditional serology test method, ELISA to validate the diagnostic capability of these peptides in another group of serum samples, which matches the sample size of peptide array screening. The ELISA result agreed with the peptide array data in terms of diagnostic ability. Compare to other research, our method would

Table 1 Statistic characteristics of pep-LppZ-1 and pep-LppZ-13 based ELISA

Peptide name	TB patients (n = 122)		Health Controls (n = 78)		P value[1]	AUC[2]
	Mean ± SD	Sensitivity	Mean ± SD	Specificity		
LppZ-1	27.03 ± 55.04	49.2%	9.49 ± 11.28	83.3%	< 0.001	0.738
LppZ-13	22.14 ± 22.11	43.4%	10.55 ± 21.77	88.5%	< 0.001	0.757
Combine		39.3%		91.0%		

[1]P value: comparison of difference between TB group and health control group using Mann-Whiney U test
[2]AUC: area under the curve according to receiver operating characteristic (ROC) indicating the discriminatory ability for TB detection from test

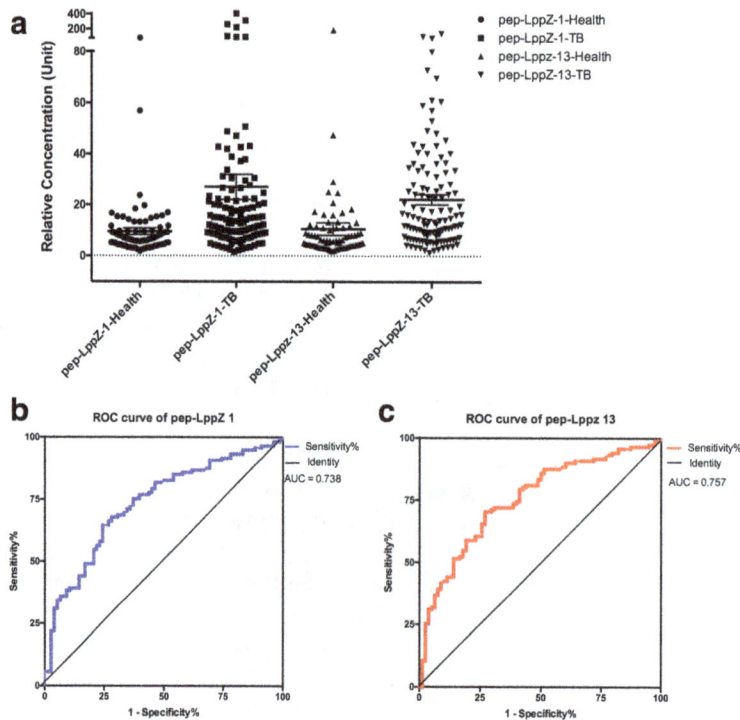

Fig. 3 Validate and evaluate the reactivity of dominated epitopes by ELISA. **a** Histogram of relative concentration of antibodies toward dominated epitopes. **b** & **c**: ROC (receiver operating characteristic) curve of pep-LppZ-1 and pep-LppZ-13 on detecting TB infection based on ELISA data

be much simpler and the verification rate is much higher [10, 16, 18]. Since the second round screening could be considered analogous to carrying out a thousand of ELISAs at one time. It would save time and cost.

According to other research findings using LppZ recombinant protein or protein fragments, the positive rate of anti-LppZ antibodies in TB patients was around 30% to 55% [11]. The specificity was not provided. In our result, one peptide was not only sufficient to obtain sensitivity similar to protein component described above, but also with a high specificity (above 90%). Combinative use of two peptides could further improve specificity, but slightly drop of sensitivity. In clinical practice, not every TB suspect is able to take sputum smear test. In our research group, only 56 of 122 TB patients could

run sputum smear test and 48 turned positive. In that case, the omission diagnostic rate was actually as high as 60.7% (74/122). In combination of smear test and peptide serology test, the detective rate could improve to 73.0% (Table 5).

In this study, we discover two derived peptides from one protein, which has a diagnostic potential in TB serology test. However, these peptides are not good enough to take place microscopy examine. The present studies provide an advanced strategy of screening TB diagnostic peptide. Integrating multiple diagnostic peptides would improve the existing performance of TB serologic test. Plenty of work had been done on using two or more markers in the form of recombination antigen or antibody groups or others to improve diagnostic

Table 2 Relationship between BCG vaccination and peptide diagnose

Subgroups	N	pep-LppZ-1		pep-LppZ-13	
		Positive N (Cutoff > 13.5)	Positive rate	Positive N (Cutoff > 16.3)	Positive rate
Health control (IGRA-)[1]					
BCG+	11	3	27.3%	1	9.1%
BCG-	20	4	20.0%	2	10.0%
TB patient					
BCG+	93	45	48.4%	39	37.5%
BCG-	8	4	50.0%	3	41.9%

[1]IGRA: IFN-γ release assay (T-SPOT.TB); [2]BCG: Bacillus Calmette- Guerin vaccine

Table 3 Diagnose consistency of peptides and traditional methods

	N	pep-LppZ-1 (cutoff > 13.5)	pep-LppZ-13 (cutoff > 16.3)
Pep-LppZ-1 vs. pep-LppZ-13	122	87.5%	–
IGRA test vs.	171	60.8%	60.8%
Sputum smear vs.	56	46.4%	44.6%
Bacteria Culture vs.	99	51.5%	50.5%

efficacy [8, 16, 20, 21]. A research using ESAT-6, CFP10 and PPE68 fusion protein in diagnosing TB could increase the sensitivity to 73.3% [22]. Chemical synthesis of peptides would be a better strategy to study TB diagnostic panel. Peptide array has already revealed application prospect in other disease area. Printed peptide microarray which covering known tumor-associated antigens could predict prognostic in glioblastoma [23]. The array consists of random sequence peptides was capable to describe serum immunosignature pattern and might have potential as a diagnostic tool in Alzheimer's disease [24]. High-density peptide array may have advanced prospect for comprehensive health monitoring [25]. In our study, we compared the peptide array as a diagnostic tool with the ELISA method. When the cutoff value was set at 4.48 and 3.0 for each pep-LppZ marker, the sensitivity and specificity of peptide array was parallel to ELISA. When we strict the cutoff of peptide arrays to 1.29 and 0.38 for each pep-LppZ marker, the sensitivity of peptide array had a remarkable improve to 75% with not much sacrifice of specificity (Additional file 1: Table S4).

Conclusions
Our study provides the proof that selected peptides can replace the target proteins in immunodiagnostic test for TB. Peptide array can be a superior tool for screening autoantibody based TB biomarker. High-throughput array technique could perform epitope mapping on a large proteome in an economic and effective way. In this study, two rounds of screening performed well and resulted in satisfactory verification rate. We recommend applying a

small amount of sample in the second round of screening. It's the key point of improving verification rate.

Methods
Patients and samples
Serum samples of 187 TB patients and 80 healthy volunteers were obtained from Beijing Chest Hospital Sample Bank (Beijing, China). The serum samples were consecutively collected between January 2012 to December 2014. The clinic characteristics of specimens were sorted in Additional file 1: Table S1. TB patients were diagnosed for pulmonary tuberculosis by either bacteria culture positive or smear positive. None of them were co-infected with HIV. Healthy controls did not have any radiological or clinical signs of TB and had negative tuberculin skin test (TST) results (< 5 mm) and negative IGRA results. Study protocol was approved by the ethics committee of Beijing Chest Hospital, Capital Medical University. The serum sample was prepared according to the standard protocol and stored at − 80 °C until used. All methods were performed in accordance with the relevant guidelines and regulations. The serum pools were consisted with equal volumes of serum from randomly selected 10 TB individuals.

SPOT synthesis and membranes immunoblotting
Peptide arrays were prepared on amino-PEG500 cellulose membrane-UC540 (Intavis, Germany) using a SPOT robot (Intavis AG, Cologne, Germany) according to standard spot-synthesis protocol. Design program provided with the instrument was used for library designing.

Table 4 Comparison of using peptides based ELISA and traditional methods in TB diagnose

TB Subgroups	N	pep-LppZ-1		pep-LppZ-13	
		Positive N (Cutoff > 13.5)	Sensitive	Positive N (Cutoff > 16.3)	Sensitive
Smear[1] +	48	22	45.8%	20	41.7%
Smear -	8	4	50.0%	3	37.5%
Culture[2] +	88	46	52.3%	43	48.9%
Culture -	11	6	54.5%	4	36.4%
IGRA[3] +	80	38	47.5%	32	40.0%
IGRA -	13	8	61.5%	6	46.2%

[1]Smear: sputum smear detection for TB bacteria
[2]Culture: bacteria culture
[3]IGRA: IFN-γ release assay (T-SPOT.TB)

Table 5 Improvement of detection rate by using pep-LppZ-1 and pep-LppZ-13

Diagnose method	N	Positive N	Detection rate
Sputum smear	122	48	39.3%
Smear + pep-LppZ-1[1]		86	70.5%
Smear + pep-LppZ-13[2]		81	66.4%
Smear + pep-LppZ-1/13		89	73.0%
Bacteria culture		88	72.1%
Culture + pep-LppZ-1		102	83.6%
Culture + pep-LppZ-13		98	80.3%
Culture + pep-LppZ-1/13		102	83.6%
IGRA test	93(29 missing)	80	86.0%
IGRA test + pep-LppZ-1		88	94.6%
IGRA test + pep-LppZ-13		86	92.5%
IGRA test + pep-LppZ-1/13		89	95.7%

[1] the threshold of pep-LppZ-1 detection is > 13.5
[2] the threshold of pep-LppZ-13 detection is > 16.3

SPOT membranes were equilibrated with PBS-T (phosphate-buffered saline, 0.1% Tween 20, pH 7.4) and blocked with 5% skim milk in PBS-T for 1 h at room temperature. Serum sample was prepared at a dilution of 1:100 in PBS-T with 5% skim milk before incubation of the membranes at 4 °C overnight. After washing with PBS-T, membranes were incubated for 1 h with HRP conjugated anti-Human-IgG (Invitrogen, USA) applied at a dilution of 1:2000 in PBS-T with 5% skim milk.

Measurements of the spot signal intensities were obtained as described [26]. Briefly, the chemiluminescent signals were measured and a digital image file generated. Signal intensities were quantified with TotalLab Software (Nonlinear Dynamics, USA) using algorithms that compared the intensity between background, spot area and negative control to define the empirical probability that the spot signal was distinct from background signal. The positive spot on the membrane was reported as having 100% density, and all other spots had their intensities values expressed as a relative percentage to this intensity. Only spots with intensity values above 30% were considered as positive.

Overlap peptide library for epitope mapping
To identify the IgG-binding epitopes, a library of 121 peptides was designed to represent and cover the entire sequence (373 amino acids) of LppZ protein (Rv3006). Each peptide was 15 amino acids in length and offset from its neighboring peptide by 3 amino acids. LppZ were assayed against 3 pools of serum samples from TB patients. Each serum pool contained an equivalence mixture of 10 TB serum samples. The peptides were assessed for reactivity with human IgG.

Dominant epitope screening
16 IgG-bound epitopes of LppZ selected by epitope mapping were integrated on a mini peptide array for dominant epitope screening. Randomly selected 170 TB serum samples and 41 health control samples were used in immunoblotting. In order to normalize between arrays, we spotted FLAG-tag peptide as reference probe on the array membrane. Data of each array was generated by image analysis software including spot gray value and background gray value. The signal value was created after normalization transformation including background correction and baseline conversion.

Narrow down peptide library for truncation assay
A truncation array of the dominated epitope was performed to determine the minimum length required and key residues for epitope activity. The truncation library was generated through a systematic truncation of the peptide's sequence from each terminus.

Quantitative measurement of serum antibodies against dominated epitope by ELISA
For further evaluate the diagnostic effect of these epitopes, ELISA assay were performed. Microtiter 96-well plates were coated with 10 ng/well of purified peptide connected with KLH in a 0.05 M carbonate/bicarbonate buffer (pH 9.6) at 4 °C overnight. The sequence of pep-LppZ-1 and pep-LppZ-13 were S-G-C-A-R-F-N-D-A-Q-S-Q-P-F-T and H-A-H-A-W-A-L-R-M-S-P-D-G-N-V. The plates were blocked with 200 µl of 5% skim milk in PBS-T for 1 h at 37 °C.

Serum sample was prepared at a dilution of 1:100 in PBS-T with 5% skim milk before incubation of the membranes at 4 °C overnight. An equivalence mixed serum pool was served as standards using gradient dilution methods. After washing with PBS-T, the plates were incubated for 1 h with HRP conjugated anti-Human-IgG (Invitrogen, USA) applied at a dilution of 1:2000 in PBS-T with 5% skim milk. Thereafter, the plates were washed with PBS-T and exposed to 100 µl TMB for 20 min at room temperature and stopped by adding 50 µl of 2 M H_2SO_4. Absorbance at 450 nm was determined using a spectrophotometer (Epoch Microplate Spectrophotometer, BioTek Laboratories, USA). Each serum sample was tested in duplicate. After normalization by the standards, the levels of serum antibody were calculated to a relative concentration to standards. The cutoff value was choosing when AUC (area under curve) reached max in ROC curve.

Statistical analysis
Receiver operating characteristic (ROC) curves was utilized to analyze the diagnostic information of each peptide by comparing the area under the curve (AUC). Comparisons of relative concentration of antibodies between

groups were preformed using Mann-Whitney U test. Histogram was plotted using GRAPHPAD Prism software (GraphPad Software, Inc., San Diego, CA, USA). Statistically significant differences were those determined to have a p value ≤0.05.

Abbreviations
AFB: Acid Fast Bacilli stain; AUC: Area under the curve; IGRA: Interferon Gamma Release Assay; LppZ: Probable conserved lipoprotein LppZ; Mtb: Mycobacterium tuberculosis; ROC: Receiver operator characteristic curve; TB: Tuberculosis; WHO: World Health Organization

Acknowledgements
The authors are grateful to the staff of Beijing Chest Hospital Sample Bank.

Funding
This study was supported by National Science and Technology Major Project of the Ministry of Science and Technology of China (2013ZX10003003003002).

Authors' contributions
HH and WY designed the study. XW performed clinical study and data analysis. JT, S. and MG performed the experimental analysis. JT and WY prepared the manuscript. All authors reviewed the manuscript.

Competing interests
The authors declare that they have no competing interests.

Author details
[1]Department of Cellular and Molecular Biology, Beijing Chest Hospital, Capital Medical University/Beijing Tuberculosis and Thoracic Tumor Research Institute, Beijing 101149, China. [2]Department of Tuberculosis, Beijing Chest Hospital, Capital Medical University, Beijing 101149, China. [3]National Clinical Laboratory on Tuberculosis, Beijing Key laboratory on Drug-resistant Tuberculosis Research, Beijing Chest Hospital, Capital Medical University/ Beijing Tuberculosis and Thoracic Tumor Institute, Beijing 101149, China. [4]Central Laboratory, Beijing Obstetrics and Gynecology Hospital, Capital Medical University, Chaoyang, Beijing 100026, China.

References
1. Zumla A, George A, Sharma V, Herbert RHN, Baroness Masham of Ilton, Oxley A, Oliver M: The WHO 2014 global tuberculosis report–further to go. Lancet Glob Health 2015; 3:e10–e12.
2. TB in China: a New Epidemic of an Old Disease [http://www.theglobalist.com/tb-in-china-a-new-epidemic-of-an-old-disease/].
3. Steingart KR, Henry M, Laal S, Hopewell PC, Ramsay A, Menzies D, Cunningham J, Weldingh K, Pai M. A systematic review of commercial serological antibody detection tests for the diagnosis of extrapulmonary tuberculosis. Postgrad Med J. 2007;83:705–12.
4. Yang Y, Wu X, Liu Y, Wang Z, Zhao W, Zhang J, Liang Y, Zhang C, Li H, Wang L. Letter to editor: comparative evaluation of four commercial serological antibody detection kits for the diagnosis of tuberculosis in China. Ann Clin Lab Sci. 2013;43:101–4.
5. Steingart KR, Flores LL, Dendukuri N, Schiller I, Laal S, Ramsay A, Hopewell PC, Pai M. Commercial serological tests for the diagnosis of active pulmonary and extrapulmonary tuberculosis: an updated systematic review and meta-analysis. PLoS Med. 2011;8:e1001062.
6. She RC, Litwin CM. Performance of a tuberculosis serologic assay in various patient populations. Am J Clin Pathol. 2015;144:240–6.
7. WHO: Commercial Serodiagnostic Tests for Diagnosis of Tuberculosis: Policy Statement. 2011.
8. Min F, Zhang Y, Huang R, Li W, Wu Y, Pan J, Zhao W, Liu X. Serum antibody responses to 10 mycobacterium tuberculosis proteins, purified protein derivative, and old tuberculin in natural and experimental tuberculosis in rhesus monkeys. Clinical and vaccine immunology: CVI. 2011;18:2154–60.
9. Herrmann JL, Delahay R, Gallagher A, Robertson B, Young D. Analysis of post-translational modification of mycobacterial proteins using a cassette expression system. FEBS Lett. 2000;473:358–62.
10. Målen H, Søfteland T, Wiker HG. Antigen analysis of mycobacterium tuberculosis H37Rv culture filtrate proteins. Scand J Immunol. 2008;67:245–52.
11. Sartain MJ, Slayden RA, Singh KK, Laal S, Belisle JT. Disease state differentiation and identification of tuberculosis biomarkers via native antigen array profiling. Molecular & cellular proteomics: MCP. 2006;5:2102–13.
12. Yang H, Sha W, Song P, Liu Z, Qin L, Huang X, Lu J, Wang J, Duthie MS, Xiao H, Hu Z. Screening and identification of immunoactive peptide mimotopes for the enhanced serodiagnosis of tuberculosis. Appl Microbiol Biotechnol. 2015:1–9.
13. Yang H, Liu Z-H, Zhang L-T, Wang J, Yang H-S, Qin L-H, Jin R-L, Feng Y-H, Cui Z-L, Zheng R-J, Hu Z-Y. Selection and application of peptide mimotopes of MPT64 protein in mycobacterium tuberculosis. J Med Microbiol. 2011;60:69–74.
14. Araujo Z, Giampietro F, Bochichio M de LA, Palacios A, Dinis J, Isern J, de WJH, Rada E, Borges R, Fernández de Larrea C, Villasmil A, Vanegas M, Enciso-Moreno JA, Patarroyo MA. Immunologic evaluation and validation of methods using synthetic peptides derived from mycobacterium tuberculosis for the diagnosis of tuberculosis infection. Mem Inst Oswaldo Cruz. 2013;108:131–9.
15. Fuchs M, Kampfer S, Helmsing S, Spallek R, Oehlmann W, Prilop W, Frank R, Dubel S, Singh M, Hust M. Novel human recombinant antibodies against mycobacterium tuberculosis antigen 85B. BMC Biotechnol. 2014;14:68.
16. Ferrara F, Naranjo LA, Kumar S, Gaiotto T, Mukundan H, Swanson B, Bradbury ARM. Using phage and yeast display to select hundreds of monoclonal antibodies: application to antigen 85, a tuberculosis biomarker. PLoS One. 2012;7:e49535.
17. Uttamchandani M, Yao SQ. Peptide microarrays: next generation biochips for detection, diagnostics and high-throughput screening. Curr Pharm Des. 2008;14:2428–38.
18. Lewinsohn DM, Swarbrick GM, Cansler ME, Null MD, Rajaraman V, Frieder MM, Sherman DR, McWeeney S, Lewinsohn DA. Human mycobacterium tuberculosis CD8 T cell antigens/epitopes identified by a proteomic peptide library. PLoS One. 2013;8:e67016–9.
19. Gaseitsiwe S, Valentini D, Mahdavifar S, Magalhaes I, Hoft DF, Zerweck J, Schutkowski M, Andersson J, Reilly M, Maeurer MJ. Pattern recognition in pulmonary tuberculosis defined by high content peptide microarray Chip analysis representing 61 Proteins from M. Tuberculosis. PLoS One. 2008;3:e3840–8.
20. Singh N, Sreenivas V, Sheoran A, Sharma S, Gupta KB, Khuller GK, Mehta PK. Serodiagnostic potential of immuno-PCR using a cocktail of mycobacterial antigen 85B, ESAT-6 and cord factor in tuberculosis patients. J Microbiol Methods. 2016;120:56–64.
21. Gonzalez JM, Francis B, Burda S, Hess K, Behera D, Gupta D, Agarwal AN, Verma I, Verma A, Myneedu VP, Niedbala S, Laal S. Development of a POC test for TB based on multiple Immunodominant epitopes of M. Tuberculosis specific Cell-Wall proteins. PLoS One. 2014;9:e106279–10.
22. Xu J-N, Chen J-P, Chen D-L. Serodiagnosis efficacy and immunogenicity of the fusion protein of mycobacterium tuberculosis composed of the 10-kilodalton culture filtrate protein, ESAT-6, and the extracellular domain fragment of PPE68. Clinical and vaccine immunology: CVI. 2012;19:536–44.
23. Mock A, Warta R, Geisenberger C, Bischoff R, Schulte A, Lamszus K, Stadler V, Felgenhauer T, Schichor C, Schwartz C, Matschke J, Jungk C, Ahmadi R,

Sahm F, Capper D, Glass R, Tonn JC, Westphal M, Deimling von A, Unterberg A, Bermejo JL, Herold-Mende C. Printed peptide arrays identify prognostic TNC serumantibodies in glioblastoma patients. Oncotarget. 2015;6(15):13579–90.

24. Restrepo L, Stafford P, Magee DM, Johnston SA. Application of immunosignatures to the assessment of Alzheimer's disease. Ann Neurol. 2011;70:286–95.

25. Legutki JB, Zhao ZG, Greving M, Woodbury N, Johnston SA, Stafford P. Scalable high-density peptide arrays for comprehensive health monitoring. Nat Commun. 2014;5:4785.

26. De-Simone SG, Napoleao-Pego P, Teixeira-Pinto LA, Melgarejo AR, Aguiar AS, Provance DWJ. IgE and IgG epitope mapping by microarray peptide-immunoassay reveals the importance and diversity of the immune response to the IgG3 equine immunoglobulin. Toxicon: official journal of the International Society on Toxinology. 2014;78:83–93.

9

Immune activation and regulatory T cells in *Mycobacterium tuberculosis* infected lymph nodes

Karima Sahmoudi[1,2], Hassan Abbassi[3], Nada Bouklata[4], Mohamed Nouredine El Alami[3], Abderrahmane Sadak[2], Christopher Burant[5], W. Henry Boom[6], Rajae El Aouad[1], David H. Canaday[6†] and Fouad Seghrouchni[1*†] (iD)

Abstract

Background: Lymph node tuberculosis (LNTB) is the most frequent extrapulmonary form of tuberculosis (TB). Studies of human tuberculosis at sites of disease are limited. LNTB provides a unique opportunity to compare local *in situ* and peripheral blood immune response in active *Mycobacterium tuberculosis* (Mtb) disease. The present study analysed T regulatory cells (Treg) frequency and activation along with CD4+ T cell function in lymph nodes from LNTB patients.

Results: Lymph node mononuclear cells (LNMC) were compared to autologous peripheral blood mononuclear cells (PBMC). LNMC were enriched for CD4+ T cells with a late differentiated effector memory phenotype. No differences were noted in the frequency and mutifunctional profile of memory CD4+ T cells specific for Mtb. The proportion of activated CD4+ and Tregs in LNMC was increased compared to PBMC. The correlation between Tregs and activated CD4+ T cells was stronger in LNMC than PBMC. Tregs in LNMC showed a strong positive correlation with Th1 cytokine production (IL2, IFNγ and TNFα) as well as MIP-1α after Mtb antigen stimulation. A subset of Tregs in LNMC co-expressed HLA-DR and CD38, markers of activation.

Conclusion: Further research will determine the functional relationship between Treg and activated CD4+ T cells at lymph node sites of Mtb infection.

Keywords: Tuberculosis, Lymphadenitis, Lymph node, Treg cells, conventional T cell, activation

Background

Mycobacterium tuberculosis (Mtb) infection is a major global health problem with approximately 10.4 million cases and 1.4 million deaths from tuberculosis (TB) in 2015 [1]. Furthermore, one-third of the world's population is thought to be infected by Mtb. Extra pulmonary TB represents approximately 20% of clinical TB disease. Lymph node tuberculosis (LNTB) is the most frequent extrapulmonary form [1].

Cellular immune responses play a pivotal role in control of Mtb infection with CD4+ T cells having the central role. After infection CD4+ T cells undergo activation manifested by expression of surface molecules including HLA-DR and CD38 [2, 3]. Functionally, CD4+ T cells control infection by producing Th1 and Th17 cytokines [4]. Polyfunctional T cells, defined by their ability to co-express more than one cytokine, have been associated with protection against Mtb disease [4–6].

At sites of infection, immune responses are modulated by T regulatory cells (Tregs) [7, 8]. Tregs express CD3, CD4, high levels of CD25, low levels of the IL-7 receptor α-chain (CD127) and the intracellular marker forkhead box p3 (FoxP3) [9].

The relationship between Tregs and immune activation at sites of Mtb disease is not clear [10, 11]. The objective of the present study was to evaluate the interaction between Tregs and the function and activation of CD4+ T cells in lymph node vs. the peripheral blood compartments in persons with LNTB.

* Correspondence: fseghrouchni@yahoo.fr
†David H. Canaday and Fouad Seghrouchni contributed equally to this work.
[1]Laboratory of Cellular Immunology, National Institute of Hygiene, 27, Avenue Ibn Batouta, PB 769, 11400 Rabat, Morocco
Full list of author information is available at the end of the article

Methods

Subjects and preparation of immune cells

Eighteen patients (5 men, 13 women, age range 17-60 years) were recruited in the Hassan II University Hospital of Fes (Morocco) among patients with cervical lymphadenitis. Active LNTB was diagnosed by history, physical examination, and lab studies by experienced clinicians. The diagnosis of LNTB was based on a combination of clinical symptoms, pathology and response to TB drug therapy. Clinical symptoms associated with lymphadenitis included local lymphadenopathy, weight loss, fever, sweats, and anorexia. Histopathological evidence consisted of the presence of a granulomatous lesion with caseation in excisional biopsy specimens. Pulmonary radiography and HIV serology were performed to exclude pulmonary TB and HIV infection respectively. All LNTB cases were newly diagnosed and none had received anti-TB chemotherapy before sample collection. Tuberculin skin test results were positive (induration ≥ 10 mm) for 15 out of 18 patients (83%). All patients were BCG vaccinated, and none reported contact with a case of pulmonary TB.

For all patients, the affected lymph node was in the neck and was surgically removed. In addition, 10 ml of peripheral blood was collected before starting anti-TB treatment. One portion of the lymph node was used for histological examination, and the other for isolation of lymph node mononuclear cells (LNMC) for immunologic studies.

Biopsy specimens were crushed gently in tissue culture medium. LNMC were spun and separated using Ficoll-Hypaque density centrifugation. Peripheral blood mononuclear cells (PBMC) were isolated from heparinized venous blood under endotoxin-free conditions by Ficoll-Hypaque (SIGMA) density centrifugation. Cells were cryopreserved and stored in liquid nitrogen until shipment by a cryoshipper to Case Western Reserve University for immunological studies.

Phenotypic and functional study of T cells

PBMC and LNMC (10^6/ tube) were stimulated with a pool of 34 overlapping peptides from Mtb-antigen ESAT6/CFP10 at 6.25 ug/ml per peptide (New England peptide, Gardner, MA), *M. tuberculosis* CDC1551 whole cells lysate (Mtb lysate) (BEI Resources) or staphylococcal enterotoxin B (SEB, 2 µg/ml, Sigma) overnight at 37 °C in 5% CO_2. Unstimulated PBMC and LNMC served as negative controls. Anti-CD28/CD49d (1 µg/ml each, eBioscience and Biolegend) was added to each tube during stimulation and brefeldin A (5 µg/ml, Sigma) was added 2 hr later. After stimulation, cells were washed with PBS and surface stained with anti-CCR7-PE-Cy7 (BD Bioscience) for 15 min at 37 °C, then live dead yellow (Invitrogen), anti-CD14-BV570, anti-CD4-APC/Cy7,

anti-CD8-BV510 (all Biolegend) and anti-CD45RA-PE/TR (Invitrogen) were added and incubated at RT for 25 min. Afterward cells were washed, permeabilized (Cytofix/Cytoperm Kit, BD Pharmingen) according to the manufacturer's instructions and stained for intracellular expression with anti-CD3-PerCP, anti-IFNγ-Alexa700, anti-IL2-APC, anti-TNFα- Pacific Blue, anti-IL17-BV711 (all Biolegend) and anti-MIP-1α-FITC (R&D). Cells were then washed, fixed in 1% paraformaldehyde and 1×10^6 total events collected from each sample on an LSR-II flow cytometer (BD). Net responding cells for each cytokine were calculated by subtracting the no antigen condition (medium only) from the antigen simulated result. The analysis of all functional markers expressed after stimulation were done on viable total memory CD4+ and CD8+ T cells. Memory phenotype was determined by CCR7 and CD45RA expression. Naïve T cells were CD45RA+/CCR7+, central memory (CM) cells were CD45RA-/CCR7+, effector memory (EM) cells were CD45RA-/CCR7-and effector cells (E) were CD45RA +/CCR7-.

To identify Tregs and activated T cells, PBMC and LNMC were surface stained with live dead yellow (Invitrogen), anti-CD3-APC/Cy7, anti-CD4-PerCP, anti-CD8 -Alexa700, anti-CD25-APC, anti-HLA-DR-FITC, anti-CD38-PE/Cy7(all Biolegend), and anti-CD127-BV6 50(BD Bioscience), and incubated at RT for 25 min. After, cells were washed, permeabilized and intracellular stained with, anti-FoxP3-PE (eBioscience) or isotype-m atched negative control for gating purposes.

Plots were analyzed using FlowJo software (version 6.1.1; Trcc Star, Ashland, OR, USA). Boolean analysis on Flow Jo and SPICE (NIAID, NIH, USA) was used to assess cytokine polyfunctionality.

Statistical analysis

Statistical analysis was performed using the paired Student's t test for comparisons of PBMC and LNMC. P value for comparison of polyfunctional profile was done using SPICE software. Significance of correlations was analyzed by the nonparametric Spearman test. A *p* value of ≤ 0.05 was considered significant. Data were analyzed by Statistical Package for the Social Sciences (SPSS) software (IBM) and the GraphPad Prism software, version 5.00 for Windows (GraphPad Software, San Diego).

Results

Phenotypic and cytokine profile of CD4+ T cells in LNMC and PBMC

We first compared memory phenotypes of T lymphocyte subsets in LNMC and PBMC. LNMC were significantly enriched for CD4+ T cells [80.7±5.6 % vs. 68.0±6.6 % ($p = 0.0015$)] (Fig. 1a). CD8+ T cells were concomitantly lower in LNMC compared to PBMC

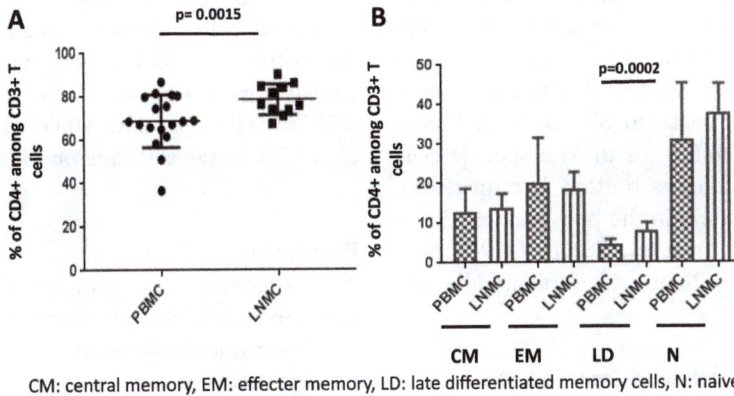

Fig. 1 Phenotypic and functional T-cell subset distribution in PBMC and LNMC. Relative frequencies of CD4+T cells (**a**) and memory subsets of CD4+ T cells (**b**) among all CD3+ T cells. Means from 18 subjects are shown and error bars represent standard deviations

[17.6±5.8 % vs. 27.4±11.7 % (*p* = 0.0055)] (Additional file 1). Memory subsets of CD4+ T cells were defined according to expression of CD45RA and CCR7 and only the effector subset was modestly increased in LNMC compared to PBMC (*p* = 0.0002) (Fig. 1b).

T cell functional profiles in response to Mtb antigens were compared between LNMC and PBMC. IFNγ, IL2,

TNFα, IL17, and MIP-1α production by CD4+ T cells in PBMC and LNMC in response to Mtb RVL were not different (Fig. 2a). Similarly CD4+ T cell responses in response to ESAT6/CFP10 peptides were not different between LNMC and PBMC (Additional file 2).

No significant differences were observed in the polyfunctionality of total memory CD4+ T cells in LNMC

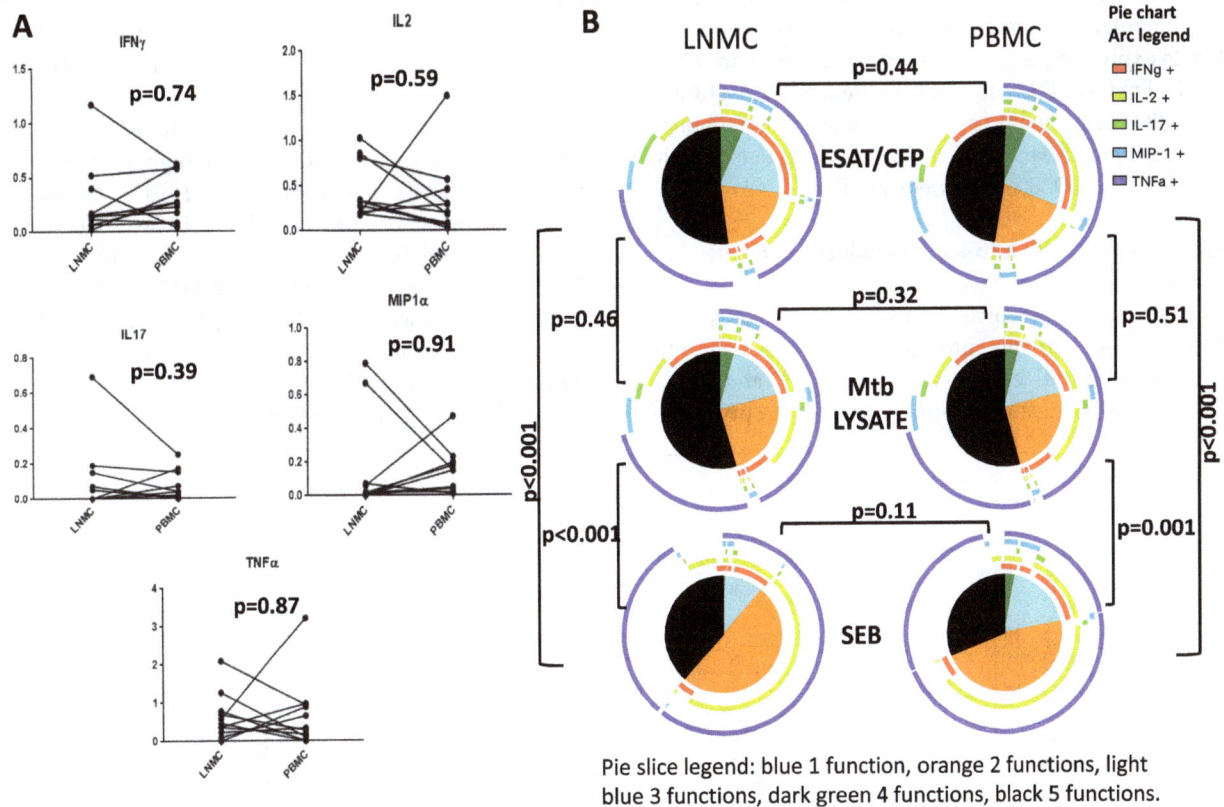

Fig. 2 Cytokine expression of memory CD4+T cells after Mtb antigen RVL stimulation (**a**) and polyfunctional composition of total memory CD4+T cells after stimulation with Mtb lysate, ESAT6/CFP10, and SEB (**b**). Results from 11 subjects are shown. Plots are gated on viable memory CD4+T cells. The pie charts depict the average polyfunctional profile of only the responding cells for each specific stimuli from all subjects. All possible combinations of responses are represented by the arcs with pie arc color legend on the figure

when compared to PBMC for the same stimuli (Fig. 2b all three rows with side to side comparison). Polyfunctionality of total memory CD4+ T cells in response to ESAT6/CFP10 peptides and Mtb lysate were significantly different from that in response to SEB in both PBMC and LNMC indicating a difference in Mtb-specific cells as a group (Fig. 2b, top 4 pies vs. bottom 2 comparison), but no differences were found in the polyfunctionality in response to Mtb-specific antigens, ESAT6/CFP10 peptides and Mtb lysate (Fig. 2b top two and middle two comparison).

Distribution of activated T cells and Tregs in LNMC and PBMC

We measured the frequency of activated conventional CD4+ T cells and Tregs in LNMC and PBMC. Activation was based on the expression of HLA-DR and CD38. Tregs were identified as CD4+, CD25+, FoxP3+ and CD127dim. An increased proportion of activated CD4+ HLA-DR+CD38+ T cells ($p < 0.0001$) and Treg CD4+ CD25+FoxP3+CD127dim ($p = 0.0089$) in LNMC compared to PBMC was observed (Fig. 3). A positive correlation between the frequency of total activated CD4+ T cells and Tregs was observed within LNMC ($r = 0.676$, $p = 0.008$) and PBMC ($r = 0.549$, $p = 0.018$) (Fig. 4).

We compared, among Tregs in LNMC, the proportion of cells expressing activation markers. More than 90% of CD25+ FoxP3+CD127dim cells expressed HLA-DR and/ or CD38. Furthermore, the predominant Treg subpopulation in both LNMC and PBMC was the one expressing HLA-DR and CD38 simultaneously (Fig. 5).

Treg correlation with Mtb-antigen induced cytokine production

We determined the correlation between the proportion of Tregs and cytokine producing CD4+ T cells after overnight Mtb-antigen activation in LNMC and PBMC. There was a positive correlation between the proportion

of Tregs and Th1 cytokine production (IL2 and IFNγ) as well as MIP-1α following stimulation by Mtb lysate antigen within LNMC but not among PBMC (Table 1). A similar correlation was found after stimulation by Mtb ESAT6/CFP10 peptides while no correlation was found after SEB mitogen stimulation (data not shown).

Discussion

The outcome of the immune response to Mtb results from the simultaneous involvement of activating and regulatory mechanisms [8, 11]. The nature of the relationship between conventional T cells and Tregs during active TB is still not clear although this interaction has been studied in different forms of TB [10, 11]. Increased expression of activation markers on T cells [12, 13] and higher levels of Tregs [7, 8] have been described in peripheral blood of patients with TB. Nevertheless, local immune responses may differ from those in peripheral blood and exploring this interaction in the site of active infection will give important clues about their involvement in protection or pathogenesis [14, 15]. The present study sought to evaluate the relationships between Tregs and conventional CD4+ T cells in lymph nodes and peripheral blood during TB lymphadenitis.

We found a higher proportion of CD4+ T cells in LNMC compared to PBMC. This is in agreement with previous studies reporting an increase in the proportion of CD4+ T cells in the blood of TB patients compared to uninfected controls and a much higher number of CD4+ T cells at the site of infection [16, 17]. Except for modest elevation in effector cells in LNMC, no difference was found in the relative frequency of memory CD4+ T cell subsets between PBMC and LNMC. Others have shown that Mtb-specific CD4+ T cells in bronchoalveolar and pleural fluids are mainly of the memory phenotype [18, 19]. In LNMC we find that up to 40% of CD4+ T cells were naïve.

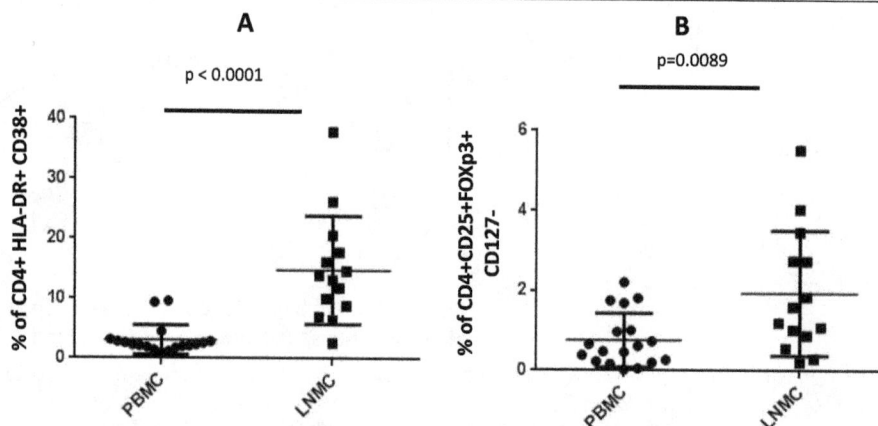

Fig. 3 Frequency distribution of HLA-DR+ CD38+ activated (**a**) and FoxP3+CD25+CD127- (**b**) regulatory CD4+T cells in LNMC and PBMC

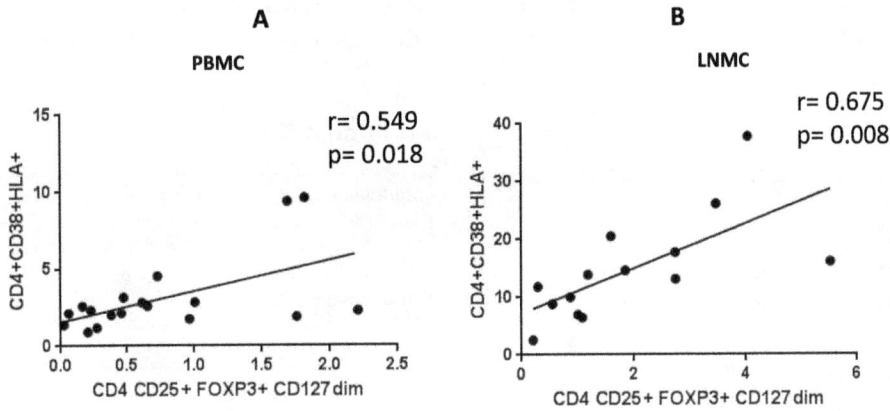

Fig. 4 Ex vivo frequencies of Tregs correlated with the ex-vivo frequencies of CD4+ activated cells in PBMC (**a**) and LNMC (**b**)

Th1 and Th17 Mtb–specific T cells contribute to the defense against progressive Mtb infection. Particularly, TB lymphadenitis was characterized by elevated frequencies of Th1 and Th17 cells in peripheral blood [20]. When we measured intracellular production of Th1 cytokines (IFNγ, IL2 and TNFα), IL17 and MIP-1α, we were surprised to not find an increase in the frequencies of Mtb-specific cytokine producing cells in LNMC vs. PBMC. LNMC were generated from a large block of excised lymph node tissue that included granulomatous and non-granulomatous areas which may have affected our ability to detect higher frequencies of Mtb-specific cells in LNMC than PBMC.

Polyfunctional T cells are correlated with protection in some studies [5, 6, 21] and with disease activity in others [22, 23]. In our case, no differences were observed in the proportion and polyfunctional qualities of the Mtb-responsive CD4+ T cells between LNMC and PBMC. Comparing polyfunctionality in CD4+ T cells responding to Mtb-antigen vs. SEB showed a significant difference with SEB eliciting a more TNFα dominated response. This supports that the Mtb-specific responses were different from those of the whole memory CD4+ T cell pool.

To analyze the interaction between conventional activated CD4+T cells and Tregs in the lymph node during active TB, we measured the frequency of CD4+T cells expressing CD38 and HLA-DR. These immune activation markers were described as substantially elevated in subjects with active TB [24]. CD4+ T cells were more activated in lymph node compared to blood. The increased proportion of activated T cells in LNMC likely reflects more exposure to Mtb antigens. The selective accumulation is likely the result of both active recruitment and local expansion of T cells at this site of Mtb replication [25, 26].

Tregs were identified by selecting CD4+ cells with high-level expression of CD25, low-level expression of CD127, and expression of FoxP3. Tregs were also increased in LNMC in response to local immune activation possibly to control immune induced damage [3, 26, 27]. In accordance with the previous study [10], our data reveal a positive correlation between Treg and CD4+ activated cells within PBMC but this correlation was stronger in LNMC. Tregs co-expressing HLA-DR and CD38

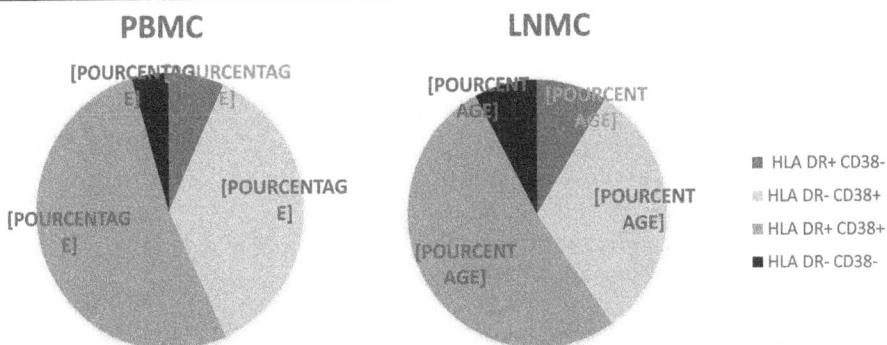

Fig. 5 Distribution of activation markers within CD4+CD25+FoxP3+CD127dim Tregs in PBMC and LNMC

Table 1 Correlation of the ex vivo frequencies of Tregs with the frequencies of CD4+T cells expressing IFNγ, IL2, TNFα, IL17 and MIP1α following Mtb lysate antigen stimulation in PBMC and LNMC

| | T reg | | | |
| | PBMC | | LNMC | |
	r	p	r	p
IFN-γ	-0.19	0.60	0.66	0.04
IL2	-0.04	0.90	0.71	0.02
TNF-α	-0.02	0.96	0.48	0.16
IL17	-0.23	0.52	0.45	0.12
MIP-1α	-0.04	0.91	0.95	<0.001

infection regulates the immune response. Whether this is advantageous to the host or not remains to be determined.

Additional files

Additional file 1: CD8+ T-cell subset distribution in PBMC and LNMC. Relatives frequencies of CD8+ T cells among all CD3+ T cells. Means from 18 subjects are shown and error bars representing standard deviations. (PPTX 51 kb)

Additional file 2: Cytokine expression of memory CD4+T cells after ESAT6/CFP10 stimulation. Results from 11 subjects are shown. Plots are gated on viable memory CD4+T cells. (PPTX 91 kb)

markers were frequent in the LNMC and PBMC. The ex-vivo MHC II expressing Tregs are believed to be a functionally mature distinct Treg subset implicated in contact-dependent *in vitro* suppression [28]. A positive correlation between Treg proportion and frequency of memory Mtb-specific CD4+ T cells expressing each individual measured Th1 function was observed in LNMC but not in PBMC. The predominance of activated Tregs in LNMC and the correlation of Tregs with activated CD4+ T cells and CD4+ T cells expressing Th1 cytokines suggests a regulatory activity specific and enhanced in the lymph node. An alternate hypothesis could be that the Treg are just expanding at tissue sites but not necessarily for regulatory purposes. The absence of an expected higher proportion of Th1 producing CD4+T cells in LNMC compared to PBMC supports the hypothesis that the Treg/CD4 correlation reflected a negative feedback for excess Th1 cytokine production by increasing suppressive Tregs. Recent data suggest that IFNγ increases Treg suppressive function for control of Th1 responses [29, 30]. A limitation of the study is that we did not have any blood or lymph node material in healthy BCG-vaccinated or latently infected individuals available to contrast to the TB lymphadenitis subjects. Contrasting these cohorts in future studies as well as further research on the function of Tregs and their modulation of immune responses in TB lymphadenitis are needed. The current study will help develop an optimal approach to such supplementary exploration.

Conclusion

This study has important original findings regarding local immune responses in active LNTB. We found no Th1, Th17 or MIP-1α production differences by Mtb-specific CD4+ T cells in total LNMC vs. PBMC. Tregs were positively correlated with Th1 expressing Mtb-specific CD4+ T cells in LNMC but not in PBMC. Activated HLA-DR +CD38+Tregs were more abundant, suggesting modulation by Tregs of immune responses in LNMC. We suggest that increased Tregs at the lymph node site of active Mtb

Abbreviations

LNTB: Lymph node TB; TB: Tuberculosis; Mtb: Mycobacterium tuberculosis; Treg: T regulatory cells; LNMC: Lymph node mononuclear cells; PBMC: Peripheral blood mononuclear cells; CD127: IL-7 receptor α-chain; FoxP3: The intracellular marker forkhead box p3; Mtb lysate: M. tuberculosis CDC1551 whole cells lysate; SEB: Staphylococcal enterotoxin B; N: Naïve T cells; CM: Central memory cells; EM: Effector memory cells; E: Effector cells

Acknowledgements

The authors would like to thank all patients for their participation. They also would like to thank all the health and laboratory professional that facilitate the realization of this work.

Funding

This study was supported by the Hassan II Academy for Sciences and techniques of Morocco (IMMGEN project), NIH AI108972, NIH AI080313, NIH P30 AI036219, NIAID Contract No. HHSN266200700022C / NO1-AI-70022, and VA GRECC.

Authors' contributions

This study was designed by KS, WHB, RE, DHC and FS. HA, NB and MN were the key investigators that assisted in design of the clinical aspects of the study then recruited, treated, and collected clinical data on the subjects. . Data analysis, interpretation and statistical analysis were performed by KS, AS, CB, DHC and FS. KS, DHC and FS wrote the first draft and AS, WHB, RE, FS and DHC contributed to the final manuscript. All authors read and approved the final manuscript.

Competing interests

The authors declare that they have no competing interests.

Author details

[1]Laboratory of Cellular Immunology, National Institute of Hygiene, 27, Avenue Ibn Batouta, PB 769, 11400 Rabat, Morocco. [2]Faculty of Sciences, University Mohammed V Agdal, Rabat, Morocco. [3]Department of ENT, Maxillo- facial, Reconstructive and Plastic Surgery, University Hospital Hassan II, Fes, Morocco. [4]National Reference Laboratory of Mycobacteriology, the National Institute of Hygiene, Rabat, Morocco. [5]Case Western Reserve

University School of Nursing, Cleveland, USA. [6]TB Research Unit and Division of Infectious Diseases, Case Western Reserve University, University Hospitals of Cleveland and Cleveland VA, Cleveland, OH, USA.

References

1. WHO, Global tuberculosis control: WHO Report 2016.
2. Rodrigues DS, Medeiros EA, Weckx LY, Bonnez W, Salomao R, Kallas EG. Immunophenotypic characterization of peripheral T lymphocytes in Mycobacterium tuberculosis infection and disease. Clin Exp Immunol. 2002; 128:149–54.
3. Hertoghe T, Wajja A, Ntambi L, Okwera A, Aziz MA, Hirsch C, Johnson J, Toossi Z, Mugerwa R, Mugyenyi P, Colebunders R, Eller J, Vanham G. T cell activation, apoptosis and cytokine dysregulation in the (co) pathogenesis of HIV and pulmonary tuberculosis (TB). Clin Exp Immunol. 2000;122:350–7.
4. Gideon HP, Phuah J, Myers AJ, Bryson BD, Rodgers MA, Coleman MT, Maiello P, Rutledge T, Marino S, Fortune SM, Kirschner DE, Lin PL, Flynn JL. Variability in tuberculosis granuloma T cell responses exists, but a balance of pro- and anti-inflammatory cytokines is associated with sterilization. PLoS Pathog. 2015;11(1):e1004603. https://doi.org/10.1371/j.ppat.1004603.
5. Day CL, Abrahams DA, Lerumo L, Janse van Rensburg E, Stone L, O'Rie T, Pienaar B, de Kock M, Kaplan G, Mahomed H, Dheda K, Hanekom WA. Functional capacity of Mycobacterium tuberculosis-specific T cell responses in humans is associated with mycobacterial load. J Immunol. 2011;187: 2222–32. https://doi.org/10.4049/j immunol.1101122.
6. Harari A, Rozot V, Enders FB, Perreau M, Stalder JM, Nicod LP, et al. Dominant TNF-α+ Mycobacterium tuberculosis-specific CD4+ T cell responses discriminate between latent infection and active disease. Nat Med. 2011;17:372–6. https://doi.org/10.1038/nm.2299 93.
7. Guyot-Revol V, Innes JA, Hackforth S, Hinks T, Lalvani A. Regulatory T-cells are expanded in blood and disease sites in patients with tuberculosis. Am J Respir Crit Care Med. 2006;7:803–10.
8. Hougardy JM, Place S, Hildebrand M, Drowart A, Debrie AS, Locht C, Mascart F. Regulatory T-cells depress immune responses to protective antigens in active tuberculosis. Am J Respir Crit Care Med. 2007;4:409–16.
9. Rodríguez-Perea AL, Arcia ED, Rueda CM, Velilla PA. Phenotypical characterization of regulatory T cells in humans and rodents. Clin Exp Imm. 2016;185(3):281–91.
10. Wergeland I, Aßmus J, Dyrhol-Riise AM. T Regulatory Cells and Immune Activation in Mycobacterium tuberculosis Infection and the Effect of Preventive Therapy. Scand J Imm. 2011;73:234–42.
11. De Almeida AS, Fiske CT, Sterling TR, Kalamsa SA. Increased Frequency of Regulatory T Cells and T Lymphocyte Activation in Persons with Previously Treated Extrapulmonary Tuberculosis. Clin Vaccine Immunol. 2012;19:45–52.
12. Baecher-Allan C, Brown JA, Freeman GJ, Hafler DA. CD4+CD25high regulatory cells in human peripheral blood. J Immunol. 2001;167:1245–53.
13. Baecher-Allan C, Wolf E, Hafler DA. Functional analysis of highly defined, FACS-isolated populations of human regulatory CD4+ CD25+ T cells. Clin Immunol. 2005;115:10–8.
14. Nemeth J, Rumetshofer R, Winkler HM, Burghuber OC, Müller C, Winkler S. Active tuberculosis is characterized by an antigen specific and strictly localized expansion of effector T cells at the site of infection. Eur J Immunol. 2012;42(11):2844–50.
15. Diedrich CR, O'Hern J, Gutierrez MG, Allie N, Papier P, Meintjes G, Coussens AK, Wainwright H, Wilkinson RJ. Relationship between HIV Coinfection, Interleukin 10 Production, and Mycobacterium tuberculosis in Human Lymph Node Granulomas. J Infect Dis. 2016;214(9):1309–18.
16. Wang T, Lv M, Qian Q, Nie Y, Yu L, Hou Y. Increased frequencies of T helper type 17 cells in tuberculous pleural effusion. Tuberculosis. 2011;91:231–7.
17. Rumetshofer R, Winkler HM, Burghuber OC, Müller C, Winkler S. Active tuberculosis is characterized by an antigen specific and strictly localized expansion of effector T cells at the site of infection. Eur J Immunol. 2012; 42(11):2844–50.
18. El Fenniri L, Toossi Z, Aung H, El Iraki G, Bourkkadi J, Benamor J, Laskri A, Berrada N, Benjouad A, Mayanja-Kizza H, Betts MR, El Aouad R, Canaday DH. Polyfunctional mycobacterium tuberculosis-specific effector memory CD4+ T cells at sites of pleural TB. Tuberculosis. 2011;91:224–30.
19. Chiacchio T, Petruccioli E, Vanini V, Butera O, Cuzzi G, Petrone L, Matteucci G, Lauria FN, Franken KL, Girardi E, Ottenhoff TH, Goletti D. Higher Frequency of T-Cell Response to M. tuberculosis Latency Antigen Rv2628 at the Site of Active Tuberculosis Disease than in Peripheral Blood. PlosOne. 2011;6:e27539. https://doi.org/10.1371/journal.pone.0027539.
20. Kumar NP, Sridhar R, Banurekha VV, Nair D, Jawahar MS, Nutman TB, Babu S. Expansion of Pathogen-Specific Mono- and Multifunctional Th1 and Th17 Cells in Multi-Focal Tuberculous Lymphadenitis. PlosOne. 2013;8(2):e57123.
21. Marín ND, Paris SC, Rojas M, Garcia LF. Functional profile of CD4+ and CD8+ T cells in latently infected individuals and patients with active TB. Tuberculosis. 2013;93:155–66.
22. Sutherland JS, Adetifa IM, Hill PC, Adegbola RA, Ota MO. Pattern and diversity of cytokine production differentiates between Mycobacterium tuberculosis infection and disease. Eur J Immunol. 2009;39:723–9.
23. Caccamo N, Guggino G, Joosten SA, Gelsomino G, Di Carlo P, Titone L, Galati D, Bocchino M, Matarese A, Salerno A, Sanduzzi A, Franken WP, Ottenhoff TH, Dieli F. Multifunctional CD4(+) T cells correlate with active Mycobacterium tuberculosis infection. Eur J Immunol. 2010;40:2211–20.
24. Adekambi T, Ibegbu CC, Cagle S, Kalokhe AS, Wang YF, Hu Y, Day CL, Ray SM, Rengarajan J. Biomarkers on patient T cells diagnose active tuberculosis and monitor treatment response. J Clin Invest. 2015;125:1827–38.
25. Wilkinson KA, Wilkinson RJ, Pathan A, Ewer K, Prakash M, Klenerman P, Maskell N, Davies R, Pasvol G, Lalvani A. Ex vivo characterization of early secretory antigenic target 6–specific T cells at sites of active disease in pleural tuberculosis. Clin Infect Dis. 2005;40:184–7.
26. Nemeth J, Winkler HM, Zwick RH, Rumetsofer R, Schenk P, Burghuber OC, Graninger W, Ramharter M, Winkler S. Recruitment of Mycobacterium tuberculosis specific CD41 T cells to the site of infection for diagnosis of active tuberculosis. J Intern Med. 2009;265:163–8.
27. Ribeiro-Rodrigues R, Resende Co T, Rojas R, Toossi Z, Dietze R, Boom WH, Maciel E, Hirsch CS. A role for CD4+CD25+ T cells in regulation of the immune response during human tuberculosis. Clin Exp Immunol. 2006;144:25–34.
28. Baecher-Allan C, Wolf E, Hafler DA. MHC Class II Expression Identifies Functionally Distinct Human Regulatory T Cells. J Immunol. 2006;176:4622–463.
29. Hall BM, Tran GT, Verma ND, Plain KM, Robinson CM, Nomura M, Hodgkinson SJ, Do Natural T. Regulatory Cells become Activated to Antigen Specific T Regulatory Cells in Transplantation and in Autoimmunity? Front Immunol. 2013;2:4–208. https://doi.org/10.3389/fimmu.2013.00208.
30. Hall AO, Beiting DP, Tato C, John B, Oldenhove G, Lombana CG, Pritchard GH, Silver JS, Bouladoux N, Stumhofer JS, Harris TH, Grainger J, Wojno ED, Wagage S, Roos DS, Scott P, Turka LA, Cherry S, Reiner SL, Cua D, Belkaid Y, Elloso MM, Hunter CA. The cytokines interleukin 27 and interferon-γ promote distinct Treg cell populations required to limit infection-induced pathology. Immunity. 2012; 37(3):511–23. https://doi.org/10.1016/j.immuni.2012.06. 014.

10

The influence of HK2 blood group antigen on human B cell activation for ABOi-KT conditions

Jingsong Cao[1,2†] (iD), Luogen Liu[2†], Yunsheng Zhang[2], Jianhua Xiao[1,2*] and Yi Wang[2,3*]

Abstract

Background: It is well known that ABO blood group system incompatible kidney transplantation (ABOi-KT) is an effective strategy for end-stage renal disease. The main barrier for ABOi-KT is how to keep host B cell activation and blood group antibody titer in low levels. Moreover, the mechanism of B cell activation induced by blood group antigen was unclear in ABOi-KT.

Results: In this study, HK2 cells were identified to express blood group B antigen when cocultured with lymphocytes of blood group A. Optical microscope observation demonstrated that HK2 cells in coculture group gradually decreased. Furthermore, flow cytometer assay identified that T cell phenotypes (CD3+, CD3+CD4+ and CD3+CD8+) had no significant change and B cell phenotypes (CD19+ and CD138+) were all significantly enhanced (3.07 and 3.02 folds) at day 4. In addition, immunoturbidimetry analysis demonstrated that blood group B antibody was significantly increased to 2.35 fold at day 4, IgG was significantly increased to 3.60 and 2.81 folds at days 4 and 8 respectively, while IgM had no significant change at the measured time points.

Conclusions: Taken together, B cells were activated and secreted blood group B antibody after treatment with HK2 expressing blood group B antigen. The results of this study maybe useful for further determination of the mechanism of B cell activation after ABO incompatible kidney endothelial cells stimulation.

Keywords: Blood group B antigen, Blood group B antibody, HK2, B cells activation, ABOi-KT

Background

ABOi-KT is an effective replacement therapy for end-stage kidney disease [1–3], in which the key for graft survival is to eliminate the host blood group antibodies prestored in peripheral blood of recipients [4, 5]. However, the allograft in part of ABOi-KT recipients survived without rejection when the blood group antibody titer was gradually increased to the preoperative level [6].

Some researchers considered the allograft survival was related to immune tolerance mediated by antibodies [7,

8]. Urschel et al. showed CD21-expressing B cells were related to ABO tolerance [9]. Chesneau et al. reported a unique B cell in vitro differentiation profile that played an important role in tolerant kidney transplant patients [10], especially the isotype of immunoglobulin (Ig) on the surface of B cells switch from IgM to IgG [11, 12]. Methot et al. [13] noted that B cell differentiation resulted in antibody diversification, which impacted the antibodies activity for binding to Fc receptors and activation of the complement system [8]. However, the mechanism of B cells activation in ABOi-KT was unclear.

In this study, HK2 cells were identified to express blood group B antigen. After coculture with lymphocytes isolated from blood group A health donors, the HK2 cells were observed by optical microscopy. Of these, the lymphocytes phenotype, such as CD3+, CD3+CD4+, CD3+CD8+, CD19+ and CD138+, were analyzed by flow cytometry. Furthermore, the blood group B antibody, IgG and IgM were detected by immunoturbidimetry assay.

* Correspondence: jhxiao223@163.com; wayne0108@126.com
†Equal contributors
[1]Institute of Pathogenic Biology, Medical College, Hunan Provincial Key Laboratory for Special Pathogens Prevention and Control; Hunan Province Cooperative Innovation Center for Molecular Target New Drug Study, University of South China, Hengyang, Hunan 421001, China
[2]Clinical research center, Institute of Pathogenic Biology, Medical College, The Second Affiliated Hospital, University of South China, Hengyang, Hunan 421001, China
Full list of author information is available at the end of the article

These results will be beneficial for further exploration of the mechanism of B cells activation after ABO incompatible kidney endothelial cells stimulation.

Methods

HK2 cell line was purchased from the Advanced Research Center of Central South University. The peripheral blood was donated from volunteers after informed consent, and subsequently approved by the Animal Welfare and Research Ethics Committee of the Institute of University of South China.

The specificity glycosyl of blood group B antigen was synthesized and coupled to keyhole limpet hemocyanin (KLH-B) at Alberta Innovates Technology Futures. The KLH-B was dissolved in phosphate buffer solution (PBS, 0.01 mol/L, pH 7.4) to 0.001 mg/ml.

Cell culture

Lymphocytes were separated from blood group A donors and cultured as Cao et al. [14] reported with some modification. Peripheral blood at 2 ml was mixed with 0.9% physiological saline ($V:V = 1:1$) for ficoll gradient separation (LymphoPrep). After centrifugation at 1800 revolutions/min for 20 min, the lymphocytes layer was collected and rinsed 2 times with 0.9% physiological saline at 1500 revolutions/min for 7 min. Then the cells were resuspended with 1640 medium (Thermo Fisher Scientific) and 15% fetal calf serum (FCS, Thermo Fisher Scientific) to 2×10^6 cells/ml.

The HK2 cells in dish culture were processed by 3 ml 0.25% trypsin (GE Healthcare Life Sciences) at room temperature for 2 minnutes, then 3 ml 1640 medium with 15% FCS added, and centrifuged at 800 revolutions/min for 10 min. Afterwards was rinsed 2 times with 0.9% physiological saline at 800 revolutions/min for 10 min, the precipitate was resuspended with 1640 medium and 15% FCS to 2×10^6 cells/ml.

Then, leukocytes and HK2 cells were divided into three groups, HK2 group was added 0.5 ml HK2 cells suspension and 0.5 ml 1640 medium with 15% FCS, PB group was added 0.5 ml lymphocytes suspension and 0.5 ml 1640 medium with 15% FCS, coculture group was added 0.5 ml HK2 cells suspension and 0.5 ml lymphocytes suspension. The three groups were all cultured in 24-well plates at 37 °C, 5% CO_2, and added 0.1 ml fresh medium to every group at day 4. The experiment was repeated for 3 times.

Immunohistochemistry assay

The process of immunohistochemistry was built as Kounelis [15] reported with some modification. HK2 cells were cultured with 1640 medium and 15% FCS at 37 °C, 5% CO_2. After rinsed with PBS (0.01 mol/L,

pH 7.2) for 2 times, the carry sheet glasses of HK2 cells were incubated with FCS at 37 °C for 20 min. Then the carry sheet glasses were divided into three groups, one group was incubated with 1 ml PBS at 37 °C for 1 h, the other two groups were respectively incubated with mouse monoclonal to anti-blood group A antibody (1: 100, Albanian Broadband Communication) and mouse monoclonal to anti-blood group B antibody (1: 100, Albanian Broadband Communication) at 37 °C for 1 h. After rinsed 3 times with PBS for 2 min, the three groups were all incubated with goat anti-mouse IgM-HRP (1: 500, ThermoFisher Scientific) at 37 °C for 20 min, followed rinsed 3 times with PBS for 2 min. Finally, the carry sheet glasses were rinsed 3 times with PBS for 2 min and analyzed with DAB Kit (BOSTER) detection method. The experiment was repeated for 3 times.

Optical microscope observation

At days 2, 4, 8, the lymphocytes were collected for further research. HK2 cells were observed by optical microscopy after two PBS rinses. The experiment was repeated for 3 times.

Flow cytometer assay

At days 2, 4, 8, the lymphocytes suspension were collected by concentrated at 1000 revolutions/min for 10 min, then the precipitate was resuspended with 1 ml 0.9% physiological saline, after centrifuged at 1000 revolutions/min for 10 min, the precipitate was resuspended with 150 μl 0.9% physiological saline, and divided into three groups. One group as isotype control was added FITC mouse IgG2α (5 μl, BD), PE mouse IgG1 (5 μl, BD) and PerCP-CyTM 5.5 mouse IgG1 (1 μl, BD), the experiment group was divided into two group and, respectively, added FITC mouse anti-human CD3 (5 μl, BD), PE mouse anti-human CD4 (5 μl, BD), PerCP-CyTM5.5 mouse anti-human CD8 (1 μl, BD) and FITC mouse anti-human CD19 (5 μl, BD), PE mouse anti-human CD138 (5 μl, BD). The three groups were all incubated at room temperature for 15 min, then resuspended with 1 ml 0.9% physiological saline and centrifuged at 1000 revolutions/min for 10 min. Finally, the precipitate was resuspended with 0.2 ml 0.9% physiological saline and prepared to analysis using BD FACSCanto II. The experiment was repeated for 3 times.

Detection of the concentration of mouse monoclonal to anti-blood group B antibody in reagent

After polyacrylamide gel electrophoresis (PAGE, 8% separation gel) of mouse monoclonal to anti-blood group B antibody reagent, the gel was transferred to a polyvinylidene fluoride (PVDF) membrane for 90 minnutes at 300 mA in transfer buffer (0.025 mol/L Tris, 0.1 mol/L glycine, and 20% methanol), and the membrane was blocked for 1 h in tween tris buffer solution (TTBS, 0.05% Tween-20, 0.02 mol/L Tris, 0.15 mol/L NaCl, pH 7.4) containing 5% skim milk at room temperate. After rinsed 3 times with tris buffer solution (TBS) for 5 min, the membrane was incubated with goat anti-mouse IgM-HRP (1: 2000) at room temperate for 40 min. Then the membrane was rinsed 2 times with TBS for 15 min and analyzed with ECL Plus (solarbio) chemiluminescence detection method.

In addition, the concentration of mouse monoclonal to anti-blood group B antibody was calculated by protein-gray value curve of bovine serum albumin (BSA). The experiment was repeated for 3 times.

Immunoturbidimetry assay

At days 2, 4, 8, the supernate was collected. Experiment group was a mixture of the supernate, buffer solution (0.01 mol/L, pH 7.4 PBS, 0.15 mol/L NaCl, 40 g/L PEG-8000) and KLH-B (V: V: V = 1: 94: 5). positive control group was a mixture of mouse monoclonal to anti-blood group B antibody, buffer solution and KLH-B (V: V: V = 1: 94: 5). Blank group was a mixture of buffer solution and KLH-B (V: V = 95: 5). All groups were incubated at room temperature for 5 min, and then detected the absorb value at λ_{340nm}.

Meanwhile, The IgM and IgG in supernate were respectively analyzed by N Antiserum to Human IgM reagent (Siemens) and N Antiserum to Human IgG reagent (Siemens). The experiments were all repeated for 3 times.

Results

Identification of blood group antigen type of HK2 cells

To research the change of B cell activation by blood group antigens of kidney endotheliocytes stimulated in vitro, the blood group antigen type of the HK2 cell line was analyzed by immunohistochemistry (Fig. 1). As for results, none of the imaged HK2 cells were stained after incubation with PBS and mouse monoclonal to anti-blood group A antibody (Fig. 1 a, b). However, the HK2 cells could specifically link with mouse monoclonal to anti-blood group B antibody (Fig. 1c).

Observation of HK2 cells proliferation

Following the results of immunohistochemistry, lymphocytes of blood group A were collected and cultured with HK2 cells. At days 2, 4, 8, HK2 cells were observed by optical microscopy (Fig. 2). Compared with PB (Fig. 2a) and HK2 groups (Fig. 2b, d), the proliferative activity of HK2 cells in coculture group was decreased and a small number of HK2 cells survived at day 8 (Fig. 2c, d).

Analysis of lymphocytes phenotype

To demonstrate the lymphocyte subtypes influencing HK2 cells proliferative activity, the T cells phenotype (CD3$^+$, CD3$^+$CD4$^+$ and CD3$^+$CD8$^+$) and B cells phenotype (CD19$^+$ and CD138$^+$) were analyzed by flow cytometer. As Fig. 3 appeared, compared with PB group, T cell phenotypes (Fig. 3a–c) had no significant change, and CD19$^+$ (Fig. 3d, f) B cells were significantly increased to 3.07 fold at day 4, CD138$^+$ (Fig. 3e, f) B cells were significantly increased to 3.02 and 1.36 folds at days 4 and 8 respectively.

Determination of the anti-blood group B mouse monoclonal antibody concentration

For further exploration of the variation of blood group B antibody secreted by B cells, the concentration of mouse monoclonal to anti-blood group B antibody in reagent was analyzed. As Fig. 4 showed, in the reagent, only the protein with a molecular weight about 181.7 kDa was specifically combined with goat anti mouse IgM-HRP. After comparison with the standard curve of BSA (Additional file 1: Figure S1), the mouse monoclonal to anti-blood group B antibody concentration was identified as 0.57 mg/ml.

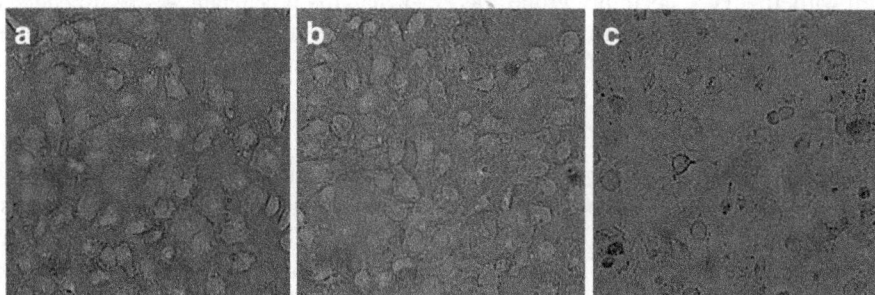

Fig. 1 Blood group antigen identified by immunohistochemistry. **a** PB group, **b** Blood group A antigen analysis, **c** Blood group B antigen analysis. All groups were repeated for 3 times

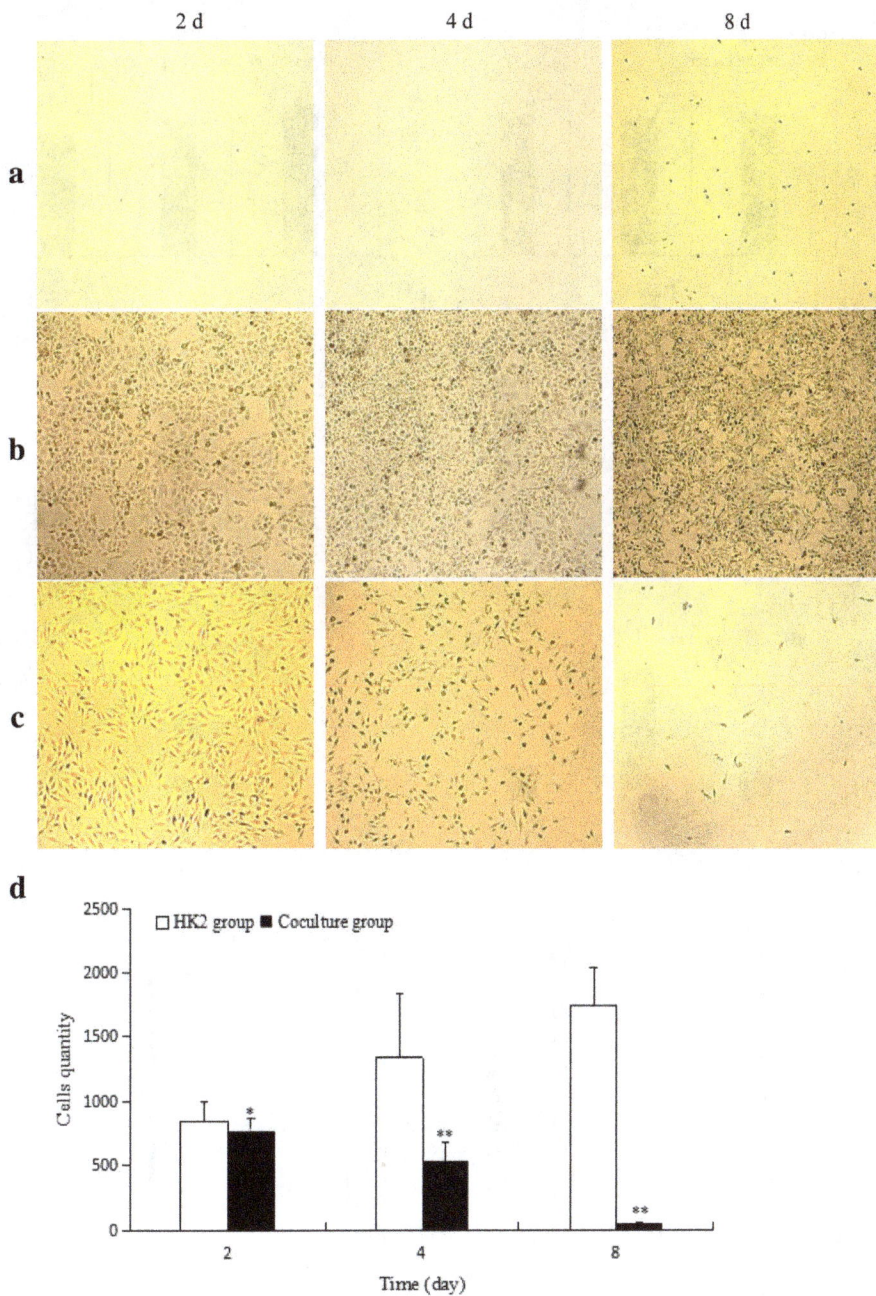

Fig. 2 Optical microscope analyzed for HK2 cells. **a** PB group, **b** HK2 group, **c** Coculture group. **d** the analysis of histogram for HK2 cell quantity. Bars represent mean ± standard deviation ($n = 3$). Significant differences between the PB and the coculture groups were indicated with one ($p < 0.05$) or two ($p < 0.01$) asterisks

Detection of the concentration of blood group antibody, IgG and IgM

Based on these results, the concentration of blood group B antibody, IgG and IgM in supernate was analyzed by immunoturbidimetry assay. As Fig. 5 showed, blood group B antibody was significantly increased to 2.35 fold at day 4 (Fig. 5a), IgG was significantly increased to 3.60 and 2.81 folds at days 4 and 8 respectively (Fig. 5b), and

IgM had no significant change between PB and coculture groups (Fig. 5c).

Discussion

ABOi-KT is an effective and important strategy to resolve the problem of kidney shortage [16–21], and the allograft in a small cohort of recipients aided survival

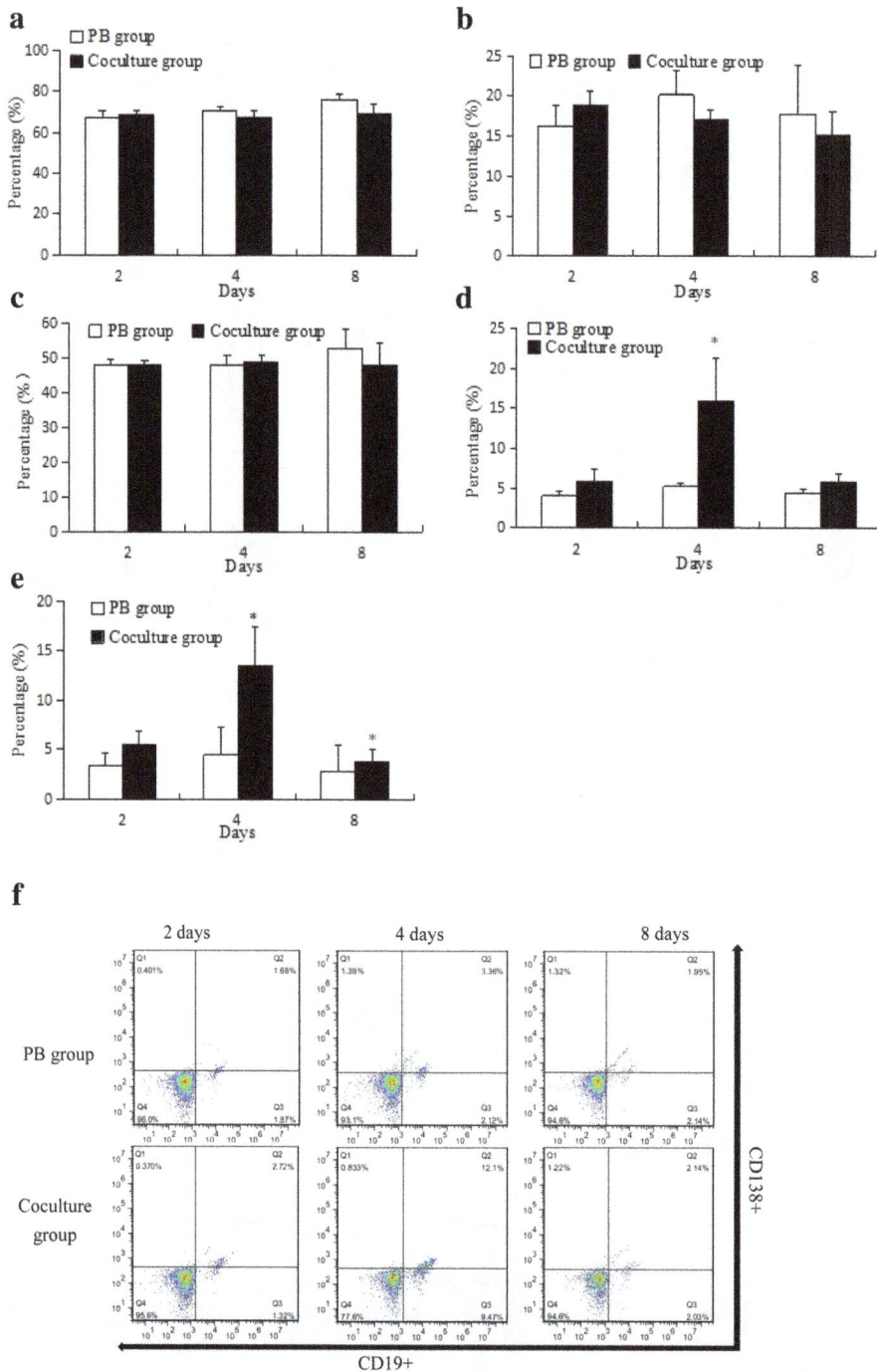

Fig. 3 The T cells and B cells subsets analyzed by flow cytometry. **a** CD3+ phenotype T cells, **b** CD3+CD8+ phenotype T cells, **c** CD3+CD4+ phenotype T cells, **d** CD19+ phenotype B cells, **e** CD138+ phenotype B cells. **f** The flow cytometry scatter plot of CD19+ and CD138+ phenotype B cells. Bars represent mean ± standard deviation (n = 3). Significant differences between the PB and the coculture groups were indicated with one (p < 0.05) asterisks

because of immune tolerance mediated by B cells activation [22, 23]. In this study, HK2 was verified to express blood group B antigen (Fig. 1) when cocultured with lymphocyte of blood group A.

Optical microscope observation shown that the proliferative activity of HK2 cells in coculture group

decreased and a small number of HK2 cells survived by day 8 (Fig. 2c, d). This phenomenon may be related to humoral immunity mediated by B cells or cell immunity mediated by T cells [24–26].

In immunoreactions mediated by lymphocytes, CD3+CD4+ and CD3+CD8+ T cells play an important role

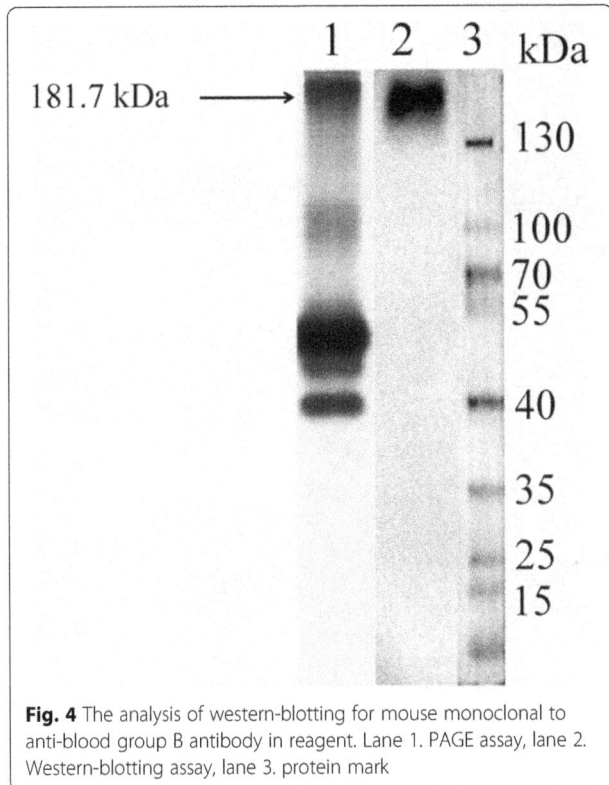

Fig. 4 The analysis of western-blotting for mouse monoclonal to anti-blood group B antibody in reagent. Lane 1. PAGE assay, lane 2. Western-blotting assay, lane 3. protein mark

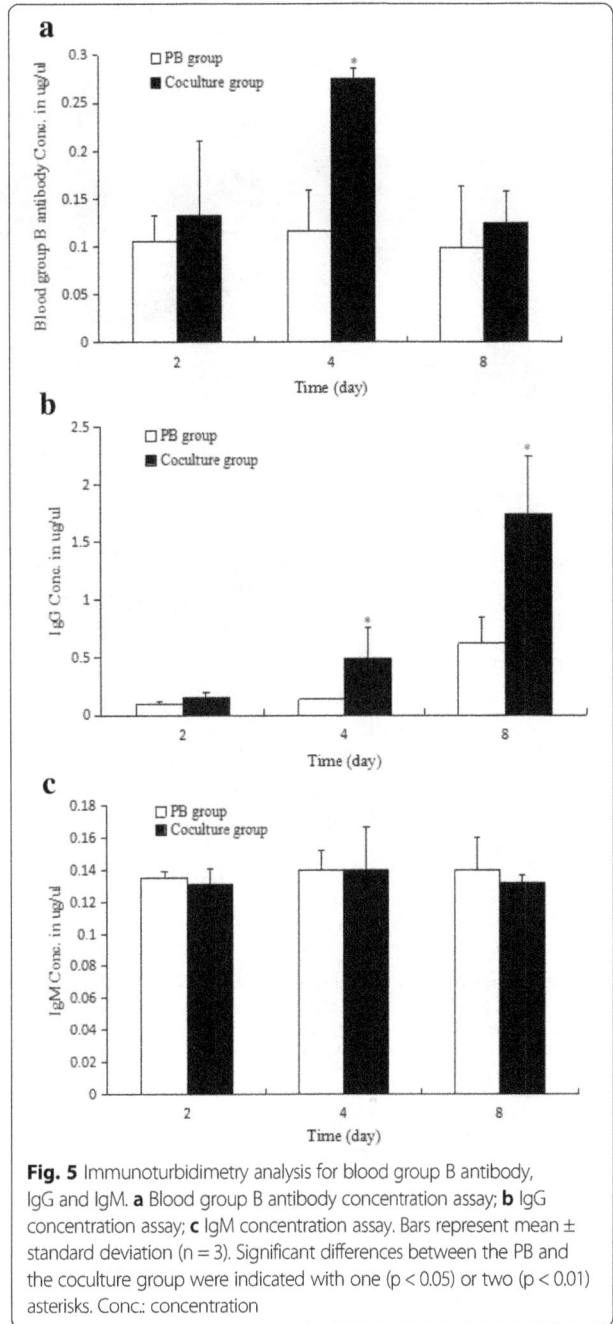

Fig. 5 Immunoturbidimetry analysis for blood group B antibody, IgG and IgM. **a** Blood group B antibody concentration assay; **b** IgG concentration assay; **c** IgM concentration assay. Bars represent mean ± standard deviation (n = 3). Significant differences between the PB and the coculture group were indicated with one ($p < 0.05$) or two ($p < 0.01$) asterisks. Conc.: concentration

as helper T cells [27] and cytotoxic T cells [28]. The $CD3^+CD4^+$ T cells, especially T follicular helper (Tfh) cells, secrete interleukin-21 [29] and express CD40 ligands and other inducible costimulator such as CD137 [30] on their surface [31], to promote B cells ($CD19^+$) class-switch and their differentiation into plasma cells ($CD138^+$) after antigen challenge [32–34] (Fig. 6) [35]. Thus, the T cells ($CD3^+$, $CD3^+CD4^+$ and $CD3^+CD8^+$) and B cells ($CD19^+$ and $CD138^+$) subset were analyzed by flow cytometry. As a result, after stimulation with HK2, the T cells phenotype had no significant variation (Fig. 3a–c), $CD19^+$ B cells (Fig. 3d, f) were significantly increased to 3.07 fold at day 4, and $CD138^+$ B cells (Fig. 3e, f) were significantly increased to 3.02 and 1.36 folds at days 4 and 8 respectively. Conjecturally, the B cells activation was induced by HK2, and it may be an important factor for the decrease of HK2 cells proliferative activity.

In addition, for further quantitative analysis the variation of blood group B antibody concentration, the mouse monoclonal to anti-blood group B antibody in reagent was detected as Eppler A et al. [36] and Yawata K et al. [37] reported with some modification. As a result, the protein with a molecular weight about 181.7 kDa was identified as mouse anti-human blood group B antibody with concentration 0.57 mg/ml in the reagent (Fig. 4 and Additional file 1: Figure S1).

Based on these results, the blood group antibody in the supernate was analyzed by immunoturbidimetry. The results showed that blood group B antibody was significantly increased to 2.35 fold at day 4 (Fig. 5a), IgG was significantly increased to 3.60 and 2.81 fold at days 4, 8 (Fig. 5b), and IgM has no significant change at the detective point (Fig. 5c). This was similar to the report that immunogloblulin was class switched to IgG4 in warthin tumor and the serum IgG4 levels were increased [7]. Consequently, it is suggested the B cells were activated by HK2 cells

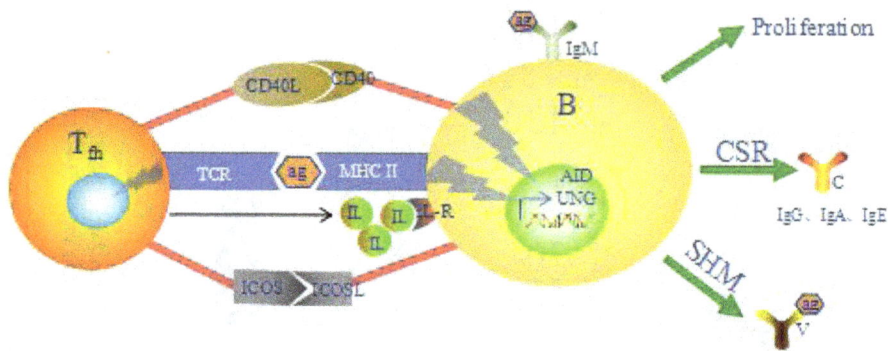

Fig. 6 The activation of T follicular helper cells for B cells*. T$_{fh}$: T follicular helper, TCR: T cell receptor, MHC II: major histocompatibility complex class II, ICOS: Inducible costimulator, ICOSL: ICOS ligand, CD40L: CD40 ligand, IL: interleukin, IL-R: interleukin receptor, CSR: class switch recombination, SHM: somatic hypermutation, AID: activation-induced cytidine deaminase, UNG: uracil-N-glycosylase. * The figure was drawn as Durandy er al [35] reported with some modification

expressing blood group B antigen and blood group B antibodies played a key role in HK2 cells apoptosis.

Conclusions

Our researches demostrated that the B cells were activated and induced differentiation to plasmocytes secreted blood group B antibody after HK2 cells treatment. This will be beneficial for further exploration of the mechanism of B cells activation after ABOi HK2 cells stimulation.

Additional file

Additional file 1: Figure S1. the establishment of protein-gray value curve of BSA. (A) PAGE assay for different concentration of BSA, lane 1. 0.5 µg BSA, lane 2. 1 µg BSA, lane 3. 2 µg BSA, lane 4. 4 µg BSA, lane 5. 8 µg BSA; (B) the relationship analysis of BSA gray value and protein. Bars represent mean ± standard deviation ($n = 3$). (PDF 611 kb)

Abbreviations
ABOi-KT: ABO blood group system incompatible kidney transplantation; AID: Activation-induced cytidine deaminase; BSA: Bovine serum albumin; CD40L: CD40 ligand; Conc.: Concentration; CSR: Class switch recombination; FCS: Fetal calf serum; ICOS: Inducible costimulator; ICOSL: ICOS ligand; Ig: Immunoglobulin; IL: Interleukin; IL-R: Interleukin receptor; KLH: Keyhole limpet hemocyanin; MHC II: Major histocompatibility complex class II; PAGE: Polyacrylamide gel electrophoresis; PBS: Phosphate buffer solution; PVDF: Polyvinylidene fluoride; S.D.: Standard deviation; SHM: Somatic hypermutation; TBS: Tris buffer solution; TCR: T cell receptor; T$_{fh}$: T follicular helper; TTBS: Tween tris buffer solution; UNG: uracil-N-glycosylase

Acknowledgments
Not applicable.

Funding
This work was supported by the Zhengxiang scholar program of the University of South China.

Authors' contributions
Laboratory experiments, data analysis and manuscript writing were accomplished by JSC; experimental design, date analysis and manuscript revise were accomplished by LGL; manuscript revise and date analysis were accomplished by YSZ; the guidance of experimental design and manuscript writing was accomplished by JHX and YW. All authors have read and approved the final manuscript.

Competing interests
The authors declare that they have no competing interest.

Author details
[1]Institute of Pathogenic Biology, Medical College, Hunan Provincial Key Laboratory for Special Pathogens Prevention and Control; Hunan Province Cooperative Innovation Center for Molecular Target New Drug Study, University of South China, Hengyang, Hunan 421001, China. [2]Clinical research center, Institute of Pathogenic Biology, Medical College, The Second Affiliated Hospital, University of South China, Hengyang, Hunan 421001, China. [3]Urinary surgery, The Second Affiliated Hospital, University of South China, Hengyang, Hunan 421001, China.

References
1.   Uchida J, Kuwabara N, Machida Y, Iwai T, Naganuma T, Kumada N, et al. Excellent outcomes of ABO-incompatible kidney transplantation: a single-center experience. Transplant Proc. 2012;44(1):204–9.
2.   Park WY, Kang SS, Park SB, Park UJ, Kim HT, Cho WH, et al. Comparison of clinical outcomes between ABO-compatible and ABO-incompatible spousal donor kidney transplantation. Kidney Res Clin Pract. 2016;35(1):50–4.
3.   Yu JH, Chung BH, Yang CW. Impact of ABO incompatible kidney transplantation on living donor transplantation. PLoS One. 2017;12(3): e0173878.
4.   Subramanian V, Gunasekaran M, Gaut JP, Phelan D, Vachharajani N, Santos RD, et al. Mohanakumar, ABO incompatible renal transplants and decreased likelihood for developing immune responses to HLA and kidney self-antigens. Hum Immunol. 2016;77(1):76–83.

5. Ferrari P, Hughes PD, Cohney SJ, Woodroffe C, Fidler S, D'Orsogna L. ABO-incompatible matching significantly enhances transplant rates in kidney paired donation. Transplantation. 2013;96(9):821–6.

6. Makroo RN, Nayak S, Chowdhry M, Jasuja S, Sagar G, Rosamma NL, et al. Role of therapeutic plasma exchange in reducing ABO titers in patients undergoing ABO-incompatible renal transplant. Apollo medicine. 2016;31(1):31–6.

7. Aga M, Kondo S, Yamada K, Wakisaka N, Yagi-Nakanishi S, Tsuji A, et al. Immunoglobulin class switching to IgG4 in Warthin tumor and analysis of serum IgG4 levels and IgG4-positive plasma cells in the tumor. Hum Pathol. 2014;45(4):793–801.

8. Kracker S, Gardes P, Mazerolles F, Durandy A. Immunoglobulin class switch recombination deficiencies. Clin Immunol. 2010;135(2):193–203.

9. Urschel S, Ryan LA, Larsen IM, Derkatz K, Rebeyka IM, Ross DB, et al. C3d plasma levels and CD21 expressing B-cells in children after ABO-incompatible heart transplantation: alterations associated with blood group tolerance. J Heart Lung Transplant. 2014;33(11):1149–56.

10. Chesneau M, Pallier A, Braza F, Lacombe G, Le Gallou S, Baron D, et al. Unique B cell differentiation profile in tolerant kidney transplant patients. Am J Transplant. 2014;14(1):144–55.

11. Urschel S, Ryan LA. M Larsen I, Biffis K, Dijke IE, west LJ. Development of B-cell memory in early childhood and the impact on antigen-specific tolerance after heart transplantation. J Heart lung transplant. 2016;35(4):491–9.

12. Batista FD, Harwood NE. The who, how and where of antigen presentation to B cells. Nat Rev Immunol. 2009;9(1):15–27.

13. Methot SP, Di Noia JM. Molecular mechanisms of somatic hypermutation and class switch recombination. Adv Immunol. 2017;133:37–87.

14. Cao J, Chen C, Wang Y, Chen X, Chen Z, Luo X. Influences of autologous dendritic cells on cytokine-induced killer cells proliferation, cell phenotype and anti-tumor activity in vitro. Oncol Lett. 2016;12(3):2033–7.

15. Kounelis S, Kapranos N, Kouri E, Coppola D, Papadaki H, Jones MW. Immunohistochemical profile of endometrial adenocarcinoma: a study of 61 cases and review of the literature. Mod Pathol. 2000;13(4):379–88.

16. Bentall A, R Barnett AN, Braitch M, Kessaris N, McKane W, Newstead C, et al. Clinical outcomes with ABO antibody titer variability in a multicenter study of ABO-incompatible kidney transplantation in the United Kingdom. Transfusion. 2016;56(11):2668–79.

17. Fadeyi EA, Stratta RJ, Farney AC, Pomper GJ. Successful ABO-incompatible renal transplantation: blood group A1B donor into A2B recipient with anti-A1 isoagglutinins. Am J Clin Pathol. 2016;146(2):268–71.

18. Koo TY, Yang J. Current progress in ABO-incompatible kidney transplantation. Kidney Res Clin Pract. 2015;34(3):170–9.

19. Shin M, Kim SJ. ABO incompatible kidney transplantation-current status and uncertainties. J Transp Secur. 2011;2011:970421.

20. Tanabe T, Ishida H, Horita S, Yamaguchi Y, Toma H, Tanabe K. Decrease of blood type antigenicity over the long-term after ABO-incompatible kidney transplantation. Transpl Immunol. 2011;25(1):1–6.

21. Abboud I, Peraldi MN, Glotz D. Renal transplantation from ABO incompatible donors. J Med Liban. 2015;63(3):159–63.

22. van de Veen W, Stanic B, OF W, Jansen K, Globinska A, Akdis M. Role of regulatory B cells in immune tolerance to allergens and beyond. J Allergy Clin Immunol. 2016;138(3):654–65.

23. Perera J, Zheng Z, Li S, Gudjonson H, Kalinina O, Benichou JI, et al. Self-antigen-driven thymic B cell class switching promotes T cell central tolerance. Cell Rep. 2016;17(2):387–98.

24. Chen C, Li J, Bi Y, Yang L, Meng S, Zhou Y, et al. Synthetic B- and T-cell epitope peptides of porcine reproductive and respiratory syndrome virus with Gp96 as adjuvant induced humoral and cell-mediated immunity. Vaccine. 2013;31(14):1838–47.

25. Montgomery RA, Cozzi E, West LJ, Warren DS. Humoral immunity and antibody-mediated rejection in solid organ transplantation. Semin Immunol. 2011;23(4):224–34.

26. Chang MC, Chiang CP, Lin CL, Lee JJ, Hahn LJ, Jeng JH. Cell-mediated immunity and head and neck cancer: with special emphasis on betel quid chewing habit. Oral Oncol. 2005;41(8):757–75.

27. Chen J, Wei Y, He J, Cui G, Zhu Y, Lu C, et al. Natural killer T cells play a necessary role in modulating of immune-mediated liver injury by gut microbiota. Sci Rep. 2014;4:7259.

28. Salaun B, Yamamoto T, Badran B, Tsunetsugu-Yokota Y, Roux A, Baitsch L, et al. Differentiation associated regulation of microRNA expression in vivo in human CD8+ T cell subsets. J Transl Med. 2011;9:44.

29. Bentebibel SE, Schmitt N, Bancherau J, Ueno H. Human tonsil B-cell lymphoma 6 (BCL6)-expressing CD4+ T-cell subset specialized for B-cell help outside germinal centers. Proc Natl Acad Sci U S A. 2011;108(33):E488–97.

30. Alfaro C, Echeveste JI, Rodriguez-Ruiz ME, Solorzano JL, Perez-Gracia JL, Idoate MA, et al. Functional expression of CD137 (4-1BB) on T helper follicular cells. Oncoimmunology. 2015;4(12):e1054597.

31. Banchereau J, Bazan F, Blanchard D, Brière F, Galizzi JP, van Kooten C, et al. The CD40 antigen and its ligand. Annu Rev Immunol. 1994;12:881–922.

32. Schmitt N, Bentebibel SE, Ueno H. Phenotype and functions of memory Tfh cells in human blood. Trends Immunol. 2014;35(9):436–42.

33. Spolski R, Leonard WJ. Interleukin-21: basic biology and implications for cancer and autoimmunity. Annu Rev Immunol. 2008;26:57–79.

34. MacLennan IC, Toellner KM, Cunningham AF, Serre K, Sze DM, Zúñiga E, et al. Extrafollicular antibody responses. Immunol Rev. 2003;194:8–18.

35. Durandy A, Kracker S. Immunoglobulin class switch recombination deficiencies. Arthritis Res Ther. 2012;14(4):218.

36. Eppler A, Weigandt M, Schulze S, Hanefeld A, Bunjes H. Comparison of different protein concentration techniques within preformulation development. Int J Pharm. 2011;421(1):120–9.

37. Yawata K, Osada S, Tanahashi T, Matsui S, Sasaki Y, Tanaka Y, et al. The significant role of cyclin D1 in the synergistic growth-inhibitory effect of combined therapy of vandetanib with 5-fluorouracil for gastric cancer. Anticancer Res. 2016;36(10):5215–26.

11

Broad induction of immunoregulatory mechanisms after a short course of anti-IL-7Rα antibodies in NOD mice

Cristina Vazquez-Mateo, Justin Collins, Michelle Fleury and Hans Dooms*

Abstract

Background: Type 1 diabetes is an autoimmune disease caused by T cell-mediated destruction of the insulin-producing β-cells in the pancreas. Therefore, approaches that effectively halt the pathogenic T cell response are predicted to have preventive or therapeutic benefit for type 1 diabetes patients. We previously demonstrated that long-term blocking of IL-7 signaling, which is critical for the survival and function of T cells, prevented and reversed type 1 diabetes in non-obese diabetic mice. However, such persistent inhibition of T cell responses raises concerns about causing immunodeficiency. Here, we asked whether a reduced duration of the treatment with anti-IL-7Rα antibodies retained efficacy in preventing diabetes. Moreover, we sought to identify immunoregulatory mechanisms induced by anti-IL-7Rα administration.

Results: Anti-IL-7Rα antibodies were administered to prediabetic NOD mice for 3 weeks and blood samples were taken at the end of treatment and 2 weeks later to analyze changes in T cell phenotypes in response to IL-7Rα blockade. We found that the co-inhibitory receptors LAG-3, Tim-3 and PD-1 were increased on peripheral blood CD4$^+$ and CD8$^+$ T cells from anti-IL-7Rα-treated mice. Expression of these receptors contributed to reduced T cell cytokine production in response to TCR stimulation. In addition, the frequency of Tregs within the circulating CD4$^+$ T cells was increased at the end of anti-IL-7Rα antibody treatment and these Tregs showed a more activated phenotype. In vitro restimulation assays revealed that effector T cells from anti-IL-7Rα-treated mice were more sensitive to co-inhibitory receptor induction after TCR stimulation. Importantly, these changes were accompanied by delayed type 1 diabetes disease kinetics.

Conclusions: Together, our data show that short-term blockade of IL-7Rα induces detectable changes in co-inhibitory receptor expression and Treg frequencies in peripheral blood of NOD mice. These changes appear to have long-lasting effects by delaying or preventing type 1 diabetes incidence. Hence, our study provides further support for using anti-IL-7Rα antibodies to modulate autoreactive T cell responses.

Keywords: Type 1 diabetes, Interleukin 7, T cells, Autoimmunity, Tregs, Inhibitory receptors, Non-obese diabetic mice

Background

Type 1 diabetes is a progressive autoimmune disease caused by infiltration of autoreactive lymphocytes in the islets of Langerhans which, ultimately, will destroy the insulin-producing β-cells. As a result of the loss of β-cells, blood sugar levels increase leading to a severe risk of secondary organ complications. Despite current advances in the understanding of type 1 diabetes,

* Correspondence: hdooms@bu.edu
Department of Medicine, Arthritis Center/Rheumatology Section, Boston University School of Medicine, 72 East Concord Street, E519, Boston, MA 02118, USA

treatment remains largely limited to insulin replacement therapy and attempts to prevent or cure the disease in humans have so far been unsuccessful [1, 2].

IL-7 is a cytokine with an important role in T cell survival and function and is an emerging target for the treatment of multiple autoimmune diseases [3]. We and others previously demonstrated that blocking IL-7 receptor alpha (IL-7Rα) prevented and reversed diabetes in non-obese diabetic (NOD) mice and hence has potential to be translated as an immunotherapy for human type 1 diabetes [4, 5]. Initial analyses of CD4$^+$ T cells in anti-IL-7Rα-treated mice revealed increased expression of the co-inhibitory receptor Programmed Death-1 (PD-1) in effector/memory CD4$^+$ T cells (T$_{E/M}$) and an increased frequency of polyclonal regulatory T cells (Tregs) in lymphoid organs [4]. These observations suggested that anti-IL-7Rα antibodies shift the balance in the immune system from active autoreactivity to a more regulated state, impacting disease progression.

Co-inhibitory receptors play critical roles in maintaining self-tolerance to autoantigens and are also associated with "T cell exhaustion", caused by chronic antigenic stimulation of virus- and tumor-specific T$_{E/M}$ cells [6–8]. Hence, increasing co-inhibitory receptor expression and "exhaustion" in autoreactive T cells are predicted to be desirable outcomes for the treatment of autoimmune diseases such as type 1 diabetes. Loss-of-function studies of the co-inhibitory receptors PD-1 and LAG-3 have demonstrated a critical role for these co-inhibitory receptors in suppressing anti-islet T cell responses in NOD mice, reflected by an accelerated kinetics of disease course [9–12]. Contributions of other co-inhibitory receptors, e.g., Tim-3 and B7x, in regulating type 1 diabetes are emerging as well [13, 14]. The role of Tregs in maintaining islet tolerance is also firmly established and defects in Tregs may underlie susceptibility for type 1 diabetes [15, 16]. Various approaches to increase Treg activity for the treatment of type 1 diabetes are intensively being developed and, in some cases, have entered clinical trials [17].

The initiation of clinical trials to use anti-IL-7Rα antibodies for the treatment of type 1 diabetes and other autoimmune diseases [18] underscores the necessity to better understand the treatment modalities and mechanisms underlying protection against type 1 diabetes provided by anti-IL-7Rα administration. Therefore, we treated prediabetic NOD mice with a short course of anti-IL-7Rα antibodies and expanded our analysis of co-inhibitory receptor expression and Tregs. We found that in addition to PD-1, LAG-3 and Tim-3 were also induced on T cells in response to IL-7Rα blockade. Importantly, changes in these receptors could be found not only in lymphoid organs but on peripheral blood T cells as well and may serve as a biomarker of treatment efficacy. Furthermore, we show that IL-7Rα blockade increases the frequency and changes the phenotype of polyclonal Tregs. Together, our data suggest that anti-IL-7Rα antibodies promote two key mechanisms of protection against autoimmunity: increased expression of co-inhibitory receptors and increased Treg activity. Moreover, short-term IL-7Rα blockade retained some capacity to alter the kinetics of the disease.

Methods

Mice

Prediabetic female NOD mice (9–11 weeks) were purchased from The Jackson Laboratory (US). All animal experiments were approved by the Institutional Animal Care and Use Committee of Boston University Medical Campus.

Diabetes assessment

Diabetes incidence was followed weekly by urine analysis (Diastix, Bayer, US) and measuring of blood glucose levels with a Contour glucose meter (Bayer; US). The percentage of diabetic mice (glucose levels >250 mg/dL) over a 32-weeks time course was calculated by the Survival Curves method using GraphPad Prism.

In vivo antibody treatment

Anti-IL-7Rα (rat IgG2a, clone A7R34) antibodies for in vivo blocking experiments were produced by a hybridoma cell line and purified with Protein G Sepharose 4 Fast Flow (GE Healthcare, US) in our laboratory. Rat IgG (Jackson ImmunoResearch Laboratories, US) was used as a control. For anti-IL-7Rα and rat IgG antibodies, 0.5 mg was administered in PBS intraperitoneally.

In vitro stimulation assays and ELISA

Cells were cultured in RPMI 1640 media (Invitrogen, US) supplemented with 1 mM each of L-glutamine, non-essential amino acids, sodium pyruvate, Hepes, penicillin, streptomycin, 50 μM 2-Mercaptoethanol (Gibco by Life Technologies, US), and 10% FCS (Omega Scientific, US), and incubated at 37 °C in 5% CO2. In vitro assays to measure cytokine production were performed by stimulating 5×10^5 cells from spleen and pancreatic lymph nodes (PLN) with soluble anti-CD3 (1 μg/ml) (clone 145-2C11; eBioscience, US) and anti-CD28 (2 μg/ml) (clone 37.51; eBioscience, US) antibodies in round-bottom 96-well plates (BD Falcon, US) in the absence or presence of blocking antibodies (10 μg/ml) for PD-L1 (clone MIH5), LAG-3 (clone C9B7W) and Tim-3 (clone RMT3-23) (Bio X Cell, US). Supernatants from the cultures were harvested after 18 h and IFN-γ and IL-2 content determined by ELISA (eBioscience, US), following the manufacturer's instructions. For assays to measure induction of co-inhibitory receptor expression, PLN cells from mice treated with anti-IL-7Rα or rat IgG antibodies were stimulated in vitro with soluble anti-CD3- (0.1 or 10 μg/ml) and anti-CD28 (1 μg/ml) antibodies. Cell cultures were set up in flat-bottom 96-well plates (BD Falcon, US) and harvested after 3 days for flow cytometric analysis.

Antibodies and staining procedures

Blood samples (50–100 μl) were drawn from mouse tail vein and an equal volume of EDTA (50 mM) (Sigma, US) was added immediately to avoid coagulation. Prior to staining, erythrocytes were lysed for spleen and blood samples. To distinguish live from dead cells, cells were preincubated with a fixable viability dye (eBioscience, US) according to manufacturer's instructions. Fc receptors were blocked with anti-CD16/CD32 antibodies for 5 min at 4 °C before any antibody staining procedures were started. The following antibodies were used for detection of murine activation and proliferation markers and co-inhibitory receptors: anti-CD4; anti-CD8; anti-PD-1; anti-Tim-3; anti-LAG-3; anti-CD44; anti-Foxp3 and anti-CD25 (eBioscience, Biolegend or BD Pharmingen, US). Extracellular staining was performed by incubating with antibodies for 15–30 min at 4 ° C. For Foxp3 intracellular staining cells were fixed and permeabilized with a Foxp3 staining buffer set (eBioscience, US) following manufacturer's instructions.

Flow cytometry

Phenotypic analysis of cell populations was performed by multiparameter flow cytometry. Fluorescence intensities were measured on a LSRII flow cytometer and data were analyzed with FlowJo software.

Statistics

Statistically significant differences between groups were determined using the Mantel–Cox log-rank test (for diabetes incidence) and one- or two-tailed paired or unpaired t tests (for flow cytometry data) using Graph Pad Prism. P values ≤ 0.05 were considered significant. Horizontal lines in graphs indicate statistical significance ($* = p \leq 0.05$, $** = p \leq 0.005$, $*** = p \leq 0.0005$, ns $= p > 0.05$).

Results

A short course of IL-7Rα blocking antibodies delays type 1 diabetes onset in NOD mice

We and others previously demonstrated that sustained, long-term treatment (14 weeks) of NOD mice with anti-IL-7Rα monoclonal antibodies (mAbs) robustly prevented diabetes incidence [4, 5]. However, such long-term treatment was accompanied by significant depletion of lymphocyte populations over time, raising concerns about broad immunosuppression and questioning the potential of translating this preventive strategy to the clinic. Therefore, we asked whether a treatment of limited duration with anti-IL-7Rα mAbs would retain benefit for long-term prevention of type 1 diabetes. Treatment was started at 11 weeks of age, when insulitis is known to be evident in NOD mice [19], hence this cohort represented a model of secondary prevention (Fig. 1a). Four doses (0.5 mg each) of anti-IL-7Rα mAbs or control rat IgG were administered intraperitoneally on days 0, 5, 15 and 19. Blood was drawn 2 and 16 days after the last dose was given to evaluate anti-IL-7Rα-induced changes in blood T lymphocytes. In the group that received rat IgG, mice started to become hyperglycemic at 12 weeks of age, whereas the mice treated with anti-IL-7Rα mAbs showed a significant delay in diabetes onset (Fig. 1b). Overall incidence was reduced from ~80% to ~60%, suggesting that in some cases secondary prevention can be achieved with temporary IL-7Rα blockade in prediabetic mice. Thus, a short treatment with blocking antibodies for IL-7Rα retains efficacy to

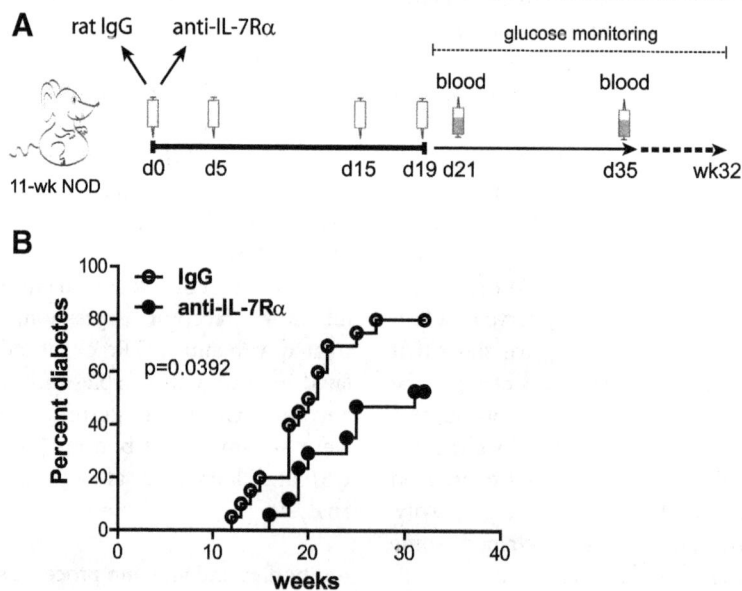

Fig. 1 A short-term treatment with anti-IL-7Rα antibodies delays and prevents diabetes in NOD mice. **a** Experimental design outline: 11-week old prediabetic female NOD mice received four doses of 0.5 mg anti-IL-7Rα ($n = 10$) or rat IgG ($n = 10$) antibodies on days 0, 5, 15 and 19. Blood was drawn at day 21 and 35 and T cell populations were analyzed by flow cytometry, and, **b** diabetes incidence was followed in mice that received anti-IL-7Rα antibodies (*black circles*) or rat IgG (*white circles*) measuring urine and blood glucose levels until 32 weeks of age. Data were pooled from two independent experiments ($n = 20$). P value is indicated in the figure

delay and, in some cases, prevent diabetes progression, supporting continued efforts to translate anti-IL-7Rα antibodies for the prevention and treatment of type 1 diabetes.

Circulating T lymphocytes from anti-IL-7Rα-treated NOD mice show enhanced expression of multiple co-inhibitory receptors

To gain insight in the changes that occur in T cell phenotypes after short-term IL-7Rα blockade, we performed a flow-cytometric analysis of peripheral blood T cell subsets from treated mice two (day 21) and sixteen (day 35) days after the final antibody administration (Fig. 2). Our previous studies showed that increased expression of the co-inhibitory receptor PD-1 in CD4$^+$ T$_{E/M}$ cells from anti-IL-7Rα-treated NOD mice contributed to protection from type 1 diabetes [4]. However, anti-PD-L1 antibodies did not efficiently restore diabetogenicity in CD4$^+$ T$_{E/M}$ cells isolated from anti-IL-7Rα-treated NOD mice, suggesting that additional protective mechanisms are induced by IL-7Rα blockade [4]. Therefore, in addition to PD-1, we analyzed the expression of the co-inhibitory receptors LAG-3 and Tim-3, which are known to play important roles in limiting autoimmunity [12, 20, 21], in CD4$^+$ and CD8$^+$ T cells (Fig. 2). Confirming our previous

observations in lymphoid organs [4], the percentage of PD-1$^+$ CD44^{high} cells within CD4$^+$Foxp3$^-$ T$_{E/M}$ cells and CD44^{high}CD8$^+$ T$_{E/M}$ cells was elevated 2 days after the end of the treatment (day 21) with anti-IL-7Rα vs. rat IgG antibodies (Fig. 3a). Interestingly, these differences were not maintained 2 weeks after the end of treatment. To the contrary, Tim-3 and LAG-3 expression in peripheral blood CD4$^+$ and CD8+ T$_{E/M}$ cells was not increased when measured immediately after treatment but was significantly increased 2 weeks after terminating anti-IL-7Rα mAb administration (Fig. 3b, c). Using a separate set of experimental mice, we analyzed the expression of Tim-3 and LAG-3 in the pancreatic lymph nodes (PLN), since this is the site where autoreactive T cells initially respond to β-cell antigens [22]. We found that the frequency of Tim-3$^+$ and LAG-3$^+$ cells within the CD4$^+$ and CD8$^+$ T$_{E/M}$ population increased after anti-IL-7Rα mAb treatment (Fig. 3d, e), thus showing that in the PLN these co-inhibitory receptors behave similarly as PD-1, whose expression in PLN was analyzed previously [4]. Taken together, these data show that T lymphocytes in anti-IL7Rα-treated NOD mice exhibit a phenotype reminiscent of T cell exhaustion, characterized by expression of multiple co-inhibitory receptors [23]. Importantly, this phenotype is not only present in the

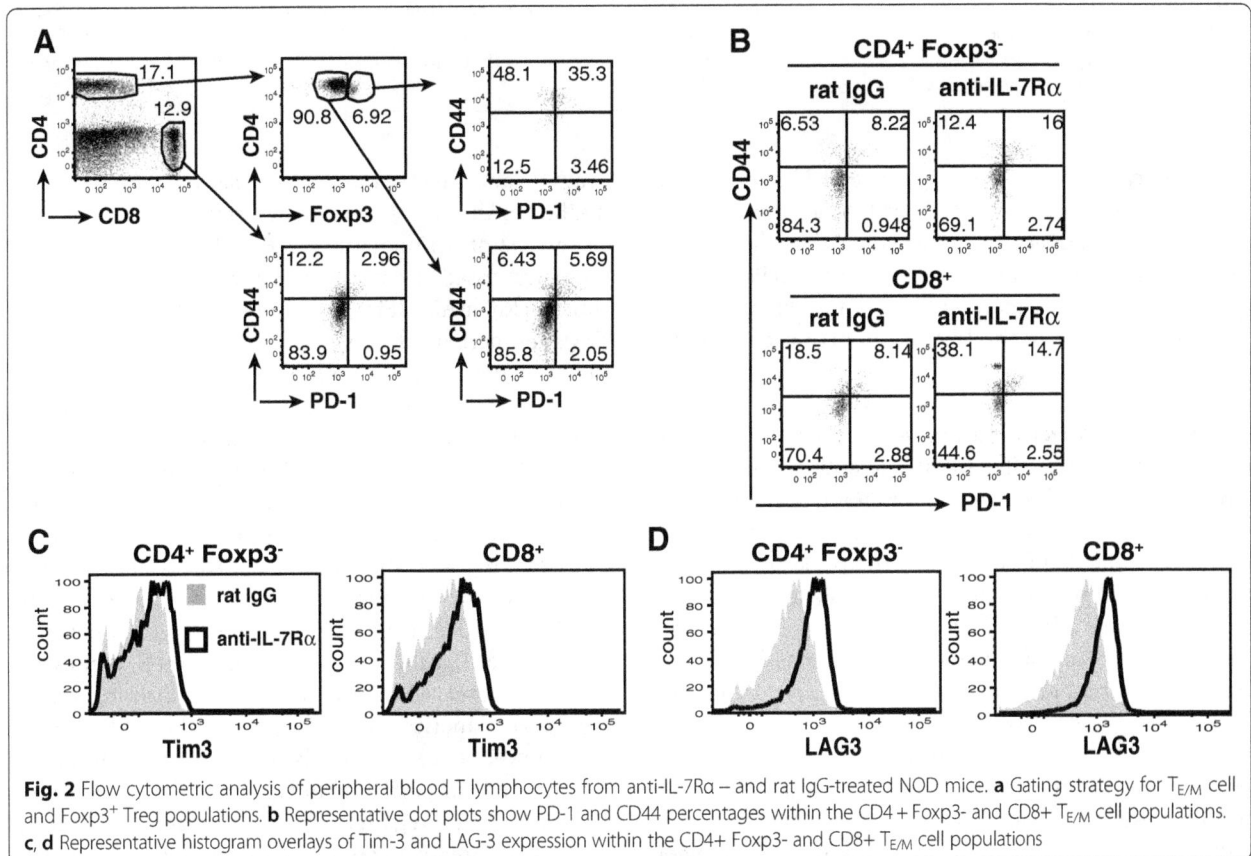

Fig. 2 Flow cytometric analysis of peripheral blood T lymphocytes from anti-IL-7Rα – and rat IgG-treated NOD mice. a Gating strategy for T$_{E/M}$ cell and Foxp3$^+$ Treg populations. b Representative dot plots show PD-1 and CD44 percentages within the CD4 + Foxp3- and CD8+ T$_{E/M}$ cell populations. c, d Representative histogram overlays of Tim-3 and LAG-3 expression within the CD4+ Foxp3- and CD8+ T$_{E/M}$ cell populations

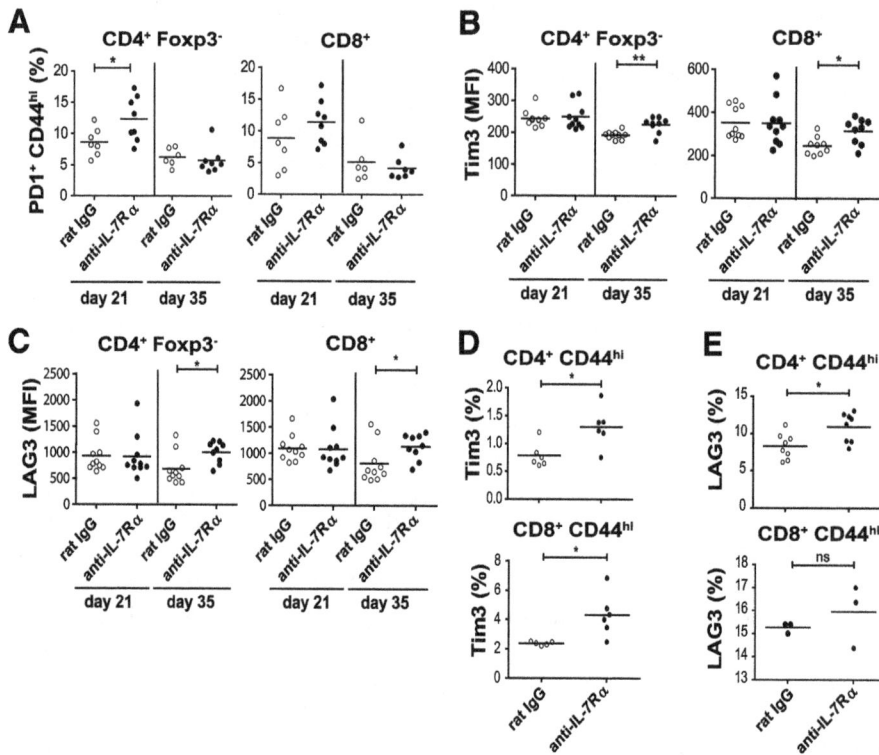

Fig. 3 IL-7Rα blockade induces multiple co-inhibitory receptors in CD4+ and CD8+ T_{E/M} cells. **a**, **b**, **c** Prediabetic female NOD mice received anti-IL-7Rα (*black circles*; n = 10) or rat IgG (*white circles*; n = 10) antibodies as in Fig. 1a and blood was drawn and analyzed as in Figs. 1a and 2. Percentage of PD-1+CD44high cells and MFI of extracellular Tim-3 and LAG-3 within the peripheral blood CD4+Foxp3− (*left*) and CD8+ (*right*) T_{E/M} cell populations were determined by flow cytometry. All data are representative for two independent experiments. Each symbol represents one individual mouse. * = p ≤ 0.05, ** = p ≤ 0.005. **d**, **e** Frequency of Tim-3+ and LAG-3+ cells within the activated (CD44high) CD4+Foxp3− and CD8+ T_{E/M} cell populations in the PLN of mice treated twice per week for two consecutive weeks with anti-IL-7Rα (*black circles*) or rat IgG (*white circles*) antibodies. Data are pooled from two or three independent experiments (n = 3–8). * = p ≤ 0.05, ns = p > 0.05

PLN but can be detected in peripheral blood samples, suggesting this could be developed as a biomarker for anti-IL-7Rα treatment. It is intriguing that the kinetics of detecting Tim-3- and LAG-3-expressing cells in blood differs from PD-1, suggesting that the former cells might be retained longer in the PLN or induction of these receptors is delayed.

Peripheral blood Tregs show increased frequency and an activated phenotype after anti-IL-7Rα antibody treatment

Tregs play a critical role in the prevention of autoimmunity and deficiencies in their frequency and function are therefore thought to contribute to the development of autoimmune diseases such as type 1 diabetes [15, 16]. In support of this, a lower frequency of Tregs has been detected in the blood of young diabetic patients [24], and it has been described that Tregs from type 1 diabetes patients and NOD mice show functional deficits, possibly related to defects in the IL-2/IL-2Rα pathway [25, 26]. To evaluate whether the frequency and phenotype of circulating Tregs was altered in NOD mice after a short treatment with anti-IL-7Rα mAbs, we analyzed peripheral blood

Tregs 2 days (day 21) and 2 weeks (day 35) after final anti-IL-7Rα mAb or rat IgG administration (Fig. 2). The percentage of peripheral blood Foxp3+ Tregs was significantly increased 2 days after the end of treatment with anti-IL-7Rα mAbs (Fig. 4a). Importantly, we found that Tregs in peripheral blood of anti-IL-7Rα-treated mice showed increased expression of Foxp3 (Fig. 4b). Increased Foxp3 expression on a per cell basis has been associated with Treg activation and improved suppressive activity [27]. PD-1 expression was also increased in activated (CD44high) Tregs from anti-IL-7Rα-treated mice (Fig. 4c), further supporting the notion that IL-7Rα blockade leads to Treg activation [28]. By 2 weeks after the end of the treatment, Treg frequencies, Foxp3 expression and PD-1 had returned to the same levels as controls. However, a significant increase in Tim-3 expression level was observed at this time, hence showing similar expression kinetics as in T_{E/M} cells (Fig. 4d). LAG-3 also showed a trend towards higher expression on day 35 (data not shown). Of note, higher levels of Tim-3 and LAG-3 in Tregs have been associated with an increased suppressive activity of this population [29–31].

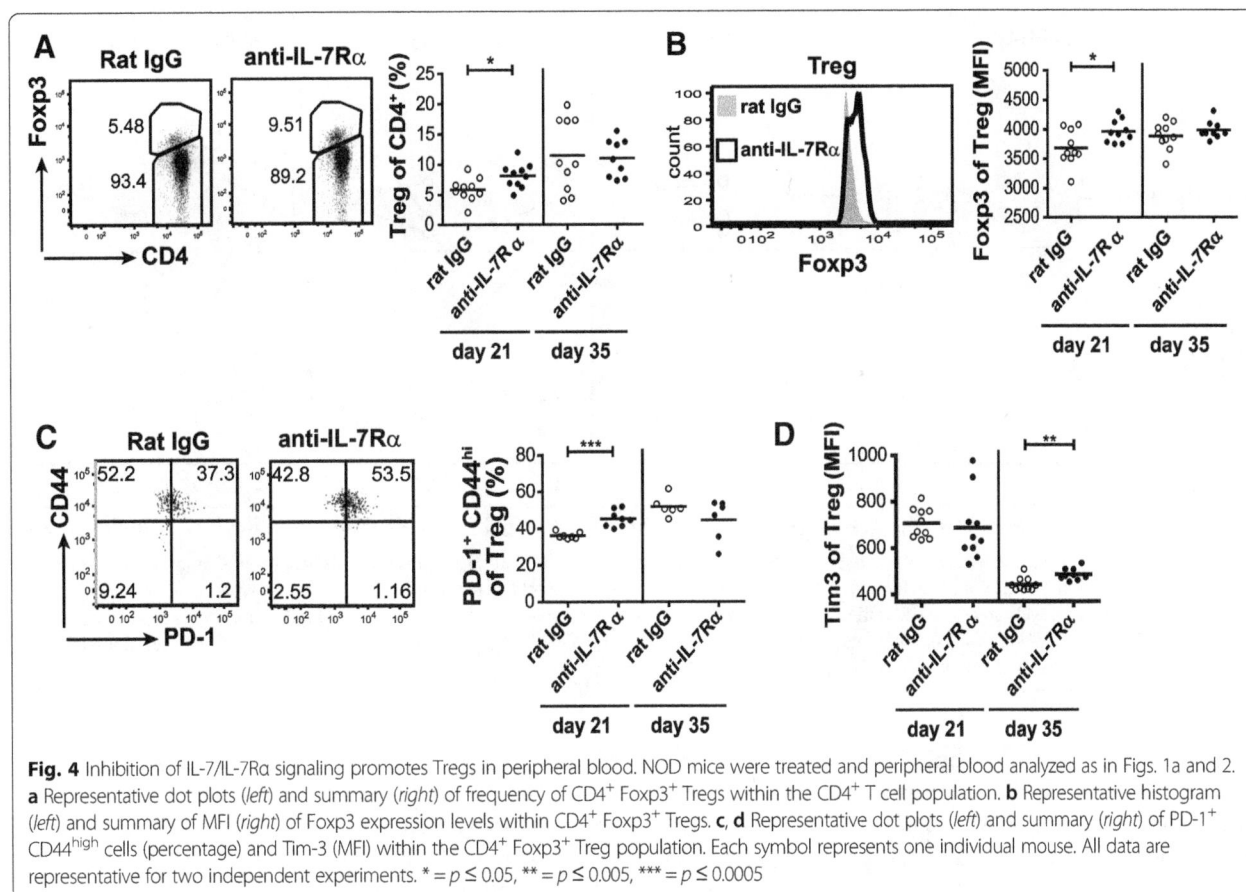

Fig. 4 Inhibition of IL-7/IL-7Rα signaling promotes Tregs in peripheral blood. NOD mice were treated and peripheral blood analyzed as in Figs. 1a and 2. **a** Representative dot plots (*left*) and summary (*right*) of frequency of CD4$^+$ Foxp3$^+$ Tregs within the CD4$^+$ T cell population. **b** Representative histogram (*left*) and summary of MFI (*right*) of Foxp3 expression levels within CD4$^+$ Foxp3$^+$ Tregs. **c, d** Representative dot plots (*left*) and summary (*right*) of PD-1$^+$ CD44^{high} cells (percentage) and Tim-3 (MFI) within the CD4$^+$ Foxp3$^+$ Treg population. Each symbol represents one individual mouse. All data are representative for two independent experiments. * = $p \leq 0.05$, ** = $p \leq 0.005$, *** = $p \leq 0.0005$

Thus, our data indicate that short-term, systemic blockade of IL-7/IL-7Rα signaling not only detectably alters the balance of Tregs/T$_{E/M}$ in peripheral blood but changes Tregs qualitatively by increasing Foxp3 expression and co-inhibitory receptors, suggesting a more activated, suppressive state.

Co-inhibitory receptor expression on T cells from anti-IL-7Rα-treated mice impairs cytokine production

To analyze whether co-inhibitory receptors functionally affected T cells from anti-IL-7Rα-treated mice, spleen and pancreatic lymph node cells were stimulated in vitro with anti-CD3 and anti-CD28 antibodies in the presence or absence of PD-L1-, Tim-3- and LAG-3-blocking antibodies (Fig. 5), and IFN-γ and IL-2 production measured. We found that anti-IL-7Rα-treated T cells produced less IFN-γ than controls, consistent with a less functional state of the T cell population. Interestingly, we found that blocking individual co-inhibitory receptors did not efficiently restore IFN-γ production, but blocking PD-L1, Tim-3 and LAG-3 simultaneously significantly increased IFN-γ secretion (Fig. 5). IL-2 production was not reduced in anti-IL-7Rα-treated T cells compared to controls but blocking PD-L1 did result in enhanced secretion.

These data demonstrate that expression of co-inhibitory receptors on T cells from anti-IL-7Rα-treated mice impacts their functionality.

Absence of IL-7 signaling sensitizes T cells to express co-inhibitory receptors in response to TCR stimulation

Co-inhibitory receptor expression is induced after T cell activation and maintained in situations of chronic antigen stimulation [6–8]. To ask how co-inhibitory receptor expression behaves in response to TCR stimulation in the absence of IL-7/IL-7Rα signals in vivo, we stimulated T cells from the PLN of anti-IL-7Rα or Rat IgG-treated NOD mice in vitro with a low (0.1 μg/ml) or high (10 μg/ml) dose of anti-CD3 mAbs in the presence of anti-CD28 (1 μg/ml) and evaluated LAG-3 and Tim-3 expression. We found that increasing TCR triggering led to higher LAG-3 expression levels in activated (CD44^{high}) CD4$^+$Foxp3$^-$ T$_{E/M}$ cells and Foxp3$^+$ Tregs from anti-IL-7Rα-treated mice vs rat IgG controls (Fig. 6a). CD8$^+$ T cells did not show increased LAG-3 expression (data not shown). Conversely, Tim-3 expression was increased after strong TCR stimulation of IL-7-deprived CD8$^+$ T cells (Fig. 6b) but remained unaffected in CD4$^+$ T cells (data not shown), albeit with significant variability between animals. These data demonstrate that T cells persisting in the

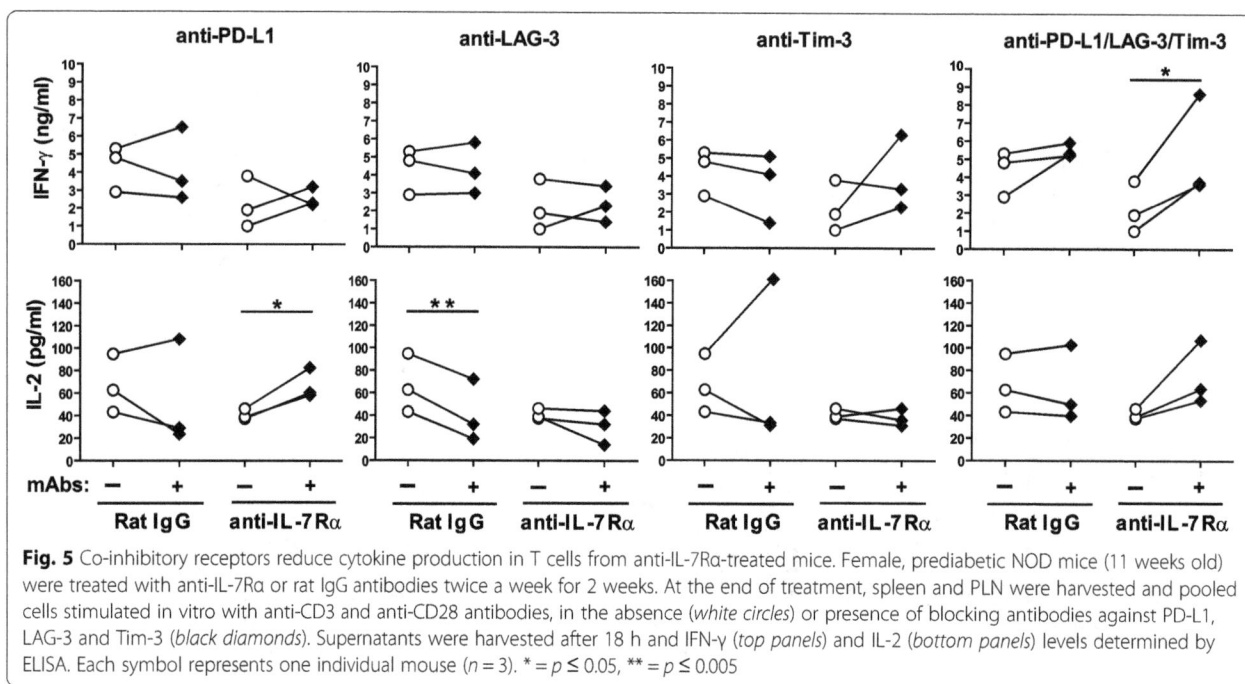

Fig. 5 Co-inhibitory receptors reduce cytokine production in T cells from anti-IL-7Rα-treated mice. Female, prediabetic NOD mice (11 weeks old) were treated with anti-IL-7Rα or rat IgG antibodies twice a week for 2 weeks. At the end of treatment, spleen and PLN were harvested and pooled cells stimulated in vitro with anti-CD3 and anti-CD28 antibodies, in the absence (*white circles*) or presence of blocking antibodies against PD-L1, LAG-3 and Tim-3 (*black diamonds*). Supernatants were harvested after 18 h and IFN-γ (*top panels*) and IL-2 (*bottom panels*) levels determined by ELISA. Each symbol represents one individual mouse (*n* = 3). * = *p* ≤ 0.05, ** = *p* ≤ 0.005

absence of IL-7 signals become more sensitive towards TCR-induced co-inhibitory receptor expression, further underscoring the idea that IL-7 protects activated T cells from various inhibitory signals, thus promoting the auto-immune response.

Discussion

In this study we sought to further characterize the protective mechanisms induced by treatment with anti-IL-7Rα antibodies during an ongoing autoreactive T cell response. We found that, in addition to PD-1, two other co-inhibitory receptors, Tim-3 and LAG-3, show increased expression in T cells from anti-IL-7Rα-treated NOD mice. Moreover, IL-7Rα blockade promoted an expansion of the polyclonal Treg population in NOD mice and, interestingly, increased their activation status, indicating enhanced suppressive potential. Our results indicate that a broad program of immunoregulation underlies the slower disease kinetics afforded by IL-7Rα blockade in type 1 diabetes and, that markers of anti-IL-7Rα antibody activity can be detected in peripheral blood following a short course of treatment.

PD-1, Tim-3 and LAG-3 are co-inhibitory receptors that are critical for controlling autoimmunity: studies with blocking antibodies as well as gene-deficient mice demonstrated that these pathways, individually or synergistically, play important roles in type 1 diabetes and other autoimmune diseases [9, 11–13, 32]. Hence, developing methods to promote activity of these pathways is a promising approach towards novel therapies for type 1 diabetes and other autoimmune diseases. Our data indicate that

this desired effect is achieved as a consequence of IL-7Rα blockade. Interestingly, such a broad increase of multiple co-inhibitory receptors in CD4+ Foxp3− and CD8+ T$_{E/M}$ cells resembles the phenotype described in previous studies for exhausted T cells responding to tumors or chronic viral infections [7, 8, 23]. In these settings, continuous antigen exposure results in inhibited, "exhausted" T cells that have lost effector functions (e.g., IFN-γ production) necessary to effectively combat tumors and chronic viral infections [8, 23, 33]. Importantly, IL-7 restored functionality in CD8+ T cells during chronic viral infections and in tumor models [34, 35]. These observations thus support the idea that IL-7 is an environmental factor promoting T cell responses during chronic antigen challenge. As a corollary, inappropriate IL-7 signaling during autoreactive T cell activation may contribute to the development of a pathogenic T cell response. In this respect, murine models of autoimmune diseases treated with inhibitors of IL-7/IL-7Rα signaling show preventive or therapeutic efficacy [4, 5, 36–38]. In many of these models, it remains to be investigated whether increased co-inhibitory receptor expression plays a role as a protective mechanism. Due to the multiple immunoregulatory pathways induced in anti-IL-7Rα-treated NOD mice, it will be a challenging endeavor to unequivocally demonstrate the contribution of each to controlling autoimmunity. In this regard, one interesting finding from our study is that cells expressing PD-1 vs Tim-3 and/or LAG-3 appear with different kinetics in the blood after anti-IL-7Rα mAb administration. This may be due to a slower kinetics of initial induction or because Tim-3 and LAG-3-expressing cells

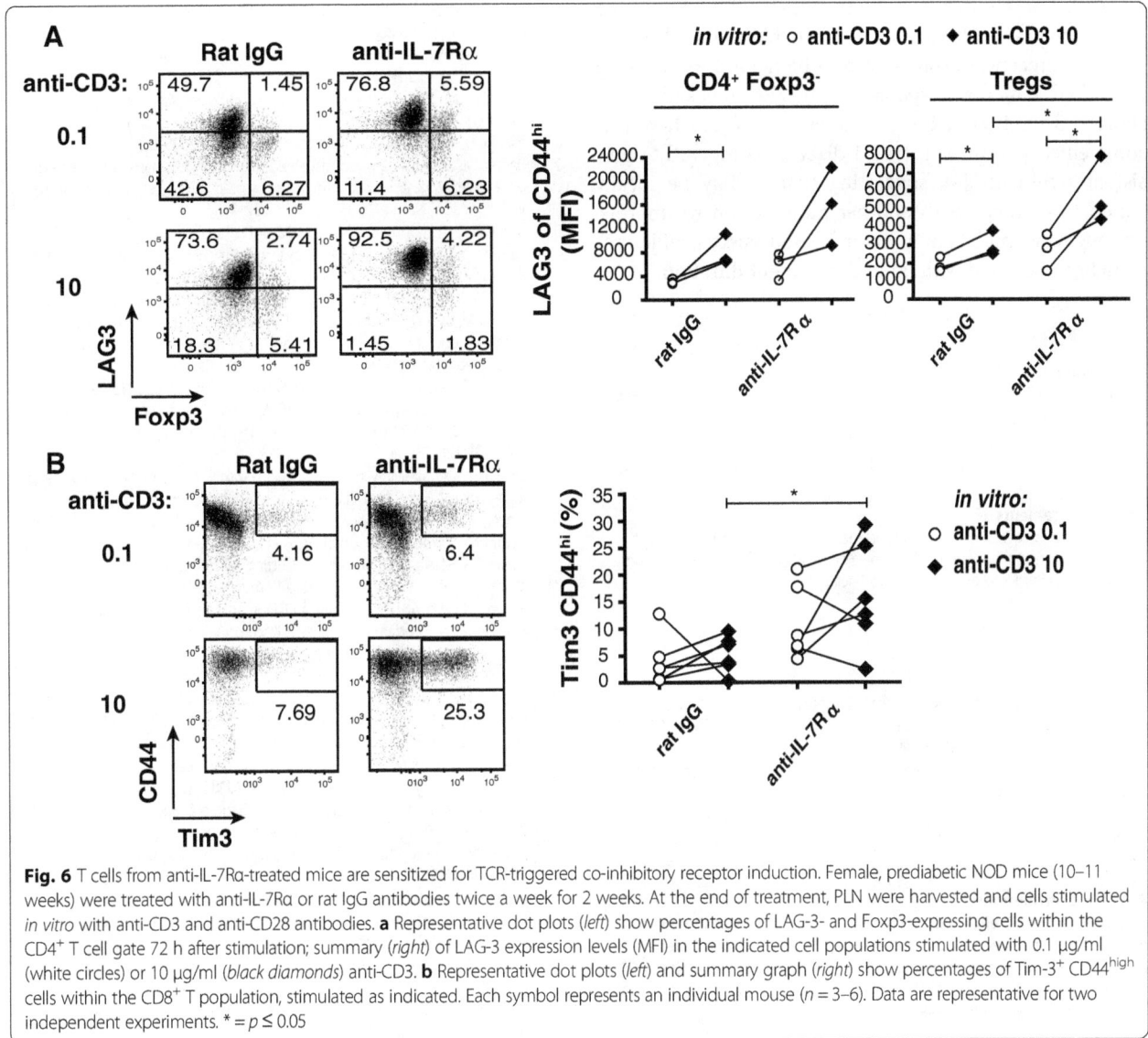

Fig. 6 T cells from anti-IL-7Rα-treated mice are sensitized for TCR-triggered co-inhibitory receptor induction. Female, prediabetic NOD mice (10–11 weeks) were treated with anti-IL-7Rα or rat IgG antibodies twice a week for 2 weeks. At the end of treatment, PLN were harvested and cells stimulated *in vitro* with anti-CD3 and anti-CD28 antibodies. **a** Representative dot plots (*left*) show percentages of LAG-3- and Foxp3-expressing cells within the CD4[+] T cell gate 72 h after stimulation; summary (*right*) of LAG-3 expression levels (MFI) in the indicated cell populations stimulated with 0.1 μg/ml (white circles) or 10 μg/ml (black diamonds) anti-CD3. **b** Representative dot plots (*left*) and summary graph (*right*) show percentages of Tim-3[+] CD44[high] cells within the CD8[+] T population, stimulated as indicated. Each symbol represents an individual mouse (n = 3–6). Data are representative for two independent experiments. * = p ≤ 0.05

are preferentially retained in the lymphoid organs while PD-1 expressing cells belong to a population that more readily enters the circulation. Besides enhanced co-inhibitory receptor expression on $T_{E/M}$ cells, PD-1, Tim-3 and LAG-3 were also increased on Tregs. Tregs expressing PD-1 [39], Tim-3 [31] and LAG-3 [30] are found at sites of active immune responses, e.g., in tumors and transplants, and are thought to possess higher suppressive activity.

The molecular mechanisms underlying increase of co-inhibitory receptors in the absence of IL-7 signaling remain to be determined. However, it is reasonable to speculate that a direct effect of IL-7 on T cells during priming is involved. For example, recent data show that IL-7 provides additional early signals (increased ERK, STAT5, Akt) during TCR engagement that promote optimal T cell activation [40, 41]. These IL-7-induced signals are important for

expression of the glucose transporter Glut1 in T cells [42] and, intriguingly, decreased Glut1 and glucose uptake have been associated with increased PD-1 and Tim-3 expression and T cell exhaustion [43]. Hence it is feasible that absence of IL-7 signaling during T cell priming promotes expression of co-inhibitory receptors, perhaps as a consequence of defective metabolic regulation.

Conclusions

Efforts to translate pre-clinical studies showing efficacy of anti-IL-7Rα antibodies for the treatment of type 1 diabetes have been initiated in the clinic [18]. Our study shows that a limited treatment with anti-IL-7Rα antibodies is sufficient to induce detectable changes in the peripheral blood T cell phenotype, increasing expression of several co-inhibitory receptors in CD4[+] and CD8[+] $T_{E/M}$ cells and promoting Treg presence. Hence, our data support the rationale for clinical trials with anti-IL-7Rα mAbs and suggest that a T cell biomarker in the blood based on co-inhibitory receptor expression may be helpful in following individual patients' response to IL-7Rα blockade. The shorter, 3-week course of treatment we tested here lost some efficacy to prevent type 1 diabetes compared to persistent treatment [4], suggesting that it may be ideally suited to combine with another intervention to improve efficacy while maintaining the increased safety profile presumably associated with limited treatment duration.

Abbreviations

IL-7: Interleukin-7; mAbs: monoclonal antibodies; NOD: Non-obese diabetic; PLN: Pancreatic lymph nodes

Acknowledgements

The authors thank Dr. Cristina Penaranda (Massachusetts General Hospital) for useful comments on the manuscript. This work was supported by the Boston University Flow Cytometry Core Facility.

Funding

This research was supported by American Diabetes Association Basic Science Grant #1-13-BS-038 (to H.D.), National Institutes of Health Grant R01 DK-102911 (to H.D.) and by the Boston University Arthritis Center. The funders had no role in the design of the study, the collection, analysis and interpretation of data, and in writing the manuscript.

Authors' contributions

CVM designed and performed experiments, analyzed data and wrote the manuscript. JC planned and conducted experiments and contributed to discussion. MF performed experiments and contributed to discussion. HD conceived the study, analyzed data and wrote the manuscript. All authors read and approved the final manuscript.

Competing interests

The authors declare that they have no competing interests.

References

1. Atkinson MA, Eisenbarth GS, Michels AW. Type 1 diabetes. Lancet. 2014; 383(9911):69–82.
2. Coppieters KT, Harrison LC, von Herrath MG. Trials in type 1 diabetes: antigen-specific therapies. Clin Immunol. 2013;149(3):345–55.
3. Dooms H. Interleukin-7: fuel for the autoimmune attack. J Autoimmun. 2013;45:40–8.
4. Penaranda C, Kuswanto W, Hofmann J, Kenefeck R, Narendran P, Walker LS, Bluestone JA, Abbas AK, Dooms H. IL-7 receptor blockade reverses autoimmune diabetes by promoting inhibition of effector/memory T cells. Proc Natl Acad Sci U S A. 2012;109(31):12668–73.
5. Lee LF, Logronio K, Tu GH, Zhai W, Ni I, Mei L, Dilley J, Yu J, Rajpal A, Brown C, et al. Anti-IL-7 receptor-alpha reverses established type 1 diabetes in nonobese diabetic mice by modulating effector T-cell function. Proc Natl Acad Sci U S A. 2012;109(31):12674–9.
6. Keir ME, Liang SC, Guleria I, Latchman YE, Qipo A, Albacker LA, Koulmanda M, Freeman GJ, Sayegh MH, Sharpe AH. Tissue expression of PD-L1 mediates peripheral T cell tolerance. J Exp Med. 2006;203(4):883–95.
7. Barber DL, Wherry EJ, Masopust D, Zhu B, Allison JP, Sharpe AH, Freeman GJ, Ahmed R. Restoring function in exhausted CD8 T cells during chronic viral infection. Nature. 2006;439(7077):682–7.
8. Sakuishi K, Apetoh L, Sullivan JM, Blazar BR, Kuchroo VK, Anderson AC. Targeting Tim-3 and PD-1 pathways to reverse T cell exhaustion and restore anti-tumor immunity. J Exp Med. 2010;207(10):2187–94.
9. Ansari MJ, Salama AD, Chitnis T, Smith RN, Yagita H, Akiba H, Yamazaki T, Azuma M, Iwai H, Khoury SJ, et al. The programmed death-1 (PD-1) pathway regulates autoimmune diabetes in nonobese diabetic (NOD) mice. J Exp Med. 2003;198(1):63–9.
10. Fife BT, Guleria I, Gubbels Bupp M, Eagar TN, Tang Q, Bour-Jordan H, Yagita H, Azuma M, Sayegh MH, Bluestone JA. Insulin-induced remission in new-onset NOD mice is maintained by the PD-1-PD-L1 pathway. J Exp Med. 2006;203(12):2737–47.
11. Okazaki T, Okazaki IM, Wang J, Sugiura D, Nakaki F, Yoshida T, Kato Y, Fagarasan S, Muramatsu M, Eto T, et al. PD-1 and LAG-3 inhibitory co-receptors act synergistically to prevent autoimmunity in mice. J Exp Med. 2011;208(2):395–407.
12. Bettini M, Szymczak-Workman AL, Forbes K, Castellaw AH, Selby M, Pan X, Drake CG, Korman AJ, Vignali DA. Cutting edge: accelerated autoimmune diabetes in the absence of LAG-3. J Immunol. 2011;187(7):3493–8.
13. Sanchez-Fueyo A, Tian J, Picarella D, Domenig C, Zheng XX, Sabatos CA, Manlongat N, Bender O, Kamradt T, Kuchroo VK, et al. Tim-3 inhibits T helper type 1-mediated auto- and alloimmune responses and promotes immunological tolerance. Nat Immunol. 2003;4(11):1093–101.
14. Wei J, Loke P, Zang X, Allison JP. Tissue-specific expression of B7x protects from CD4 T cell-mediated autoimmunity. J Exp Med. 2011;208(8):1683–94.
15. Tritt M, Sgouroudis E, d'Hennezel E, Albanese A, Piccirillo CA. Functional waning of naturally occurring CD4+ regulatory T-cells contributes to the onset of autoimmune diabetes. Diabetes. 2008;57(1):113–23.
16. Tang Q, Adams JY, Penaranda C, Melli K, Piaggio E, Sgouroudis E, Piccirillo CA, Salomon BL, Bluestone JA. Central role of defective interleukin-2 production in the triggering of islet autoimmune destruction. Immunity. 2008;28(5):687–97.
17. Bluestone JA, Buckner JH, Fitch M, Gitelman SE, Gupta S, Hellerstein MK, Herold KC, Lares A, Lee MR, Li K, et al. Type 1 diabetes immunotherapy using polyclonal regulatory T cells. Sci Transl Med. 2015;7(315):315ra189.
18. Vignali D, Monti P. Targeting homeostatic T cell proliferation to control beta-cell autoimmunity. Curr Diabet Reports. 2016;16(5):40.
19. Anderson MS, Bluestone JA. The NOD mouse: a model of immune dysregulation. Annu Rev Immunol. 2005;23:447–85.
20. Morimoto K, Hosomi S, Yamagami H, Watanabe K, Kamata N, Sogawa M, Machida H, Okazaki H, Tanigawa T, Nagahara H, et al. Dysregulated upregulation of T-cell immunoglobulin and mucin domain-3 on mucosal T helper 1 cells in patients with Crohn's disease. Scand J Gastroenterol. 2011;46(6):701–9.
21. Koguchi K, Anderson DE, Yang L, O'Connor KC, Kuchroo VK, Hafler DA. Dysregulated T cell expression of TIM3 in multiple sclerosis. J Exp Med. 2006;203(6):1413–8.
22. Mathis D, Vence L. Benoist C: beta-Cell death during progression to diabetes. Nature. 2001;414(6865):792–8.
23. Wherry EJ. T cell exhaustion. Nat Immunol. 2011;12(6):492–9.
24. Szypowska A, Stelmaszczyk-Emmel A, Demkow U, Luczynski W. Low frequency of regulatory T cells in the peripheral blood of children with type 1 diabetes diagnosed under the age of five. Arch Immunol Ther Exp (Warsz). 2012;60(4):307–13.
25. Long SA, Rieck M, Sanda S, Bollyky JB, Samuels PL, Goland R, Ahmann A, Rabinovitch A, Aggarwal S, Phippard D, et al. Rapamycin/IL-2 combination therapy in patients with type 1 diabetes augments Tregs yet transiently impairs beta-cell function. Diabetes. 2012;61(9):2340–8.
26. Kukreja A, Cost G, Marker J, Zhang C, Sun Z, Lin-Su K, Ten S, Sanz M, Exley M, Wilson B, et al. Multiple immuno-regulatory defects in type-1 diabetes. J Clin Invest. 2002;109(1):131–40.
27. Yamaguchi T, Wing JB, Sakaguchi S. Two modes of immune suppression by Foxp3(+) regulatory T cells under inflammatory or non-inflammatory conditions. Semin Immunol. 2011;23(6):424–30.

28. Francisco LM, Sage PT, Sharpe AH. The PD-1 pathway in tolerance and autoimmunity. Immunol Rev. 2010;236:219–42.
29. Liang B, Workman C, Lee J, Chew C, Dale BM, Colonna L, Flores M, Li N, Schweighoffer E, Greenberg S, et al. Regulatory T cells inhibit dendritic cells by lymphocyte activation gene-3 engagement of MHC class II. J Immunol. 2008;180(9):5916–26.
30. Camisaschi C, Casati C, Rini F, Perego M, De Filippo A, Triebel F, Parmiani G, Belli F, Rivoltini L, Castelli C. LAG-3 expression defines a subset of CD4(+)CD25(high)Foxp3(+) regulatory T cells that are expanded at tumor sites. J Immunol. 2010;184(11):6545–51.
31. Gautron AS, Dominguez-Villar M, de Marcken M, Hafler DA. Enhanced suppressor function of TIM-3(+) FoxP3(+) regulatory T cells. Eur J Immunol. 2014;44(9):2703–11.
32. Monney L, Sabatos CA, Gaglia JL, Ryu A, Waldner H, Chernova T, Manning S, Greenfield EA, Coyle AJ, Sobel RA, et al. Th1-specific cell surface protein Tim-3 regulates macrophage activation and severity of an autoimmune disease. Nature. 2002;415(6871):536–41.
33. Wherry EJ, Ha SJ, Kaech SM, Haining WN, Sarkar S, Kalia V, Subramaniam S, Blattman JN, Barber DL, Ahmed R. Molecular signature of CD8+ T cell exhaustion during chronic viral infection. Immunity. 2007;27(4):670–84.
34. Pellegrini M, Calzascia T, Elford AR, Shahinian A, Lin AE, Dissanayake D, Dhanji S, Nguyen LT, Gronski MA, Morre M, et al. Adjuvant IL-7 antagonizes multiple cellular and molecular inhibitory networks to enhance immunotherapies. Nat Med. 2009;15(5):528–36.
35. Pellegrini M, Calzascia T, Toe JG, Preston SP, Lin AE, Elford AR, Shahinian A, Lang PA, Lang KS, Morre M, et al. IL-7 engages multiple mechanisms to overcome chronic viral infection and limit organ pathology. Cell. 2011;144(4):601–13.
36. Hartgring SA, Willis CR, Alcorn D, Nelson LJ, Bijlsma JW, Lafeber FP, van Roon JA. Blockade of the interleukin-7 receptor inhibits collagen-induced arthritis and is associated with reduction of T cell activity and proinflammatory mediators. Arthritis Rheum. 2010;62(9):2716–25.
37. Willis CR, Seamons A, Maxwell J, Treuting PM, Nelson L, Chen G, Phelps S, Smith CL, Brabb T, Iritani BM, et al. Interleukin-7 receptor blockade suppresses adaptive and innate inflammatory responses in experimental colitis. J Inflamm. 2012;9(1):39.
38. Gonzalez-Quintial R, Lawson BR, Scatizzi JC, Craft J, Kono DH, Baccala R, Theofilopoulos AN. Systemic autoimmunity and lymphoproliferation are associated with excess IL-7 and inhibited by IL-7Ralpha blockade. PLoS One. 2011;6(11):e27528.
39. Park HJ, Kusnadi A, Lee EJ, Kim WW, Cho BC, Lee IJ, Seong J, Ha SJ. Tumor-infiltrating regulatory T cells delineated by upregulation of PD-1 and inhibitory receptors. Cell Immunol. 2012;278(1-2):76–83.
40. Deshpande P, Cavanagh MM, Le Saux S, Singh K, Weyand CM, Goronzy JJ. IL-7- and IL-15-mediated TCR sensitization enables T cell responses to self-antigens. J Immunol. 2013;190(4):1416–23.
41. Lawson BR, Gonzalez-Quintial R, Eleftheriadis T, Farrar MA, Miller SD, Sauer K, McGavern DB, Kono DH, Baccala R, Theofilopoulos AN. Interleukin-7 is required for CD4(+) T cell activation and autoimmune neuroinflammation. Clin Immunol. 2015;161(2):260–9.
42. Wofford JA, Wieman HL, Jacobs SR, Zhao Y, Rathmell JC. IL-7 promotes Glut1 trafficking and glucose uptake via STAT5-mediated activation of Akt to support T-cell survival. Blood. 2008;111(4):2101–11.
43. Siska PJ, van der Windt GJ, Kishton RJ, Cohen S, Eisner W, MacIver NJ, Kater AP, Weinberg JB, Rathmell JC. Suppression of Glut1 and glucose metabolism by decreased Akt/mTORC1 signaling drives T cell impairment in B cell leukemia. J Immunol. 2016;197(6):2532–40.

12

Blood handling and leukocyte isolation methods impact the global transcriptome of immune cells

Brittany A. Goods[1*], Jacqueline M. Vahey[2†], Arthur F. Steinschneider[3†], Michael H. Askenase[3], Lauren Sansing[3†] and J. Christopher Love[1,4,5*†]

Abstract

Background: Transcriptional profiling with ultra-low input methods can yield valuable insights into disease, particularly when applied to the study of immune cells using RNA-sequencing. The advent of these methods has allowed for their use in profiling cells collected in clinical trials and other studies that involve the coordination of human-derived material. To date, few studies have sought to quantify what effects that collection and handling of this material can have on resulting data.

Results: We characterized the global effects of blood handling, methods for leukocyte isolation, and preservation media on low numbers of immune cells isolated from blood. We found overall that storage/shipping temperature of blood prior to leukocyte isolation and sorting led to global changes in both CD8+ T cells and monocytes, including alterations in immune-related gene sets. We found that the use of a leukocyte filtration system minimized these alterations and we applied this method to generate high-quality transcriptional data from sorted immune cells isolated from the blood of intracerebral hemorrhage patients and matched healthy controls.

Conclusions: Our data underscore the necessity of processing samples with comparably defined protocols prior to transcriptional profiling and demonstrate that a filtration method can be applied to quickly isolate immune cells of interest while minimizing transcriptional bias.

Keywords: Immune profiling, Peripheral blood mononuclear cells, Transcriptome, RNA-seq

Background

Transcriptional profiling can yield valuable insights into cellular states and phenotypes across tissues and diseases [1, 2]. This approach is especially useful when applied to study cells and tissues in the context of perturbations such as drugs or disease state. These data allow for the inference of target pathways of interest [3], unique functional states [4], correlates of disease state [5], and novel subtype classifications [6].

Sequencing methods such as Smart-Seq2 to assess the transcriptome using RNA isolated from very low numbers of cells (~ 1–1,000) has enabled profiling of clinical samples containing very low numbers of cells, rare cell types, or rely on previously biobanked materials [7]. Many studies have identified optimal processing procedures and analysis methods for low-input or degraded RNA samples [8–11]. The availability of preservatives and stabilizing reagents for whole blood has also allowed the generation of high-quality data from ultra-low volumes of blood [12]. The application of transcriptional profiling to clinical samples, such as tissues and sorted populations of cells, however, presents unique and significant challenges associated with sample acquisition, sample processing, and tissue isolation. For example, multi-center studies often require centralized processing of patient samples; this transfer risks introducing bias. Additionally, RNA quality can vary widely between tissues [13], which can confound study design. Simply relying on acquiring enough high-quality samples to reach target

* Correspondence: bagoods@mit.edu; clove@mit.edu
†Jacqueline M. Vahey, Arthur S. Steinschneider, Lauren Sansing and J. Christopher Love contributed equally to this work.
1Department of Biological Engineering, Koch Institute for Integrative Cancer Research at the Massachusetts Institute of Technology, Cambridge, MA 02139, USA
Full list of author information is available at the end of the article

cohort sizes with high RNA quality is not always practical with rare or difficult to procure samples.

Few previous studies have sought to identify artifacts introduced into transcriptional data by sample handling in the context of RNA-sequencing. For expression profiles generated by microarrays or quantitative PCR, studies have identified several factors that can affect resulting data. One such study found that incubation time prior to standard procedures for leukocyte collection can rapidly change blood transcriptomics [14]. Shipping at 4 °C may mitigate these changes, but does not completely abrogate the effects. Another study, using microarrays, investigated the effect of time, temperature, and preservation on the transcriptome of isolated peripheral blood mononuclear cells (PBMCs) [15]: each preservation material tested had an effect on the transcriptome, but relied on large volumes of blood. To date, there has been a paucity of studies that have characterized artifacts introduced by the method of leukocyte isolation method followed by low input RNA-sequencing.

Here, we characterized the global effects of blood handling, method of leukocyte isolation, and preservation on low numbers of immune cells isolated from blood. We found overall that the storage/shipping temperature of blood prior to leukocyte isolation and sorting led to global changes in both CD8$^+$ T cells and monocytes, including alterations in immune-related gene sets. We found these alterations could be minimized through the use of a leukocyte filtration system, and we applied this method to generate high-quality transcriptional data from sorted immune cells isolated from the blood of patients with acute intracerebral hemorrhage and matched healthy controls.

Our data demonstrate the utility of our filtration approach and underscore the necessity of processing samples with defined and closely matched protocols prior to transcriptional profiling.

Results
Simulated approach for sample handling
We first sought to determine how methods for sample handling impact transcriptional data quality, composition, and downstream biological interpretation. We used blood since it is a readily available biological material that is often used for biomarker discovery and transcriptional profiling. To this end, we simulated several sample handling conditions that are typically encountered when profiling immune cells, and emphasized methods and handling techniques often associated with clinical trials or multi-site studies that require sample transport prior to analysis or tissue analysis (Fig. 1). Handling conditions included the effect of overnight shipping, various methods of leukocyte isolation, and the effect of a transcriptome preservation medium called CellCover. First, we compared processing over a Ficoll gradient directly after collection (freshly isolated) to whole blood shipped overnight at 20 °C or 4 °C (1 day at 20 °C and 1 day at 4 °C, respectively). Second, we tested the effect of the method used to isolate leukocytes from blood samples. Methods tested included i) Ficoll gradient isolation since this is typically used for blood (Ficoll), ii) collagenase/DNase digestion and subsequent isolation by percoll gradient since this is typically used for tissue (collagenase plus percoll), iii) RBC lysis as this is typically used for small amounts of aspirate or tissue

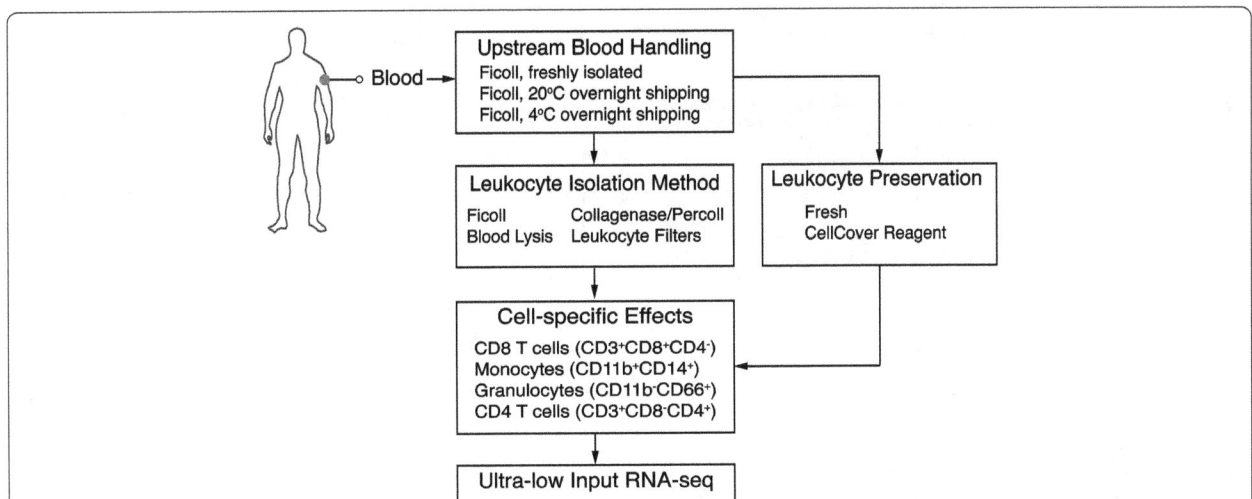

Fig. 1 Simulated sample handling methods. Diagram outlines methods used to simulate various sample handling techniques representative of those encountered in clinical immunology, including: blood shipping temperature (20 °C or 4 °C), peripheral blood mononuclear cell isolation method (Ficoll gradient, collagenase plus percoll gradient, whole blood lysis, leukocyte filtration), and immune cell types of interest (CD8$^+$ T cells, CD4$^+$ T cells, granulocytes or monocytes)

(whole blood lysis), and iv) a modified method for leukocyte filtration (whole blood filtration). The filtration method used was an adaptation of the LeukoLock filter system where whole blood is applied to the filter, which captures leukocytes while allowing red blood cells and platelets to pass through. The filters are then washed to further remove red blood cells and platelets and leukocytes are subsequently isolated by back flushing the filter. The comparison of Ficoll to collagenase plus percoll or whole blood lysis was particularly important, since many studies aim to compare blood and tissue compartments. Finally, we wanted to quantify the effect of CellCover, a solution that stabilizes RNA and other biomolecules in live cells and tissue by inhibiting enzymatic hydrolysis. This media was added after leukocyte isolation and has the advantage of allowing for antibody and live cell staining. After leukocyte isolation for each condition, cells were stained (Additional file 1: Table S1) and analyzed by flow cytometry.

Effects of blood shipping temperature, leukocyte isolation method, and preservation on percentage of cell types isolated

First we wanted to determine how storage/shipping, isolation, and preservation (Fig. 1) affected the percentage of immune cell types isolated. For each donor, we examined the percentage of the following immune cell types across each condition (Additional file 1: Figure S1): monocytes (CD11b$^+$CD66$^-$), granulocytes (CD11b$^-$CD66$^+$), CD4$^+$ T cells (CD3$^+$CD4$^+$CD8$^-$), and CD8$^+$ T cells (CD3$^+$CD4$^-$CD8$^+$). We found that shipping temperature, isolation method, and preservation all had some effect on the percentages of immune cell types isolated (Fig. 2), with some methods having a more significant impact than others (Additional file 1: Table S2). Globally, we found that shipping at 4 °C resulted in a statistically significant higher percentage of live granulocytes but a lower percentage of CD4$^+$ T cells isolated (Fig. 2a). Shipping temperature did not significantly affect CD8$^+$ T cells or monocytes. We also found that both

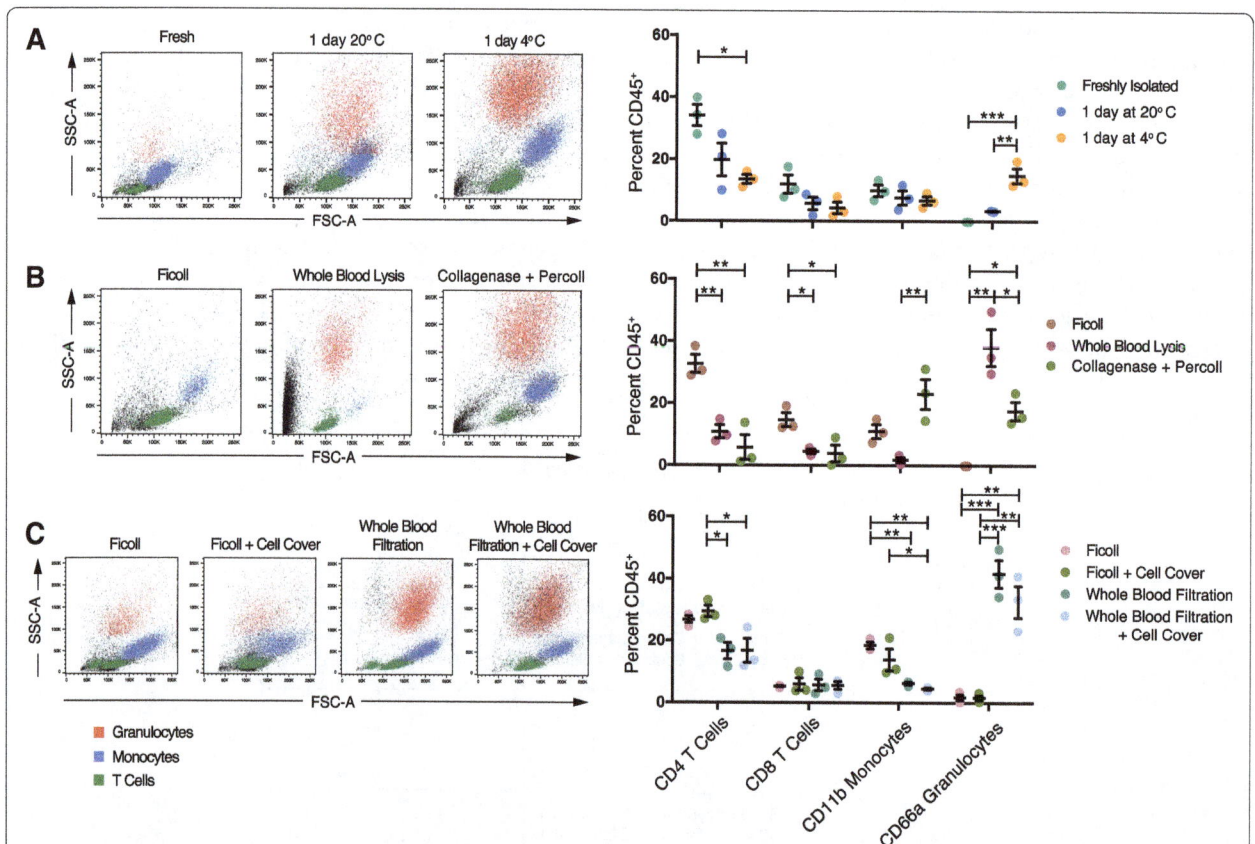

Fig. 2 Sample handling has differential effects on the percent of immune cell types isolated. Blood was processed according to the sample simulation schematic for (**a**) blood handling (fresh, 1 day at 4 °C, or 1 day at room temperature (20 °C) followed by Ficoll isolation), (**b**) PBMC isolation method (Ficoll, whole blood lysis, or collagenase plus percoll gradient), or (**c**) PBMC shipping method (fresh versus CellCover reagent) for Ficoll or filtration isolation methods. For each, example plots on the left are colored according to T cells (CD4$^+$, green), monocytes (CD11b$^+$CD66a$^-$, blue), granulocytes (CD11$^+$CD66a$^+$, red), or debris (black). Quantification of percentages of total CD45$^+$ PBMCs are shown for each replicate (*n* = 3) on the right. Statistical analyses were performed by one-way ANOVA with Tukey's multiple comparisons test within each cell type. Summary significance is shown in each panel and exact *P* values are reported in Additional file 1: Table S2

whole blood lysis and the collagenase plus percoll gradient resulted in more debris overall; the latter resulted in a significantly higher yield of monocytes compared to whole blood lysis (Fig. 2b). Overall, both whole blood lysis and collagenase plus percoll methods resulted in a lower yield of CD4$^+$ and CD8$^+$ T cells. Finally, we found that the addition of the CellCover reagent did not significantly impact either ficoll or whole blood-filtered protocols (Fig. 2c). Additionally, we found that whole blood filtration led to significantly greater yields of granulocytes with less debris, while still enabling isolation of comparable frequencies of T cells and monocytes. Together, these data suggest that the method chosen for upstream cell isolation could have a large impact on the percentages of desired cell types, which will significantly impact the isolation of rare populations of cells.

Blood handling and conventional leukocyte isolation methods alter the global transcriptome of monocytes and CD8$^+$ T cells

Given that immune cells are poised to quickly react to their surroundings, we sought to determine how each sample handling condition could affect the global transcriptome of isolated immune cells. We sorted two populations of immune cells representative of the T cell (CD8$^+$ T cells CD3$^+$CD8$^+$) and the innate (monocytes, CD11b$^+$CD66a$^-$) immune compartments into lysis buffer for low-input RNA-sequencing. RNA-sequencing libraries were generated as previously described [16]. In total, we profiled three healthy donors for each condition, resulting in 64 total libraries that were sequenced to a depth greater than 10 million reads (Additional file 2: Table S3). We found that the quality of libraries generated was not significantly affected by incubation temperature processing method, or preservation method, but that whole blood filtration resulted in slightly higher quality libraries for both T cells and monocytes (Additional file 1: Figure S2).

To determine global effects of upstream handling and processing on the transcriptome, we performed principal component analysis (PCA) on all coding genes across each condition for monocytes (Fig. 3a) and CD8$^+$ T cells (Fig. 3b) and are showing data projected along principal components 1 and 2 (PC1 and PC2). We also plotted pair-wise scatter plots of the average transcriptome (Fig. 3c and d) and each individual transcriptome (Additional file 1: Figures. S3 and S4) for each condition and performed linear regression. We found that for both monocytes and CD8$^+$ T cells, the fresh ficoll-isolated conditions clustered closely (Fig. 3 a, b), suggesting good correlation between independent experiments. Unsurprisingly, we found that for both monocytes and CD8$^+$ T cells, shipping at 20 °C resulted in transcriptomes that differed the most from the freshly-obtained Ficoll controls (Fig. 3b, d). We also found

that collagenase plus percoll and whole blood lysis isolation methods had a large effect on the monocytes, whereas shipping at 4 °C resembled the freshly-obtained controls (Fig. 3a). Pair-wise scatter plots across all donors (Additional file 1: Figure S3) also showed that collagenase plus percoll and whole blood lysis methods led to induced alterations in biological reproducibility as compared to Ficoll controls for the monocytes. For the CD8$^+$ T cells, the collagenase plus percoll and whole blood lysis methods did not have as large of an effect, with correlations remaining high across biological replicates (Additional file 1: Figure S4A) and on average (Fig. 3d). Overall, our data suggests that for monocytes, isolation with collagenase plus percoll or through whole blood lysis, and shipping at room temperature prior to isolation can induce global changes in the resulting transcriptome. For CD8$^+$ T cells, our data suggests that shipping at room temperature induced the largest global transcriptional changes.

In order to determine the biological nature of detected alterations, we performed single sample gene set enrichment analysis (ssGSEA) [17]. This method allows for comparison of enriched gene sets across all conditions of interest by generating individual enrichment scores for each gene set. Significantly different gene sets ($p < 0.05$) were identified through pair-wise comparisons of each condition tested to the freshly-isolated leukocytes obtained by Ficoll gradient as control for each processing condition (Additional file 3: Table S4). Gene sets that were significant for any comparison were merged and enrichment scores were hierarchically clustered across rows and columns, with gene sets as rows and samples as columns (Fig. 4). The top five significant gene sets are highlighted in each clustergram, where the color of each arrow indicates from which comparison it derives its significance to allow for global comparison. Overall, we found that each processing condition clustered together, indicating that sample processing alone can drive sample clustering. We also found that processing condition altered many gene sets, including immune-related gene sets. In general, temperature induced fewer changes than the method of leukocyte isolation. For monocytes, there was a cluster of gene sets that included Vascular endothelial growth factor (VEGF)-related signaling and RXR VDR pathway (retinoic acid related), that were significantly different between the shipping at 4 °C and fresh Ficoll conditions (Fig. 4a). This result may indicate that shipping at 4 °C could alter monocyte migration pathways and homeostasis pathways. For CD8$^+$ T cells, shipping at 20 °C induced alterations in cell cycle (circadian clock), ecosanoid ligand binding, and prolactin receptor signaling, all of which contribute to immune homeostasis (Fig. 4b) [18]. We also found that leukocyte isolation method induced alterations in immune-cell related signaling pathways. For monocytes, isolation by collagenase plus percoll led to increased

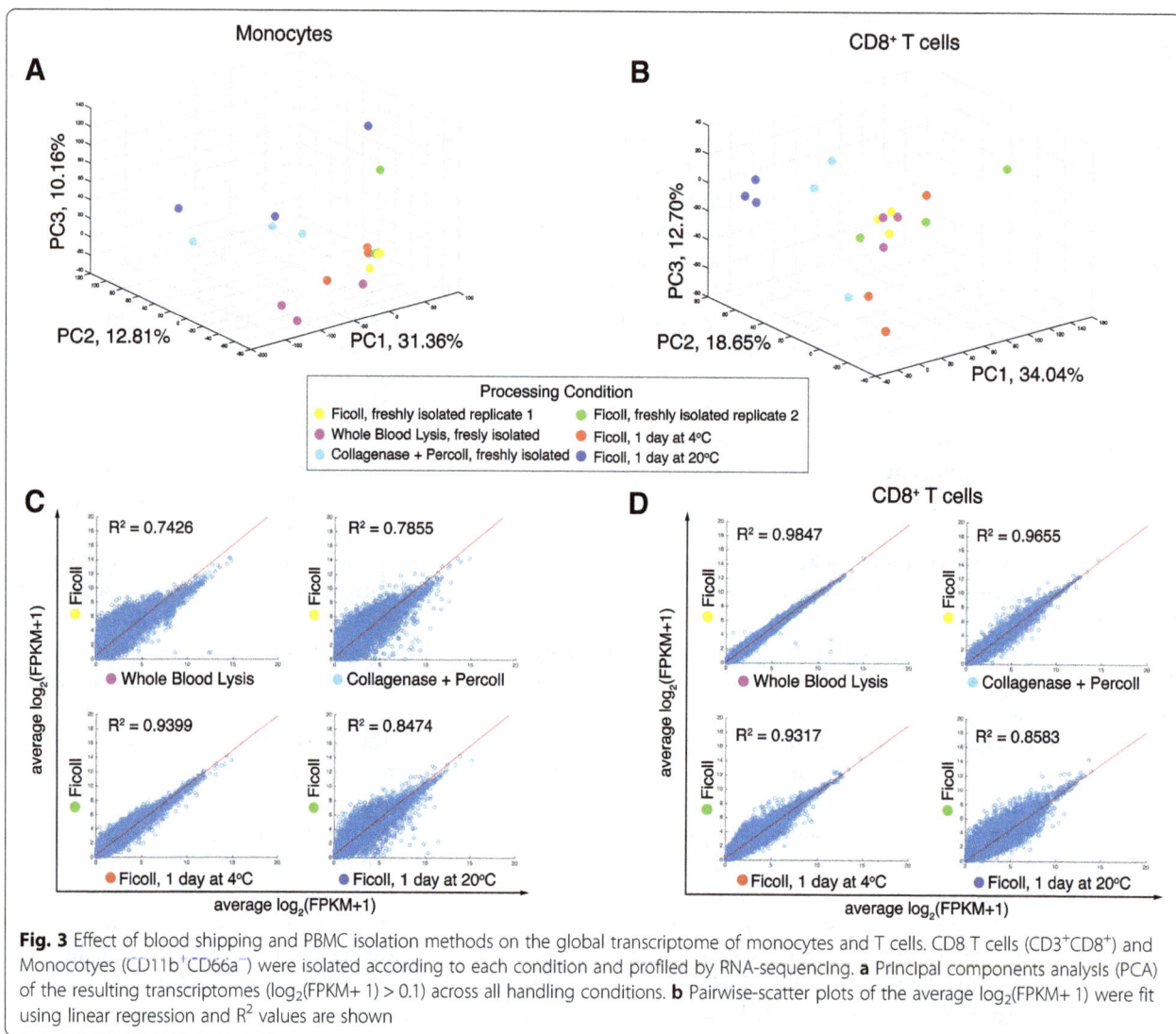

Fig. 3 Effect of blood shipping and PBMC isolation methods on the global transcriptome of monocytes and T cells. CD8 T cells (CD3⁺CD8⁺) and Monocotyes (CD11b⁺CD66a⁻) were isolated according to each condition and profiled by RNA-sequencing. **a** Principal components analysis (PCA) of the resulting transcriptomes (log₂(FPKM+ 1) > 0.1) across all handling conditions. **b** Pairwise-scatter plots of the average log₂(FPKM+ 1) were fit using linear regression and R² values are shown

enrichment in cytokine pathways, IL-23, and VEGF receptor interaction (Fig. 4c). Conversely, isolation by whole blood lysis or collagenase plus percoll actually abrogated a distinct set of gene sets enriched in the Ficoll control, including Phosphatidylinositol-4,5-bisphosphate 3-kinase/protein kinase B (PI3K/AKT) signaling, lagging strand synthesis, and nitric oxide 1 (NO1) signaling, the latter of which plays a key role in monocyte migration [19]. For CD8⁺ T cells, isolation with collagenase plus percoll led to enrichment of a distinct set of gene sets, including those that are relevant to T cell functionality, including cytotoxic-T-lymphocyte-associated protein 4 (CTLA-4) pathway, IL-7 signaling, and TNF Receptor Superfamily Member 1A (TNFR1) pathway (Fig. 4d). The effect of whole blood lysis on T cells is less clear, but there was a cluster of enriched gene sets abrogated in this condition, which included neurotrophin receptor p75 (p75 NTR) signaling. Taken together,

our data suggest that each isolation method induced specific alterations in gene signatures that may impact biological interpretation.

Mechanical isolation by filtration has minimal effect on the global transcriptome of CD8⁺ T cells and monocytes

Given that we found striking differences induced by conventional methods for sample handling, we sought to determine the effect of a mechanical isolation (filtration) method on the global transcriptome. We also sought to determine if preservation with CellCover, a transcriptome preservation reagent, could minimize effects of temporal delays during sample processing. As above, we generated pairwise scatter plots of the average across replicates for each comparison (Fig. 5a) and performed PCA (Fig. 5b). We found that mechanical isolation by whole blood filtration had no significant effect on the quality, and in some

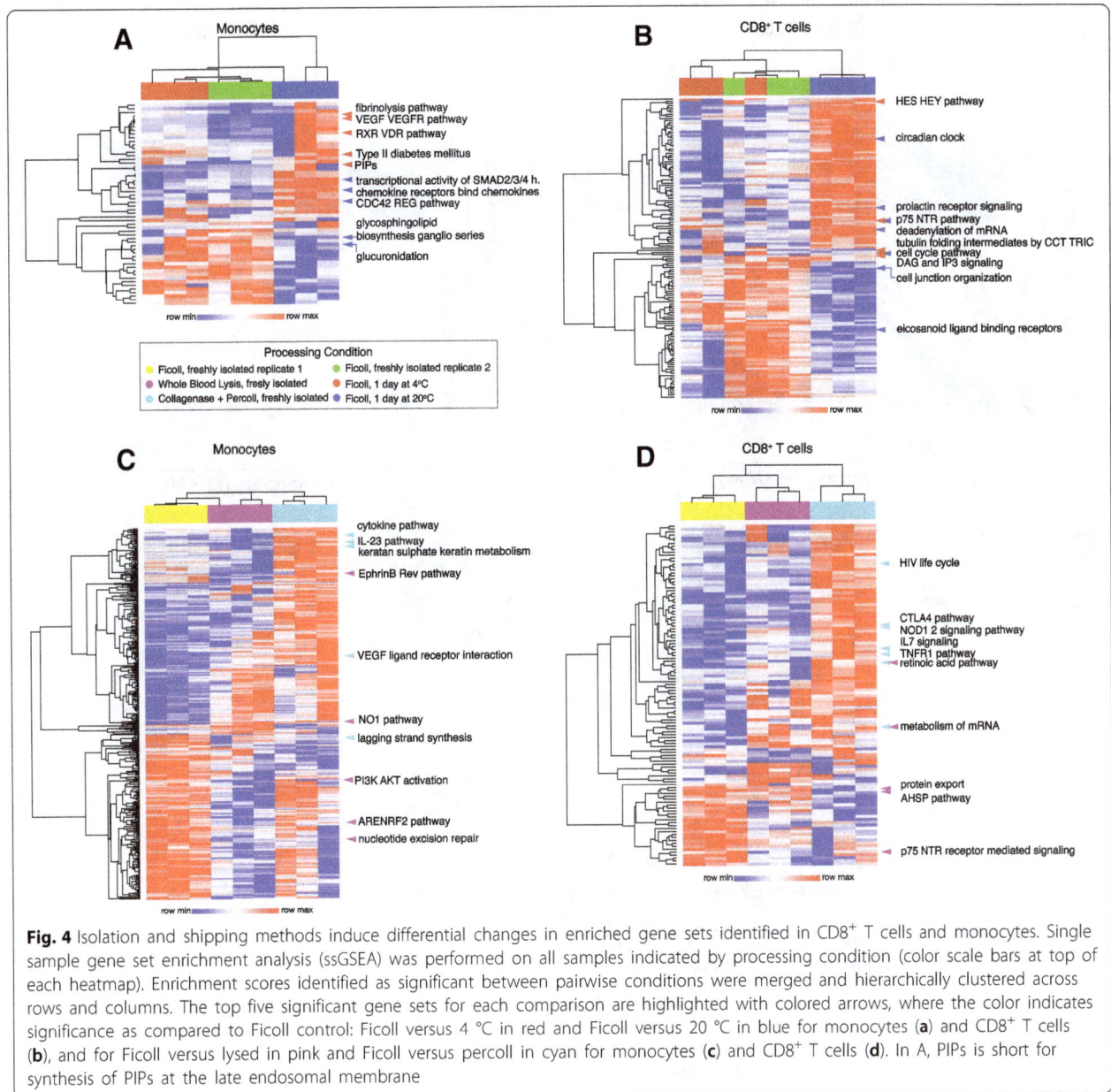

Fig. 4 Isolation and shipping methods induce differential changes in enriched gene sets identified in CD8[+] T cells and monocytes. Single sample gene set enrichment analysis (ssGSEA) was performed on all samples indicated by processing condition (color scale bars at top of each heatmap). Enrichment scores identified as significant between pairwise conditions were merged and hierarchically clustered across rows and columns. The top five significant gene sets for each comparison are highlighted with colored arrows, where the color indicates significance as compared to Ficoll control: Ficoll versus 4 °C in red and Ficoll versus 20 °C in blue for monocytes (**a**) and CD8[+] T cells (**b**), and for Ficoll versus lysed in pink and Ficoll versus percoll in cyan for monocytes (**c**) and CD8[+] T cells (**d**). In A, PIPs is short for synthesis of PIPs at the late endosomal membrane

cases actually improved the quality metrics of the resulting library (Additional file 1: Figure S2C, Table S1). We also found that the global transcriptome for both CD8[+] T cells and monocytes remained similar when isolated with filters, with high correlation values to the Ficoll control (Fig. 5a).

The inclusion of CellCover may actually induce variability in both monocytes and CD8[+] T cells. We observed clear outliers, regardless of filtration or Ficoll processing (Fig. 5b). We also performed ssGSEA and found overall fewer total gene sets altered (Additional file 4: Table S5). Of the top gene sets that were altered, surprisingly there were few related directly to immune function (Additional file 1: Figure S5A). For monocytes, unlike previous methods, we did not find alterations in VEGF or migration pathways, but did find

maintained alterations in P75NTR signaling (Additional file 1: Figure S5A). For CD8[+] T cells, we did not see induction of cytokine-related pathways, but did see alterations in pathways related to the cell matrix and platelets (Additional file 1: Figure S5B). Taken together, these data suggest that mechanical filtration, without CellCover, results in consistent transcriptomes generated by RNA-seq for both monocytes and CD8[+] T cells.

Application of leukocyte filtration to patient samples retains unique cell-type biology

Given that we found leukocyte filtration had minimal effect on the global transcriptome and allowed for fast processing of low volumes of biological material, we applied this

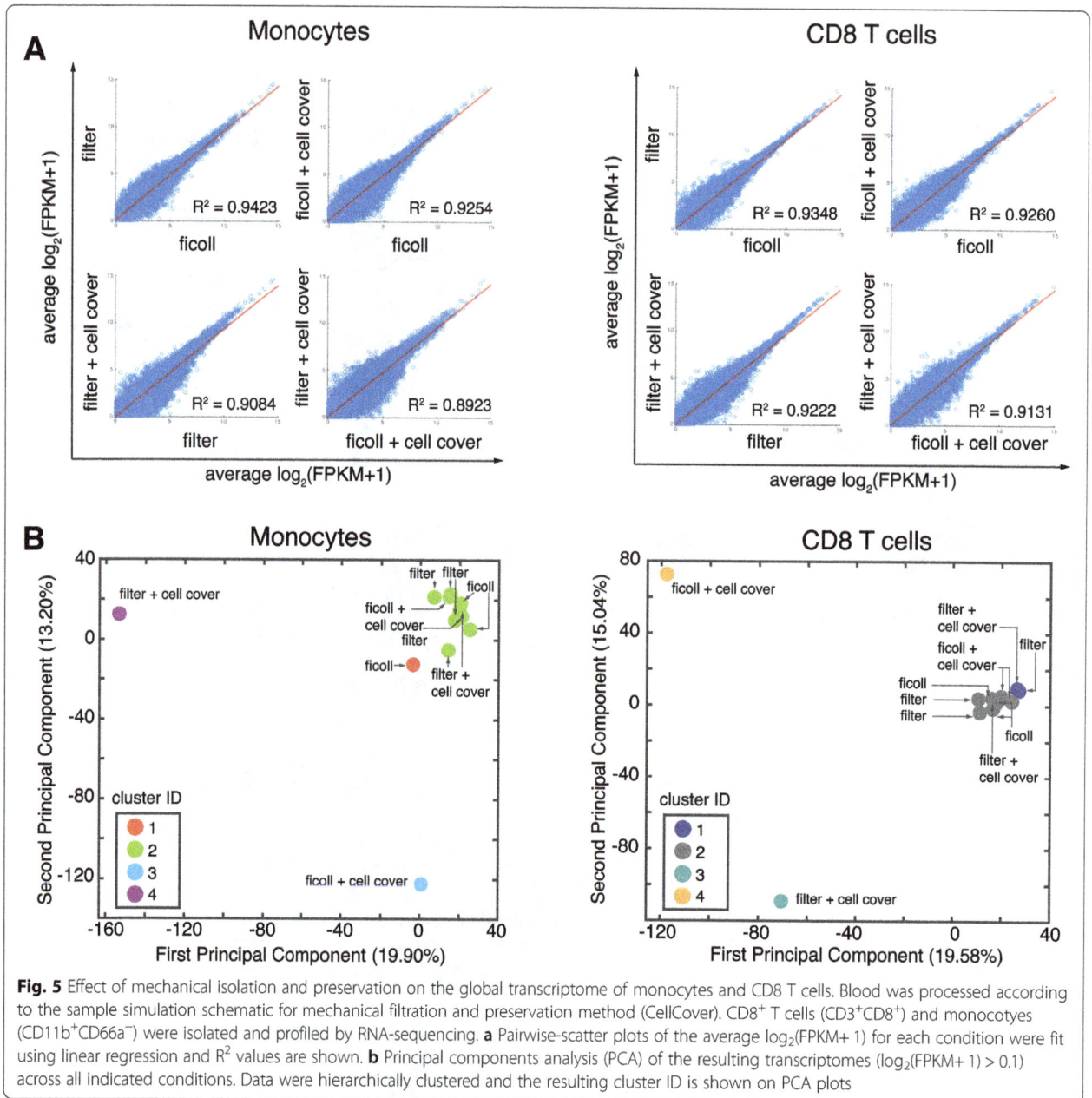

Fig. 5 Effect of mechanical isolation and preservation on the global transcriptome of monocytes and CD8 T cells. Blood was processed according to the sample simulation schematic for mechanical filtration and preservation method (CellCover). CD8$^+$ T cells (CD3$^+$CD8$^+$) and monocotyes (CD11b$^+$CD66a$^-$) were isolated and profiled by RNA-sequencing. **a** Pairwise-scatter plots of the average log$_2$(FPKM+ 1) for each condition were fit using linear regression and R^2 values are shown. **b** Principal components analysis (PCA) of the resulting transcriptomes (log$_2$(FPKM+ 1) > 0.1) across all indicated conditions. Data were hierarchically clustered and the resulting cluster ID is shown on PCA plots

method to low volumes of blood from intracerebral hemorrhage patients (ICH) and matched healthy donors (HD) to mimic material and workflows that would be obtained as part of a clinical study. We isolated leukocytes by filtration, stained for flow cytometry, and isolated monocytes, CD8$^+$ T cells and granulocytes (Additional file 1: Figure S6). Each isolated subset yielded high-quality data by RNA-sequencing (Additional file 1: Figure S7), including granulocytes. PCA across all data showed that cell types clustered together, and within each cluster separation between ICH and healthy-derived subsets were evident (Fig. 6a). Notably, CD8$^+$ T cells and CD66$^+$ granulocytes primarily segregated along PC1, with little separation

along PC2; CD14$^+$ monocytes were distinct from these populations along both PC1 and PC2. We next wanted to look at the highest-ranking genes driving separation between cell types (Fig. 6b). We found several genes that drive separation along PC1 that are characteristic of CD8$^+$ T cell identity (*Cd3d, Cd3e, Lck, CD8a*) or granulocyte identity (*S100a8, S100a9, Fpr1, Cxcr1*), agreeing with the observed separation of cells and granulocytes along this principal component. High-ranking genes driving separation along PC2 included several important for monocyte function (*Lyz, CD36, CD68*), in agreement with the separation of monocytes from other cell types along this principal

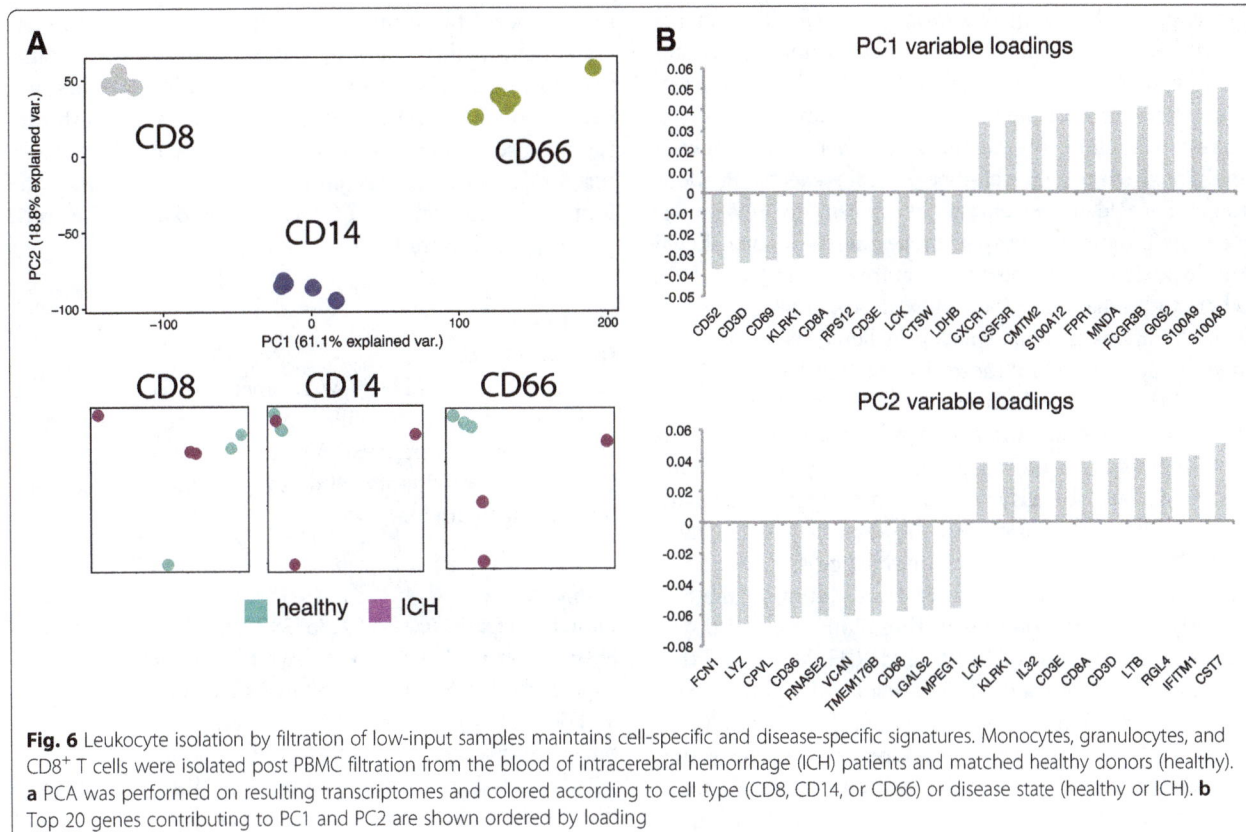

Fig. 6 Leukocyte isolation by filtration of low-input samples maintains cell-specific and disease-specific signatures. Monocytes, granulocytes, and CD8+ T cells were isolated post PBMC filtration from the blood of intracerebral hemorrhage (ICH) patients and matched healthy donors (healthy). **a** PCA was performed on resulting transcriptomes and colored according to cell type (CD8, CD14, or CD66) or disease state (healthy or ICH). **b** Top 20 genes contributing to PC1 and PC2 are shown ordered by loading

component. Taken together, our data suggest that leukocyte filtration retains cell specific biology in clinical samples while providing a fast workflow that is compatible with low volumes of material.

Discussion

Few studies have characterized artifacts that can be introduced into transcriptional data, especially data generated by sensitive methods like low-input RNA-sequencing. We sought to quantify how sample handling and leukocyte isolation method affects the global transcriptome of isolated immune cells, with emphasis on conditions that may be encountered when profiling blood and tissue (ie: solid tissue) associated with clinical trials and multi-center studies with the goal of providing data and guidance for early stage experimental design. We simulated upstream blood handling conditions (fresh, shipment of whole blood at 20 °C, or 4 °C overnight, where all were compared to fresh as a control), leukocyte isolation methods (Ficoll gradient isolation, collagenase/DNase digestion and subsequent Percoll gradient isolation, whole blood lysis, or a modified leukocyte filtration method, where Ficoll gradient isolation was used as a control), and leukocyte preservation methods (CellCover, where the absence of CellCover was used as a control).

We found that shipping temperature of blood prior to leukocyte isolation and sorting led to unique global

changes in both CD8+ T cells and monocytes. These included biologically meaningful alterations in immune-related gene sets, such as monocyte migration and homeostasis pathways in monocytes at 4 °C and cell cycle pathways at 20 °C in T cells. Our data also show that each method for leukocyte isolation can significantly impact the percent of isolated immune cells. This outcome can have a large impact on transcriptional studies, especially when starting from low-input material, including small volume blood draws, tissue biopsies, or aspirates. Thus, it is critical when designing clinical studies to choose a method that maximizes the cell type of scientific interest for the study. For example, if the main interest is to isolate granulocytes, processing with whole blood lysis or the newly described filtration method would yield the greatest fraction of granulocytes from a sample. Conversely, if the main interest were T cells, isolation with a Ficoll gradient from a fresh sample would yield the greatest fraction of T cells in the immune compartment.

We also observed global alterations in the transcriptome due to leukocyte isolation method, suggesting that each handling and leukocyte isolation condition induces distinct alterations in the global transcriptome of monocytes and CD8+ T cells. Isolation by collagenase plus percoll led to alterations in cytokine pathways in monocytes and T cell signaling, like the CTLA-4 pathway, in T cells. The latter is crucial because inhibitory pathways are biologically meaningful in many contexts, including cancer [20]. Transcriptome alterations are unique to the immune cell type of interest, with little overlap in altered gene sets between conditions, suggesting cell-type specific effects. Previous studies have identified alterations in gene expression induced by a temporal delay in processing, and have shown that hypoxia and apoptosis signatures are induced [15]. Other studies have also found that delays in processing induce alterations in RNA-splicing in liquid biopsies across large cohorts, including those derived from public repositories [14]. Here, we found that differences in processing can induce significant alterations in immune-related signatures that could lead to misinterpretation of resulting data sets. To account for this effect, our data suggests that samples must be processed comparably, especially when comparing blood and tissue-derived immune cells.

Finally, we applied a novel leukocyte filtration method to study the transcriptomes of three immune cell populations in the context of health and ICH. We found that leukocyte filtration leads to high-quality global transcriptomes across different immune cell types, results in retained disease-specific information, and suggests that cell identities are preserved in transcriptional space through enrichment in well-studied immune cell gene signatures. Importantly, transcriptomes generated using this filtration approach were highly correlated with those derived from Ficoll isolation, allowing comparison to previous studies that have used Ficoll. The filtration method, however, additionally allows for the collection of high-quality transcriptional data from granulocytes, even after overnight shipping at 4 °C. Together with our data from healthy donors, this suggests that processing samples with filtration allows for the recovery of high quality transcriptomes from a broad range of leukocytes and preserves biologically meaningful contexts of the original samples.

Conclusion
We found that the shipping temperature of blood and the method of isolation have global effects on the transcriptome of both immune cell types we studied. Specifically, our data suggests that isolation of immune cells from blood with collagenase plus percoll or through whole blood lysis, and shipping at room temperature prior to isolation can induce meaningful global alterations in monocyte transcriptomes. Similarly, for CD8+ T cells, shipping blood at room temperature prior to isolation induced the greatest global changes. These findings suggest that care should be taken when designing studies to ensure samples, both blood and tissue, are processing comparably. Strikingly, we found these alterations could be minimized through the use of a system

for leukocyte filtration. We applied this method to generate high-quality transcriptional data from sorted immune cells isolated from the blood of ICH patients and healthy donors. Taken together, our data suggest that sample processing has drastic effects on resulting transcriptional data across immune cell types, and the immune-related effects of these methods may be mitigated through filtration.

Methods
Human subjects
A total of nine subjects were analyzed for cell sorting and transcriptional profiling by RNA-seq according to IRB approved protocols. A total of six subjects were healthy blood donors and three were intracerebral hemorrhage patients.

Reagents
Lithium Heparin (catalog # 367886) and ACD-A (catalog # 364606) were obtained from BD Biosciences. Erythrocyte hypotonic lysis buffer was prepared by mixing 8.6 g NH4Cl in 1 L MilliQ water, and 0.2 um filtered. Azide-free FACS buffer was prepared with a final concentration of 2% BSA *w/v* and 1 mM EDTA. PBS (catalog # 14190144) was obtained from Gibco. BD Pharm Lyse (catalog # 555899) was purchased from BD Biosciences. Ficoll Paque PLUS (catalog # 17–1440-03) and Percoll (catalog # 17–0891-01) was obtained from GE Healthcare. Collagenase/displace (catalog # 10269638001) and DNAse (catalog # 10104159001) were obtained from Roche. The EasySep Human CD3 Positive Selection Kit II (catalog # 17851) was obtained from STEMCELL technologies. The monoclonal antibodies used to identify leukocyte subpopulations for cell sorting are listed in Additional file 1: Table S1.

Shipping conditions
In order to test the effect of sample transport temperature, two commercially available shipping container systems for biological samples were utilized: 4 °C in an activated cold shipping container (medium size, standard duration, nanoCool©) and 20 °C in a controlled room temperature shipping container with two phase change material insulators (Saf-T-Temp® CRT 10/30 (2) in a STP-302, Saf-T-Pak™). Each was shipped FedEx® Priority Overnight.

Leukocyte isolation by Ficoll gradient
Density gradient centrifugation was used to isolate leukocytes from a peripheral blood sample by spinning blood over Ficoll Paque Plus in a SepMate-50 (STEMCELL technologies, Inc., Canada) tubes following the manufacturer's protocol. Isolated cells were resuspended

in 1 ml of PBS and 1×10^6 cells were aliquoted for cell sorting.

Leukocyte isolation by whole blood lysis (RBC lysis)

Whole blood lysis was performed by mixing 1 ml of whole blood with 10 ml of erythrocyte hypotonic lysis buffer (161 μM NH$_4$Cl in MilliQ water) and incubating for 5 min at room temperature. The blood samples were then spun and the supernatants were removed by vacuum aspiration. An additional 10 ml of erythrocyte hypotonic lysis buffer was added to each blood sample, incubated for 5 min at room temperature, and spun again. The cell pellets were washed three times with PBS, resuspended in 1 ml of PBS and 1×10^6 cells were aliquoted for cell sorting.

Leukocyte isolation by DNAse/collagenase digestion and Percoll gradient

Whole blood was processed in a modified brain mononuclear cell preparation described previously [21]. Briefly, peripheral blood samples were passed through an 18-gauge needle. Then, 200 μl of collagenase/dispase (10 mg/ml) and 600 μl DNAse (10 mg/ml) were added to each vacutainer and incubated at 37 °C for 1 h. Samples were then diluted to 14 ml with PBS and spun at 500 RCF for 5 min. The plasma layer was discarded by aspirating with a vacuum, and then 1 ml of the packed formed blood elements was mixed with 70% Percoll solution (3.1 ml isotonic Percoll mixed with 0.9 ml HBSS) and layered under a 30% Percoll solution (2.6 ml isotonic Percoll mixed with 5.4 ml RPMI). The Percoll gradient was centrifuged at 500 RCF for 20 min without brakes. The cells were harvested from the 30:70 interface using a transfer pipette. The cells were washed three times with PBS, resuspended in 1 ml of PBS, and 1×10^6 cells were aliquoted for cell sorting.

Leukocyte isolation by filtration and subsequent hypotonic lysis

LeukoLock filters were used with a modified protocol from the manufacturer's instructions. The filters were sterilized by incubating the filters in 1.0 M NaOH and 2.0 M NaCl for 48 h at room temperature and were then washed by flushing twice with MilliQ water and twice with 70% ethanol. The filters were then vacuum dried and stored prior to use. Immediately prior to use the filters were flushed with 10 ml sterile PBS. After flushing, undiluted blood (6 mL) was pipetted directly from the vacutainer with a transfer pipette into the barrel of the syringe and allowed to pass through the filter by gravity. After the blood had passed through, the filters were rinsed by flushing with 3 ml of PBS. Leukocytes were harvested from the filter by connecting a female Luer coupler to the opposite end of the filter, and

backflushing with 20 mL PBS into a new tube. The cell suspensions were pelleted at 300 RCF for 8 min and then resuspended in 5 mL Pharm Lyse buffer (BD) and incubated for 15 min. The cell suspensions were then washed twice with PBS, counted, and then resuspended in 1 ml of PBS and 1×10^6 cells were aliquoted for cell sorting.

Cell cover

When indicated, cells were lightly fixed in CellCover (Anacyte) after isolation but before staining for FACS by resuspending the cells in 1 ml ice-cold CellCover and incubating on ice for 10 min. The cells were spun at 300 RCF for 8 min and then stained for cell sorting. After staining, the cells were resuspended in 300 μl of ice-cold CellCover instead of azide-free FACS buffer and kept on ice before sorting.

Isolation of leukocytes from intracerebral hemorrhage patients and healthy controls

Peripheral blood (8.5 mL) was collected from ICH patients and healthy controls in BD Vacutainer collection tubes with acid citrate dextran (Fisher Scientific) as an anti-coagulant and shipped overnight at 4 °C as described above. Leukocytes were isolated as described in the methods section titled "Leukocyte Isolation by Filtration and Subsequent Hypotonic Lysis". Leukocytes were incubated in CellCover for 10 min on ice and then washed with HBSS. T cells were separated from other leukocytes by magnetic selection prior to FACS using an EasySep™ Human CD3 Positive Selection Kit II (Stem Cell) according to the manufacturer's instructions and subsequently, the CD3$^+$ and CD3$^-$ fractions were stained individually. Briefly, cells were washed in ice-cold EasySep buffer (2% FBS, 1 mM EDTA in PBS) and subsequently stained with antibodies detailed in Additional file 1: Table S1 on ice for 15 min. Cells were incubated on ice prior to sorting on a BD FACS Aria II for CD8$^+$ T cells and CD14$^+$ monocytes.

Fluorescence-activated cell sorting

Leukocyte populations were labeled with fluorescent conjugated antibodies and processed for fluorescence activation cell sorting (FACS). Antibodies used for each sorting panel and target cell population in this study are shown in Additional file 1: Table S1. Briefly: 1×10^6 cells washed with 1 ml of PBS and centrifuged at 500 RCF for 5 min. The supernatants were aspirated, and the cell pellets were resuspended in 50ul human AB serum for 10 min to block Fc receptors. After Fc Block, 50 μl of the antibody cocktail was added to each sample and incubated for 20 min. The cells were washed with 1 ml PBS and centrifuged at 500 RCF for 5 min. The cells were then stained for dead cell exclusion by resuspending them in LIVE/DEAD Fixable Red Dead Cell Stain solution diluted 1:10,000 in PBS and incubated for 20 min. The samples were then washed with 1 ml of azide-free FACS buffer (2% BSA *w/v* and 1 mM EDTA in PBS) and spun at 500 RCF for 5 min. The supernatants were removed, and the cells were resuspended in 300 ul azide-free FACS buffer and kept on ice until cell sorting. All cell populations were isolated using fluorescent-activated cell sorting FACS Aria II (BD Biocsciences). The cells were sorted directly into 100 μl lysis buffer (RA1 spiked with 10 mM TCEP) and frozen at − 80 °C.

Preparation of RNA-seq libraries

RNA was extracted using the NucleoSpin RNA XS Kit (Macherey-Nagel) according to the manufacturers instructions. cDNA synthesis and amplification were performed using SMARTer Ultra Low Input RNA V3 or V4 as indicated for Illumina Sequencing (Clontech) according to the manufacturers instructions. The input RNA was normalized prior to cDNA generation by diluting to ~ 1,000 cells per reaction. Paired-end sequencing libraries were prepared using the Nextera XT DNA sample Prep Kit (Illumina) according to the manufacturers instructions. Libraries were pooled in an equimolar ratio and sequenced on a NextSeq500 sequencer with 200 cycles per lane (Illumina).

Transcriptional analysis

All samples were processed with STAR (v2.4.1d) and RSEM (v1.2.30). STAR was run on eight threads to align reads to a previously constructed transcriptome, with a reduced number of "spurious" junctions. A maximum number of 20 different alignments were allowed for each read. If this maximum was exceeded, the read was considered unmapped. A minimum overhang of 8 was permitted for unannotated junctions and a minimum overhang of 1 was permitted for annotated junctions. The maximum number of allowed mismatches per pair was 999, and the allowable intron length was between 10 and 1,000,000. The maximum genomic distance between mates was 1,000,000 and most of these settings used were the default according to the STAR manual provided by the developer (STAR --runThreadN 8 --runMode alignReads --genomeDir /home/Genomes/ hg19_75_STAR/ --readFilesIn $read1 $read2 --outFilterType BySJout --outFilterMultimapNmax 20 --alignSJoverhangMin 8 --alignSJDBoverhangMin 1 --outFilterMismatchNmax 999 --alignIntronMin 10 --alignIntronMax 1000000 --alignMatesGapMax 1000000 --outFileNamePrefix STAR_output/ ${sampleprefix} --outSAMtype BAM SortedByCoordinate --quantMode TranscriptomeSAM). RSEM was run on paired-end reads, calculating 95% credibility intervals and posterior mean estimates (rsem-calculate-expression --paired-end --calc-ci -bam −p 8). FPKMs were log

transformed post adding pseudocount of 1 and all down-stream analyses were performed on coding genes.

Principal component analysis, clustering, and ssGSEA

Principal component analysis (PCA) was performed on interquartile-normalized data filtered for $\log_2$ (FPKM+ 1) > 0.1 using custom scripts in MATLAB (vR2015a) using the pca() function. Clustering was performed using Morpheus (hierarchical, one minus Pearson correlation) available through the Broad Institute or custom scripts in MATLAB. To enable global comparison across conditions to infer biological changes induced or masked by sample handling, single sample gene set enrichment (ssGSEA, v7) was performed [17] using the following settings: C2CPv5.1 gene sets, rank, weighting at 0.75, and minimum gene set size of 10. Significant gene sets were identified by paired t tests (with and without Benjamini-Hochberg FDR) of each condition to Ficoll isolated or fresh isolated, then merged and clustered hierarchically.

Statistical analysis

Statistical analysis, including one-way ANOVA with Tukeys multiple comparisons test and students t test, was performed in Prism (v 7.0c). Statistical tests performed are indicated in the figure legends where data is presented.

Additional files

Additional file 1: Supplemental Material contains the following data: **Figure S1.** Sorting strategy used to profile peripheral blood mononuclear cells (PBMCs) from blood of healthy donors across all conditions tested. Antibodies are listed in Table 1. **Figure S2.** Exon/intergenic ratios are plotted for each indicated condition for (**A**) monocytes, (**B**) T cells and (**C**) for filtration as compared to ficoll. Statistically significant comparisons are indicated and were calculated by one-way ANOVA with Tukey's multiple comparisons test. **Figure S3.** Pairwise scatter plots of coding transcriptomes generated from monocytes for each indicated comparison. Regression lines and R^2 values are shown on each plot for (**A**) ficoll, percoll and lysis processing conditions, and (**B**) ficoll, 4 °C for 1 day or 20 °C for 1 day conditions. **Figure S4.** Pairwise scatter plots of coding transcriptomes generated from CD8+ T cells for each indicated comparison. Regression lines and R^2 values are shown on each plot for (**A**) ficoll, percoll and lysis processing conditions, and (**B**) ficoll, 4 °C for 1 day or 20 °C for 1 day conditions. **Figure S5.** ssGSEA results for ficoll and filter methods for isolation of PBMCs. Forest plots of top 15 significantly altered gene sets when PBMCs are isolated using filters for monocytes (**A**) and CD8+ T cells (**B**). **Figure S6.** Flow cytometry isolation scheme for sequencing data generated from cells isolated from intracerebral hemorrhage (ICH) and matched healthy donors (HD). **Figure S7.** Quality control metrics for sequencing data generated from cells isolated from intracerebral hemorrhage (ICH) and matched healthy donors (HD). (**A**) Exon/intergenic ratio for each indicated condition. No statistically significant differences were found when comparing healthy to ICH within each cell type by students t test. (**B**) Percent mapped reads for each indicated condition. No statistically significant differences were found when comparing healthy to ICH within each cell type by students t test for each percent metric plotted. **Table S1.** Antibodies used for cell sorting in this study. **Table S2.** Summary statistics performed by one-way ANOVA with Tukey's multiple comparisons test for data shown in Fig. 2. (DOCX 3717 kb)

Additional file 2: Table S3. Quality control metrics for each library generated. Sample names, figure corresponding to data, cell type, and condition are indicated. (XLSX 65 kb)

Additional file 3: Table S4. ssGSEA results and significant comparisons. (XLSX 86 kb)

Additional file 4: Table S5. *P* values for each comparison of ssGSEA results for Fig. 5. Gene sets for which any comparison yielded a significant (*p* < 0.05) value is shown. (XLSX 52 kb)

Abbreviations
CTLA-4: Cytotoxic-T-lymphocyte-associated protein 4; HD: Healthy donor; ICH: Intracerebral hemorrhage; NO1: Nitric oxide 1; p75 NTR: Neurotrophin receptor p75; PBMCs: Peripheral blood mononuclear cells; PCA: Principal component analysis; PCR: Polymerase chain reaction; PI3K AKT: Phosphatidylinositol-4,5-bisphosphate 3-kinase/protein kinase B; RBC: Red blood cell; RNA: Ribonucleic acid; ssGSEA: Single sample gene set enrichment analysis; TNFR1: TNF Receptor Superfamily Member 1A; VEGF: Vascular endothelial growth factor

Acknowledgements
We would like to thank the Koch Institute Swanson Biotechnology Center for technical support, specifically the BioMicroCenter for assistance with RNA sequencing and data processing.

Funding
This work was supported by a National Institutes of Health Grant through the National Institute of Neurological Disorders and Stroke (Project Number: 5R01NS097728–02). This work was also supported in part by the Koch Institute Support (core) Grant P30-CA14051 from the National Cancer Institute. B.A.G is supported in part by a fellowship from the National Science Foundation and the Siebel Scholars Foundation.

Authors' contributions
BAG, AS, LHS, and JCL conceived of and designed the study. BAG, JV, AS, and MA generated and analyzed data. BAG, AS, LS, JV, MA, and JCL interpreted results. BAG, AS, LHS and JCL wrote the manuscript with input from all authors. All authors have read and approve the current manuscript.

Competing interests
The authors declare that they have no competing interests.

Author details
[1]Department of Biological Engineering, Koch Institute for Integrative Cancer Research at the Massachusetts Institute of Technology, Cambridge, MA 02139, USA. [2]Department of Electrical Engineering and Computer Science, Massachusetts Institute of Technology, Cambridge, MA 02139, USA. [3]Department of Neurology, Yale School of Medicine, New Haven, CT 06520, USA. [4]Department of Chemical Engineering, Koch Institute for Integrative Cancer Research at the Massachusetts Institute of Technology, Cambridge, MA 02139, USA. [5]The Broad Institute of the Massachusetts Institute of Technology and Harvard, Cambridge, MA 02142, USA.

References
1. McGettigan PA. Transcriptomics in the RNA-seq era. Curr Opin Chem Biol Elsevier Ltd. 2013;17:4–11.
2. Chaussabel D, Pascual V, Banchereau J. Assessing the human immune system through blood transcriptomics. BMC Biol. 2010;8:84–14.
3. Melas IN, Sakellaropoulos T, Iorio F, Alexopoulos LG, Loh W-Y, Lauffenburger DA, et al. Identification of drug-specific pathways based on gene expression data: application to drug induced lung injury. Integr Biol. Royal Society of Chemistry. 2015:1–17.
4. Simeoni O, Piras V, Tomita M, Selvarajoo K. Tracking global gene expression responses in T cell differentiation. Gene. Elsevier B.V; 2015;:1–8.
5. Ottoboni L, Keenan BT, Tamayo P, Kuchroo M, Mesirov JP, Buckle GJ, et al. An RNA Profile Identifies Two Subsets of Multiple Sclerosis Patients Differing in Disease Activity. Sci Transl Med. 2012;4:153ra131.
6. Doucette T, Rao G, Rao A, Shen L, Aldape K, Wei J, et al. Immune heterogeneity of glioblastoma subtypes: extrapolation from the Cancer genome atlas. Cancer Immunol Res. 2013;1:112–22.
7. Picelli S, Faridani OR, ASKBO R, GOS W, Sagasser S, Sandberg R. full-length RNA-seq from single cells using smart-seq2. Nat Protoc. Nat Publ Group. 2014;9:171–81.
8. Adiconis X, Borges-Rivera D, Satija R, DeLuca DS, Busby MA, Berlin AM, et al. Comparative analysis of RNA sequencing methods for degraded or low-input samples. Nat Meth. 2013;10:623–9.
9. Chen EA, Souaiaia T, Herstein JS, Evgrafov OV, Spitsyna VN, Rebolini DF, et al. Effect of RNA integrity on uniquely mapped reads in RNA-Seq. 2014;7:1–3.
10. Janes J, Hu F, Lewin A, Turro E. A comparative study of RNA-seq analysis strategies. Brief Bioinform. 2015;16(6):932–40. https://doi.org/10.1093/bib/bbv007.
11. Rapaport F, Khanin R, Liang Y, Pirun M, Krek A, Zumbo P, et al. Comprehensive evaluation of differential gene expression analysis methods for RNA-seq data. Genome Biol. BioMed Central Ltd. 2013;14:R95.
12. Robison EH, Mondala TS, Williams AR, Head SR, Salomon DR, Kurian SM. Whole genome transcript profiling from fingerstick blood samples: a comparison and feasibility study. BMC Genomics. 2009;10:617–9.
13. GTEx Consortium. Human genomics. The Genotype-Tissue Expression (GTEx) pilot analysis: Multitissue gene regulation in humans. Science. 2015; 348(6235):648–60. https://doi.org/10.1126/science.1262110.
14. Dvinge H, Ries RE, Ilagan JO, Stirewalt DL, Meshinchi S, Bradley RK. Sample processing obscures cancer-specific alterations in leukemic transcriptomes. Proc Natl Acad Sci. 2014;111:16802–7.
15. Debey S, Schoenbeck U, Hellmich M, Gathof BS, Pillai R, Zander T, et al. Comparison of different isolation techniques prior gene expression profiling of blood derived cells: impact on physiological responses, on overall expression and the role of different cell types. Pharmacogenomics J. 2004;4:193–207.
16. Cao Y, Goods BA, Raddassi K, Nepom GT, Kwok WW, Love JC, et al. Functional inflammatory profiles distinguish myelin-reactive T cells from patients with multiple sclerosis. Science Transl Med. American Association for the Advancement of Science. 2015;7:287ra74.
17. Barbie DA, Tamayo P, Boehm JS, Kim SY, Moody SE, Dunn IF, et al. Systematic RNA interference reveals that oncogenic KRAS-driven cancers require TBK1. Nature Nature Publishing Group. 2009;461:108–12.
18. Radhakrishnan A, Raju R, Tuladhar N, Subbannayya T, Thomas JK, Goel R, et al. A pathway map of prolactin signaling. J Cell Commun Signal. 2012;6:169–73.
19. Wink DA, Hines HB, Cheng RYS, Switzer CH, Flores-Santana W, Vitek MP, et al. Nitric oxide and redox mechanisms in the immune response. J Leukoc Biol. 2011;89:873–91.
20. Sharma P, Allison JP. The future of immune checkpoint therapy. Science. 2015;348:56–61.
21. Wilson EH, Wille-Reece U, Dzierszinski F, Hunter CA. A critical role for IL-10 in limiting inflammation during toxoplasmic encephalitis. J Neuroimmunol. 2005;165:63–74.

13

Renal allograft rejection, lymphocyte infiltration, and de novo donor-specific antibodies in a novel model of non-adherence to immunosuppressive therapy

Louisa Kühne[1]*, Bettina Jung[1], Helen Poth[1], Antonia Schuster[1], Simone Wurm[1], Petra Ruemmele[2], Bernhard Banas[1] and Tobias Bergler[1]

Abstract

Background: Non-adherence has been associated with reduced graft survival. The aim of this study was to investigate the immunological mechanisms underlying chronic renal allograft rejection using a model of non-adherence to immunosuppressive therapy. We used a MHC (major histocompatibility complex) -mismatched rat model of renal transplantation (Brown Norway to Lewis), in which rats received daily oral cyclosporine A. In analogy to non-adherence to therapy, one group received cyclosporine A on alternating days only. Rejection was histologically graded according to the Banff classification. We quantified fibrosis by trichrome staining and intra-graft infiltration of T cells, B cells, and monocytes/macrophages by immunohistochemistry. The distribution of B lymphocytes was assessed using immunofluorescence microscopy. Intra-graft chemokine, chemokine receptor, BAFF (B cell activating factor belonging to the TNF family), and immunoglobulin G transcription levels were analysed by RT-PCR. Finally, we evaluated donor-specific antibodies (DSA) and complement-dependent cytotoxicity using flow cytometry.

Results: After 28 days, cellular rejection occurred during non-adherence in 5/6 animals, mixed with humoral rejection in 3/6 animals. After non-adherence, the number of T lymphocytes were elevated compared to daily immunosuppression. Monocyte numbers declined over time. Accordingly, lymphocyte chemokine transcription was significantly increased in the graft, as was the transcription of BAFF, BAFF receptor, and Immunoglobulin G. Donor specific antibodies were elevated in non-adherence, but did not induce complement-dependent cytotoxicity.

Conclusion: Cellular and humoral rejection, lymphocyte infiltration, and de novo DSA are induced in this model of non-adherence.

Keywords: Donor specific antibodies, Humoral rejection, Renal transplantation, Non-adherence, Leukocyte infiltration, BAFF

Background

Although short-term renal allograft survival has improved over the past decades, long-term graft survival is still limited with overall 5- and 10-year graft survival rates of 77 and 56% respectively in Europe [1]. Research efforts have therefore focused on identifying ways to prolong graft survival. A multitude of factors are responsible for chronic allograft failure, including concomitant disease, calcineurin-inhibitor (CNI) toxicity, recurrent or de novo renal disease, as well as chronic allograft rejection [2]. Among these factors, chronic rejection most frequently causes graft failure [2, 3]. In this context, subclinical inflammation in renal allografts [4–6] and the serological appearance of de novo donor-specific antibodies (dnDSA) have been strongly implicated as factors for reduced graft survival [3, 7–9]. A major cause for the formation of de novo DSA is non-adherence to immunosuppressive therapy [3], and

* Correspondence: Louisa.Kuehne@ukr.de
[1]Department of Nephrology, University Hospital Regensburg, Franz-Josef-Strauß Allee 11, D-93053 Regensburg, Germany
Full list of author information is available at the end of the article

numerous studies show that non-adherence itself is a risk factor for reduced graft survival [10–12].

Antibody mediated rejection (ABMR) is known to be a major contributor to graft loss [3]. Histologically, the hallmark feature of chronic antibody mediated rejection is transplant glomerulopathy (TG), which has been shown to correlate with the formation of DSA and specific patterns of C4d deposition [13]. Interstitial fibrosis and tubular atrophy (IF/TA), though non-specific, frequently accompany TG in chronic ABMR. Another histopathological feature, which has been observed in chronically rejected grafts, are B cell rich tertiary lymphoid organs (TLO) [14], which have also been found in other types of chronically inflamed tissues.

Since dnDSA and ABMR are prominent causes of graft failure, increasing attention has been drawn to B cells, due to their function as antibody-producers, as well as regulatory functions, such as cytokine production. However, so far B cells have not been specifically targeted by standard immunosuppressive protocols in renal transplantation, apart from some special applications, such as ABO-incompatible renal transplantation. Furthermore, the benefit of B cell depleting agents, such as Rituximab, in the treatment of ABMR remains controversial [15]. Other B cell targeted therapies have been developed for chronic inflammatory and autoimmune diseases [16, 17], but their contribution in allogeneic solid organ transplantation is still under scrutiny.

Previously, we reported on a notable difference in the relative infiltration of B-lymphocytes in the context of allogeneic vs. syngeneic transplantation in a rat kidney transplant model [18]. In the current study, we used a rat model reflecting non-adherence to immunosuppressive therapy, to answer to following questions: 1.) to what extent can non-adherence cause rejection 2.) what effect does non-adherence have on infiltrating leukocyte populations 3.) how are chemokine transcription patterns affected 4.) how are intra-renal B-cells affected and 5.) does non-adherence result in the development of donor specific antibodies?

To this end, we used a MHC-mismatched rat model of allogeneic renal transplantation.

Methods
Animals/experimental renal transplantation
Animal experiments were performed according to German animal protection laws and NIH's laboratory animal care principles. Study approval was granted by the inspecting authority (Regierung der Oberpfalz). A MHC-mismatched rat kidney transplantation model was used, as previously described [19]. Male Brown Norway rats (BN) served as donors and male Lewis rats (LEW) as recipients (Charles River Laboratories, Sulzfeld, Germany, 200–250 g). Kidney transplantation was either

syngeneic (Lewis-to-Lewis) or allogeneic (Brown-Norway-to-Lewis).

Kidney transplantation (Tx) was performed as previously described [19]. In brief, left BN kidneys were explanted, flushed with cold saline and transplanted orthotopically in Lewis rats by end-to-end anastomosis of the ureter and blood vessels. Cold and warm ischemia times were approximately 35 and 30 min, respectively. Nephrectomy of the right kidney was performed at the end of the surgery.

All animals with allogeneic transplantation were treated with cyclosporine A (CyA 5 mg/kg body weight; Neoral, Novartis, Basel, Switzerland), administered once daily by gavage. In one group, CyA was administered only on alternating days after day 6, in analogy to non-adherence to immunosuppressive therapy ("Tx d28 CyA alt."). Rats were sacrificed 6 and 28 days after transplantation. In general, syngeneic transplantation was used as a control, except for complement-dependent-cytotoxicity assay, where Lewis rat serum from day 0 was used.

Groups were abbreviated as follows:
Syngeneic transplantation sacrificed on day 6 (SynTxd6), allogeneic transplantation with daily CyA sacrificed on day 6 or day 28 (Txd6CyA, Txd28CyA), and allogeneic transplantation with CyA administered on alternating days, sacrificed on day 28 (Txd28CyAalt). Groups consisted of 6 to 11 animals.

Harvested organs were divided into quarters and either fixed in paraffin or snap-frozen in N_2 and stored at −80 °C, or processed for flow cytometry.

Histology, Immunohistochemistry and Immunofluorescence
Paraffin sections were prepared from rat kidneys as previously described [20]. After staining with hematoxylin and eosin (HE) and periodic acid schiff (PAS) stains, the histomorphological alterations were classified according to the Banff classification [21] by an experienced pathologist.

Immunohistochemistry was performed on 3 μm formalin-fixed, paraffin-embedded sections as previously described [18]. Primary antibodies included polyclonal rabbit anti-rat CD3 antibody (1:100, Abcam, ab5690, Cambridge, UK), polyclonal goat anti-rat CD20 antibody (1:100, Santa Cruz, sc-7735, Heidelberg, Germany), monoclonal mouse anti-rat CD68 antibody (1:150, Serotec, MCA341GA, Oxford, UK), rabbit anti-rat C4d antibody (Hycultec, HP8034, Beutelsbach, Germany), goat polyclonal anti-CCL21 / SLC antibody (aa24–133) (LS-C150160, Lifespan Biosciences, Seattle, USA), rabbit monoclonal anti-CCR7 antibody (Y59, ab32527, Abcam, Cambridge, UK). Secondary antibodies were goat anti-rabbit-biotin (Dianova, 111–065-144, Hamburg, Germany), mouse anti-goat-biotin (Dianova, 205–065-108, Hamburg,

Germany), donkey anti-mouse-biotin (Dianova, 715–065-150, Hamburg, Germany). Staining was done using DAB (0.4 mg/ml, Sigma, D5637, St. Louis, USA) and AP-RED (Zytomed, ZUC001–125, Berlin, Germany). For CCL21 staining, anti-goat-Polymer-HRP Kit (Vector laboratories, Immpress Reagent Anti-Goat Ig HRP, MP-7405, Peterborough, UK) was used as a secondary antibody. C4d staining was enhanced using AP-One-Step Polymer (Zytomed, ZUC068–006, Berlin, Germany) with Permanent AP RED Kit (Zytomed, ZUC001–125, Berlin, Germany) as secondary antibody. For CCL21 and CCR7, two to three sections from randomly selected rats from each group were stained.

CD20, CD3, and CD68 staining was analyzed using Histoquest® software. Digital pictures were taken and 10 high power fields (HPF) per specimen were examined for analysis (original × 400, covering an area of 296 μm × 222 μm) of each graft as previously described [18]. Using Histoquest® software, the number of CD68$^+$, CD20$^+$, and CD3$^+$ cells were counted in relation to all cells within a defined area. Furthermore, we used immunofluorescence to better visualize the distribution of CD20$^+$ cell population within the grafts on formalin-fixed, paraffin-embedded materials.

Immunofluorescence staining for CD20 was performed as previously described [20] on 1–2 randomly selected sections from each experimental group. Sections (4 μm) were deparaffinized and rehydrated. Antigen retrieval was performed in a decloaking chamber (Biocare Medical, Pacheco, USA) by treatment in citrate buffer and Antigen Unmasking Solution (Linaris, H-3300, Dossenheim, Germany). Sections were blocked using Superblock Solution (Pierce Technology, 37,515, Rockford, USA). The polyclonal goat anti-rat CD20 antibody (1:100, Santa Cruz, sc-7735, Heidelberg, Germany) was used at 1:100 in PBS overnight. After subsequent washing steps, the tissue was incubated with the donkey anti-goat-FITC antibody (1:500 in PBS, Dianova, 705–095-147, Hamburg, Germany) for 1 h at room temperature. Cell nuclei were stained using Hoechst 33,342 (Molecular Probes H-1399, Waltham, USA) 1:50,000 in PBS for 2 min. at room temperature. Sections were assessed and images taken using a Zeiss observer Z.1 Fluorescence microscope at 20× magnification. Staining specificity of anti-CD20, anti-CD3, and anti-CD68 antibodies was confirmed by anatomical staining pattern of B, and T cells, and monocytes/macrophages respectively in immunofluorescence of rat spleen sections, showing CD20-positive B cell zones and CD3-positive T cell zones in splenic follicles, as well as dispersed distribution of CD68-positive macrophages in the splenic red pulp (Additional file 1 and Additional file 2). A facs co-stain of rat monocyte/macrophage marker CD11b/c (mouse anti-rat CD11b/c-PE, eBiosciences 12–0110-82, San Diego, USA) and CD68 is also presented in the additional files section (Additional file 3). T cells were stained using rabbit anti-rat/hu/ms CD3 (5690, Abcam, Cambridge, UK) and donkey anti-rabbit-Cy5 (Dianova, 711–175-152) as secondary antibody (Additional file1) or donkey anti-rabbit-biotin (Dianova, 711–065-152) and Strep-594 (Dianova, 016–580-084) (Additional file 2). B-cells were stained using mouse anti-rat CD20 (SantaCruz, sc-393,894) and goat anti-mouse(IgM)-biotin (ThermoFisher, 31,804) as a secondary antibody with strep-Cy3 (Dianova, 016–160-084) (Additional file 1) or using goat anti-rat CD20 (SantaCruz, sc-7735) and donkey anti-goat-FITC (Dianova, 705–095-147) (Additional file 2). Macrophages were stained using mouse anti-rat CD68 (BioRad, MCA341GA) and donkey anti-mouse-DyLight 650 (Abcam, ab98797) as a secondary antibody.

Flow Cytometry

Rat spleen was mechanically macerated to yield single cell suspensions for antibody staining and flow cytometry. Spleen was coarsely chopped using a scalpel, then passed through a 70 μm cell strainer, washed, and then passed through a 30 μm filter. The cell suspension was further separated using ficoll gradient centrifugation. The white cell layer (buffy coat) was collected and used for FACS staining. Cells were blocked using 10% BSA PBS. The following antibodies were used: mouse anti-rat CD11b/c-PE (eBiosciences 12–0110-82, San Diego, USA) and mouse anti-rat CD68 (BioRad, MCA341GA) with secondary antibody donkey anti-mouse-DyLight 650 (Abcam, ab98797).

Masson Trichrome staining

Renal tissues were fixed in 4% paraformaldehyde and embedded in paraffin, cut into 4-μm thick sections and stained with hematoxylin and eosin (HE) and Masson's trichrome (MT) staining as follows. First, sections were deparaffinized and rehydrated by treatment with decreasing percentages of ethanol and rinsing in deionized water. Sections were then treated with Bouin's solution containing Pikrin acid, 5% acetic acid and 10% formaldehyde overnight and then rinsed. This was followed by 5 min. of Weigerts iron-hematoxylin solution in order to stain cell nuclei dark blue. Then Bieberich-Scarlet red acid-fuchsin was applied for 5 min. to stain cytoplasms red. Phosphorus tungsten and phosphorus molybdenic acid was applied for 5 min., followed by Anilin blue solution for 15 min., 1 min of 1% acetic acid, and after rinsing with water, sections were dehydrated using ethanol treatments in increasing concentrations. The morphological changes were examined under a Zeiss Axiostar microscope equipped with a digital camera and analyzed by Metamorphe software (Metamorph 4.6 Universal Imaging Corporation). Depending on the size of the tissue section 10 to 20 images per section (×20 magnification) were captured along the renal cortex, in order to calculate the total percentages of the fibrotic areas for each section.

Real-time PCR

After homogenization of frozen tissue sections using RNeasy MiniKit® (cat. 74,106, Qiagen, Hilden, Germany) total RNA was extracted, with additional DNase digestion to remove all traces of genomic DNA. Total RNA was reverse transcribed into cDNA: cDNA probes were synthesized in 20 µL reaction volume with 1 µg total RNA, 0.5 µg oligo(dT) primer (Promega, Mannheim, Gemany), 40 units of RNasin (Promega, Mannheim, Germany), 0.5 mM dNTP (Biolabs, Frankfurt am Main, Germany), 4 µL 5× transcription buffer and 200 units of Moloney murine leukemia virus (M-MLV) reverse transcriptase (Promega, Mannheim, Germany) for 1 h at 37 °C. In parallel, no-RT and no-template controls were performed. RT-PCR was performed on ViiA7 detection system in triplicates (Applied Biosystems, Darmstadt, Germany) using QuantiTect SYBR Green PCR Kit (Qiagen, Hilden, Germany). Hypoxanthine-guanine-phosphoribosyl-transferase (HPRT) was used as reference gene. All water controls were negative for target and housekeeper. The sequences of the primers were: rHPRT forw: 5'-CTTTGGTCAAGCAGTACAGCC-3'; rHPRT rev: 5'-TCCGCTGATGACACAAACATGA-3'; r CCL2 forw: 5'-ATGCAGTTAATGCCCCACTC-3'; rC CL2 rev: 5'-TTCCTTATTGGGGTCAGCAC-3'; rCCL5 forw: 5'-CTGCCCCTACTTGTCATGGT-3'; rCCL5 rev: 5'-AGATGAGCCTCACAGCCCTA-3'; rCCR5 forw: 5'-CTATGCCCTTGTTGGGGAGA-3'; rCCR5 rev: 5'-TC CTGTGGACCGGGTATAGA-3', rCXCL13 forw: 5'-GC AAAAATCAGGCTTCCAGA -3'; rCXCL13 rev: 5'-GG GTCACAGTGCAAAGGAAT-3'; rCCL19 forw: 5'-AG ACTGCTGCCTGTCTGTGA-3'; rCCL19 rev: 5'-GC TGGTAGCCCCTTAGTGTG-3'; rCCL20 forw: 5'-CA ACTTTGACTGCTGCCTCA-3, rCCL20 rev: 5'-CGG ATCTTTTCGACTTCAGG-3; rCCR7 forw: 5'-GGTC ATTTTCCAGGTGTGCT-3, rCCR7 rev: 5'-AGTTCCG-CACATCCTTCTTG-3; rLymphotoxin-β forw: 5'-TAT-CAC TGTCCTGGCTGTGC-3', rLymphotoxin-β rev: 5'-GAGATGCACGAGGGTTTGTT-3'; rCCL21 forw: 5'-ACTGCAGGAAGAATCGAGGA-3'; rCCL21 rev: 5'-TGGACTGTGAACCACTCAGG-3'; rBAFF-R forw: 5'-GTGGGTCTGGTCAGTCTGGT -3'; rBAFF-R rev: 5'-C ATTTTCCAGGGACTCTTGG-3'; rBAFF forw: 5'-CT GGAAACTGCCATGCTTCT-3'; rBAFF rev: 5'-TTC GTATAGTCGGCGTGTTG-3'; rIgG forw: 5'-CATT CCCTGCCCCCATC-3'; rIgG rev: 5'-CCGTTCATCTT CCACTCCGT-3'. rCXCL12 forw: 5'-CTGCCGATTCT TTGAGAGCC-3'; rCXCL12 rev: 5'-TTCGGGTCAAT GCACACTTG-3'; rCXCR4 forw: 5'- TCTGAGGCGT TTGGTGCT-3'; rCXCR4 rev: 5'-CAGACCCTACTTCT TCGGA-3'. cDNA quantity was determined using a standard curve. Quantity values of target genes were normalized to the house-keeping gene HPRT, and x-fold change of normalized target gene values compared to syngeneic Tx d6 (used as calibrator) was calculated.

Quantification of donor-specific antibodies (DSA)

Donor (Brown Norway) splenocytes were isolated by macerating spleen through a 100 µm and 40 µm cell strainer, followed by ficoll centrifugation and collection of the white cell layer. Recipient serum was heat-inactivated (56 °C for 30 min.) in order to disable complement factors. Donor splenocytes were incubated with recipient serum for 30 min at 4 °C and then washed. Cells were then stained using either monoclonal mouse anti-rat IgM-PE (eBioscience, 12–0990, San Diego, USA) or polyclonal chicken anti-rat IgG-AlexFluor647 antibody (Invitrogen/Thermo Fischer, A21472, Waltham, USA). As positive controls, we incubated donor splenocytes with heat-inactivated goat or rabbit serum and stained for either goat (donkey anti-goat IgG-DyLight 650, Abcam 96,938, Cambridge, UK) or rabbit (donkey anti-rabbit IgG-Cy5, Dianova, 711–175-152, Hamburg, Germany) antibody. Finally, cells were stained for CD3-FITC (eBioscience 11–0030, San Diego, USA) and measured by flow cytometry. Data is shown for CD3+-gated cells, in order to avoid skewing of data by Fc-receptor binding of non-specific antibodies.

Complement-dependent Cytotoxicity assay (CDC)

Donor splenocytes were isolated as above and resuspended in RPMI1640 Medium (Gibco/Thermo Fischer, Waltham, USA) containing 10% inactivated FCS and 1%Penicillin/Streptomycin. Heat-inactivated recipient serum and donor splenocytes (200,000 cells/well) were incubated at 4 °C for 30 min. Rabbit complement (BAG 7018, Lich, Germany) was added and incubated for 2 h at 24 °C. Goat (DAKO X0907, Hamburg, Germany) or rabbit (DAKO X0902, Hamburg, Germany) serum were used as positive control. Cells were washed and stained with propidium iodide (PI) (Invitrogen/Thermo Fischer, Waltham, USA) to distinguish dead cells and then measured by flow cytometry. Complete lysis was measured using FixPerm (Thermo Fischer, Waltham, USA). Percent cytotoxicity was calculated using the formula: ("PI+cells in sample" – "PI+cells in medium")/("PI+cells in FixPerm" – "PI+cells in Medium") ×100.

Statistical analysis

Values are provided as mean ± SEM. Statistical analysis was performed by the non-parametric Mann-Whitney U-test. $p < 0.05$ was considered to be statistically significant.

Results

Pronounced rejection and acceleration of chronic interstitial damage under conditions simulating non-adherence

Syngeneic transplantation did not lead to any relevant histological changes (Table 1). Allogeneic transplantation lead to mixed cellular and humoral rejection at day 6 (Txd6CyA). In this group, cellular rejection occurred primarily in the form of tubulitis (Table 1), although 1/11 allografts also had signs of vascular rejection (Banff class 4 IIA). Ten of 11 grafts from this group showed specific features of humoral rejection, including discrete to moderate peritubular capillaritis and C4d-positive staining along peritubular capillaries (Table 1, Fig. 1a-b). After continued daily immunosuppression until day 28 (Txd28CyA), 3/6 grafts showed normal histology, but 3/6 grafts still showed cellular rejection with beginning endothelialitis and predominantly perivascular infiltrates, but without signs of additional humoral rejection (Table 1, Fig. 1c-d). When cyclosporine was only administered on alternating days simulating non-adherence (Txd28CyAalt.), graft histology showed moderate cellular rejection in 5/6 grafts, with endothelialitis and perivascular infiltrates, and 3/6 grafts from this group also showed signs of humoral rejection with ongoing peritubular capillaritis, but negative C4d staining (Table 1, Fig. 1e-f). In addition, trichrome staining showed a significant increase of interstitial fibrosis in the non-adherent group in comparison to the adherent group as shown in Fig. 2a-c (Txd28CyA vs. Txd28CyAalt. $p = 0.0043$) demonstrating an acceleration of chronic interstitial changes induced by intermittent immunosuppression.

Infiltration of inflammatory cell populations

Immunohistochemical staining of CD3, CD68, and CD20 in kidney sections showed that, as expected, allogeneic transplantation led to a significant infiltration of CD68[+] monocytes/macrophages, and CD3[+] and CD20[+] lymphocytes by day 6 when compared to syngeneic transplantation (Fig. 3 a-c). When daily cyclosporine treatment was continued until day 28 (Txd28CyA), intra-renal infiltration of all 3 cell populations was strongly reduced in comparison to day 6 after allogeneic transplantation (CD3 $p = 0.004$, CD20 $p = 0.06$, CD68 $p = 0.002$). However, after

simulation of "non-adherence" (Txd28CyAalt.), strong CD3[+] cell infiltration was sustained ($p = 0.0047$ for CD3[+] cell infiltration in TxCyAd28 vs. Txd28CyAalt.). CD20[+] cell infiltration in non-adherence was similar to infiltration after daily immunosuppression, but was significantly elevated compared to syngeneic transplantation. Monocyte/macrophage numbers were as low after non-adherence as after syngeneic transplantation.

Distribution of B cells in clusters after non-adherence

Although the total number of intra-renal CD20[+] B lymphocytes only showed a slight increase after non-adherence compared to daily immunosuppression, which did not reach statistical significance at this group size, analysis of B cell distribution by immunofluorescent staining showed a remarkable trend towards more organized clusters of B cells. As shown in representative sections in Fig. 4, infiltrating CD20[+] cells are randomly scattered in allograft tissue at day 6 (Fig. 4a) and moved into a distinctly grouped distribution after continued daily immunosuppression until day 28 (Fig. 4b). When immunosuppression was intermittently omitted in analogy to non-adherence, B cells formed dense clusters as shown in Fig. 4c. Fully matured tertiary lymphoid follicles were not observed at this time-point.

Chemokines recruit adaptive immunity during non-adherence

Intra-graft chemokine transcription was compared to infiltrating leukocyte populations. Fittingly, a strong induction of chemokines attracting lymphocytes (CCL19/CCL20/CCL21/Lymphotoxin-β/CCL5), rather than monocytes (CCL2), was seen under conditions simulating non-adherence (Fig. 5); p-values for the difference in "non-adherence" compared to standard immunosuppression at day 28 were: $p = 0.009$ for CCL19, $p = 0.03$ for CCL20, $p = 0.019$ for CCL21, $p = 0.004$ for Lymphotoxin-β, $p = 0.03$ for CCL5, and $p = 0.90$ for CCL2. However, an induction of corresponding chemokine receptors CCR7 (CCL19/CCL21 receptor) and CCR5 (CCL5 receptor) was not observed after "non-adherence" (Fig. 5). However, immunohistochemical staining of CCR7 of renal allograft sections revealed positive staining of leukocyte infiltrates, and this was increased in the groups Txd6CyA and Txd28CyAalt.

Table 1 Histopathological classification of allograft rejection in analogy to the Banff classification. Group sizes ranged from 6 to 11 rats per group

Group	No rejection	Class 2 I-II C4d-positive	Class 2 I-II C4d-negative	Class 4 IA	Class 4 IB	Class 4 IIA	Class 4 IIB	Mixed Rejection
Syn Tx d6 ($n = 8$)	8							
Tx d6 CyA ($n = 11$)		10		2	8	1		10
Tx d28 CyA ($n = 6$)	3					3		
Tx d28 CyA alt. ($n = 6$)	1		3			5		3

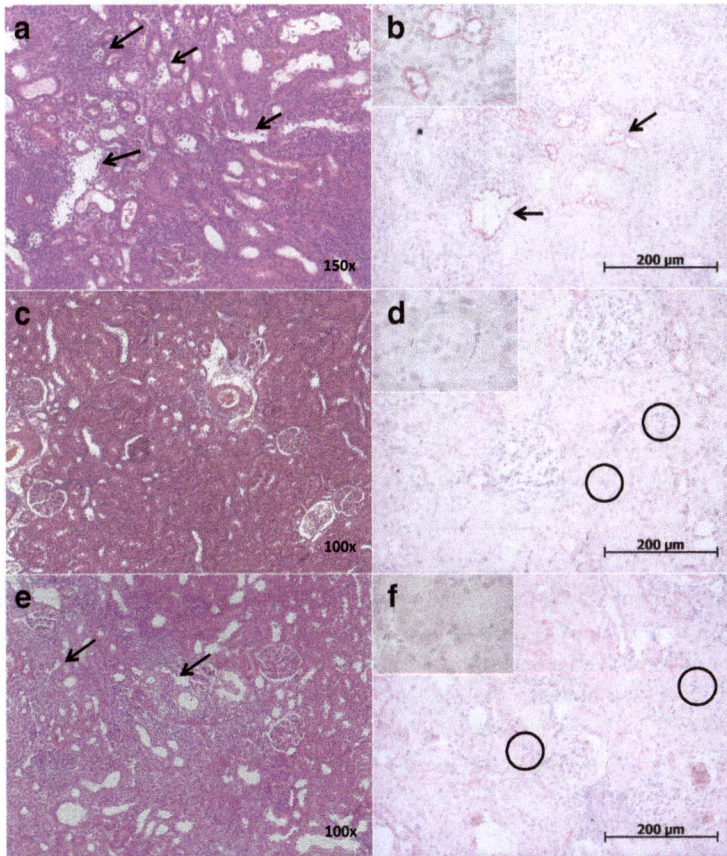

Fig. 1 a-f Representative renal allograft sections are shown from each group of transplanted rats ($n = 6–11$) (**a-b**) Txd6CyA (**c-d**) Txd28CyA, and (**e-f**) Txd28CyAalt. The left shows hematoxylin & eosin staining with arrows showing peritubular capillaritis. The right shows anti-rat C4d staining (brown) with arrows pointing out dilated peritubular capillaries containing marginated mononuclear cells and neutrophils and C4d-positivity and black circles showing negative anti-rat C4d staining in peritubular capillaries

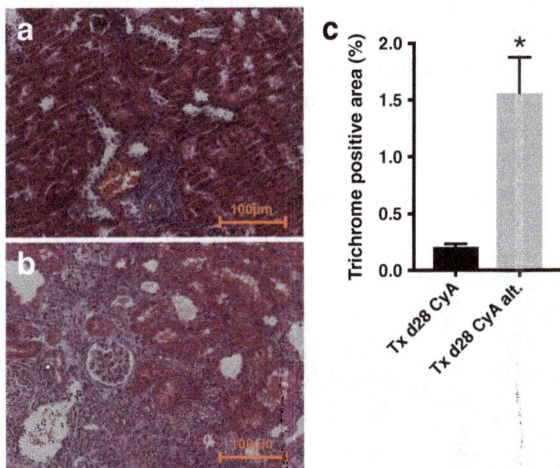

Fig. 2 a-c Trichrome staining was used to quantify interstitial fibrosis. Representative sections are shown (**a**) Txd28CyA and (**b**) Txd28Cyalt. In (**c**) quantitative analysis of percent trichrome positive area is shown. 6 rats per group were analyzed. The mean and standard error is shown. Significance (Mann-Whitney U Test) is shown as * $p < 0.05$ compared to "Txd28CyAalt"

(Fig. 6) compared to synTxd6 and Txd28CyA. In the non-adherence group CCR7-staining of infiltrates was more pronounced than in infiltrates from group Txd6CyA. Notably, tubular epithelial cells were also CCR7-positive, which has previously been reported in the context of renal transplantation [22]. Overall, the intensity of CCR7 staining reflected the pattern of mRNA expression in the different experimental groups. Interestingly, transcription of CCL19, CCL20, and CCL21 was not induced early after transplantation (day 6), but strongly induced after a period of "non-adherence" (Txd6CyA vs. Txd28CyAalt: $p = 0.0001$ for CCL19, $p = 0.005$ for CCL20, $p = 0.008$ for CCL21, Fig. 5). In order to confirm mRNA expression on a protein level, immunohistochemical staining of CCL21 was performed in 2–3 randomly selected allograft sections from each group (Fig. 7). The intensity of CCL21 staining correlated well with PCR data, where expression was low in all groups except the non-adherence group (Fig. 7d). Here, strong CCL21 expression was localized in areas of lymphocyte infiltration. Transcription of the B cell specific chemokine CXCL13 was not significantly induced after "non-

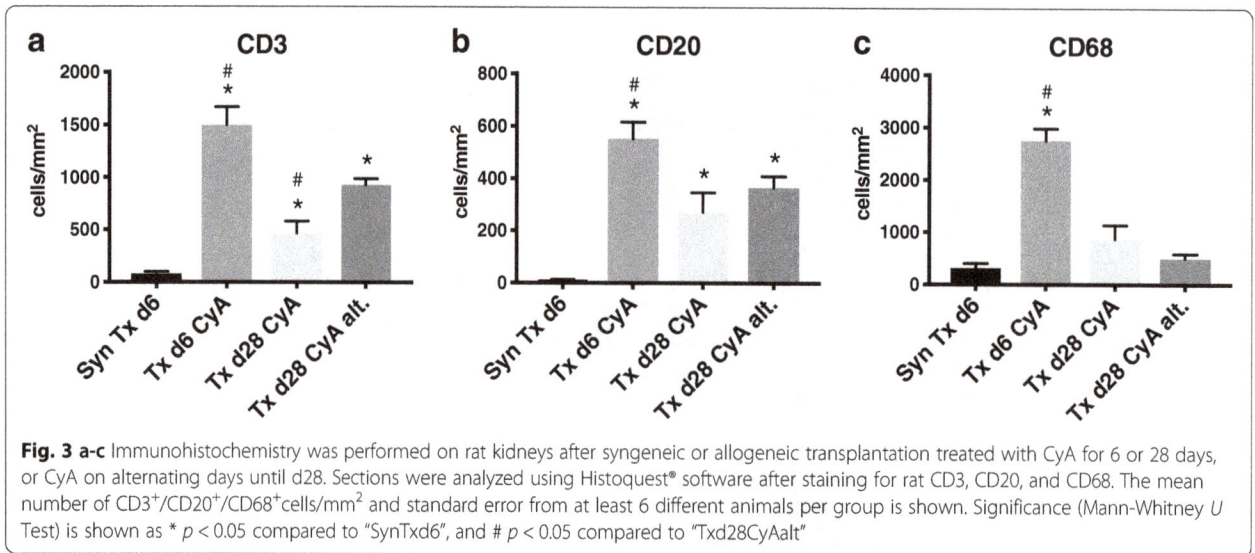

Fig. 3 a-c Immunohistochemistry was performed on rat kidneys after syngeneic or allogeneic transplantation treated with CyA for 6 or 28 days, or CyA on alternating days until d28. Sections were analyzed using Histoquest® software after staining for rat CD3, CD20, and CD68. The mean number of CD3$^+$/CD20$^+$/CD68$^+$cells/mm^2 and standard error from at least 6 different animals per group is shown. Significance (Mann-Whitney U Test) is shown as * p < 0.05 compared to "SynTxd6", and # p < 0.05 compared to "Txd28CyAalt"

adherence". CXCL12 and its receptor CXCR4 represent an important axis for migration of T, B, and plasma cells, as well as dendritic cells [23], and have been shown to induce dendritic cell rich TLOs in mice [24], however the mRNA expression of CXCR4 and CXCL12 was relatively low. Intra-graft CXCR4 expression was increased in Txd6CyA, but no other group compared to syngeneic Tx d6 (Additional file 4). CXCL12 expression was low and did not differ in the different experimental groups (Additional file 4).

Non-adherence increases intra-renal B cell activating factor (BAFF) and IgG transcription

Intra-graft BAFF (B cell activating factor belonging to the TNF family) transcription is induced early after allogeneic transplantation (p = 0.0003 for Txd6CyA vs. SynTxd6) and is additionally significantly increased in non-adherence compared to standard immunosuppression at day 28 (p = 0.026 for Txd28CyAalt. vs. Txd28CyA, Fig. 8a). BAFF-receptor transcription levels are also significantly increased after non-adherence (p = 0.0007 compared to control n = 6, Fig. 8b). A significant rise of intra-graft Immunoglobulin G

(IgG) transcription was observed in the non-adherence group in comparison to all other groups (Txd28CyAalt. vs. Txd28CyA p = 0.004, vs. Txd6 p = 0.0028, vs. SynTxd6 p = 0.0007, Fig. 8c).

Development of de novo donor-specific antibodies

To test for DSA, recipient serum was incubated with donor splenocytes and stained for rat IgM (immunoglobulin M) and IgG (immunoglobulin G). Goat and rabbit serum were expected to contain xenoantibodies and were used as positive controls showing robust and titratable positive signals for the anti-rat IgG and IgM FACS stain (data not shown) and also complement-dependent cytotoxicity (Fig. 10a). Recipient sera after syngeneic transplantation did not show positive anti-rat IgG or IgM staining on donor splenocytes (Fig. 9a-b). However, allogeneic transplantation led to the appearance of high levels of donor-specific IgM and IgG early after transplantation (day 6) (p = 0.004 for Txd6CyA vs. SynTxd6 for IgM and p = 0.002 for IgG). As expected, donor-specific IgM disappeared by day 28 (Fig. 9a). IgG

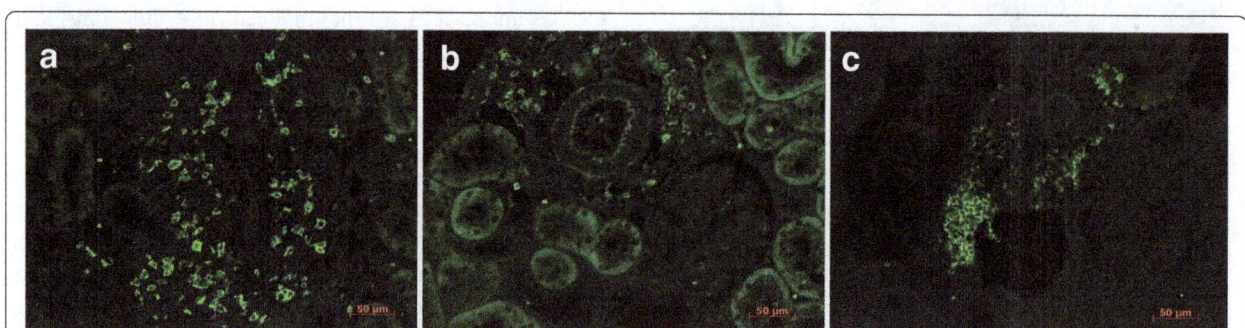

Fig. 4 a-c Immunofluorescent staining of CD20 in renal allograft was performed. Representative sections from Txd6CyA (**a**), Tx28CyA (**b**), and Txd28CyAalt. (**c**) are shown. Anti-CD20 was labeled with a fitc-conjugated secondary antibody (bright green)

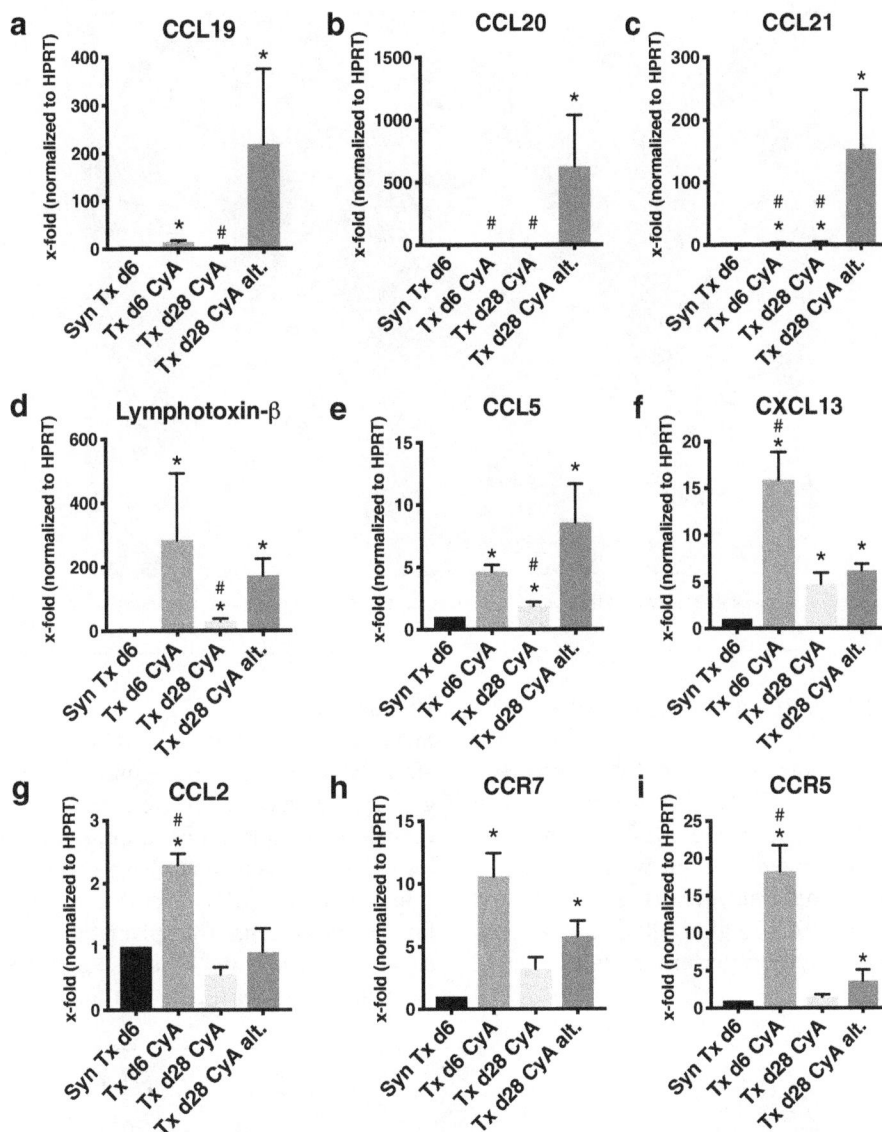

Fig. 5 a-i Quantitative RT-PCR analysis of chemokine and chemokine receptor expression from renal grafts after syngeneic or allogeneic transplantation treated with CyA for 6 or 28 days, or CyA on alternating days until d28. mRNA expression of target genes was normalized to the house-keeping gene HPRT and x-fold expression in comparison to syngeneic Tx d6 is shown. In (**a**) CCL19, (**b**) CCL20, (**c**) CCL21, (**d**) Lymphotoxin-β, (**e**) CCL5, (**f**) CXCL13, (**g**) CCL2, (**h**) CCR7, and (**i**) CCR5. Data is shown as mean ± SEM. Groups consisted of at least 6 animals. Statistical analysis is shown (Mann-Whitney U Test). Significance is shown as *$p < 0.05$ compared to "SynTxd6", and # $p < 0.05$ compared to "Txd28CyAalt"

levels also markedly decreased by day 28 under daily immunosuppression in 3/6 subjects, but remained elevated in another 3/6 (Fig. 9b, Txd28CyA). A highly relevant observation was, that the same 3/6 rats from the group showing virtually no DSA also lacked histological signs of rejection; in contrast, the remaining 3/6 rats which did show histological signs of rejection (Table 1), also displayed measurable amounts of DSA in serum. In the non-adherence group, donor-specific IgG was elevated in all measured samples ($p = 0.004$ for SynTxd6 vs. Txd28CyAalt.), and this corresponded with histological signs of C4d-negative ABMR in 3/6 animals in this group.

In order to rule out any binding of non-specific immunoglobulins, we incubated recipient sera, which had previously shown IgG-binding on donor splenocytes (Txd6CyA) with recipient Lewis rat splenocytes (data not shown). There was no staining of rat-IgG or IgM on Lewis splenocytes, confirming that the observed anti-rat IgG are donor-specific. Similarly, Lewis rat serum from day 0 did not show any specific binding of anti-rat IgG on BN splenocytes (data not shown).

Using a complement-dependent cytotoxicity assay, we found that only DSA produced early after transplantation (Txd6CyA) activated complement-mediated

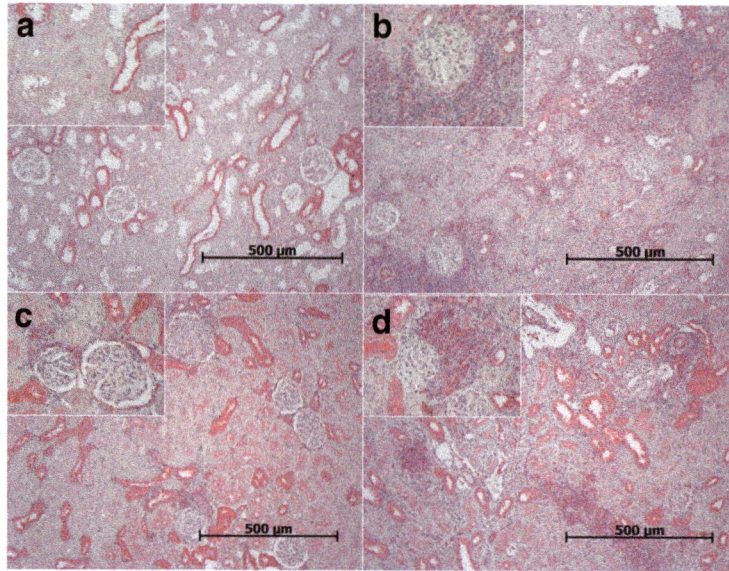

Fig. 6 a-d CCR-7 expression in renal allografts. Two to three randomly selected sections per group were stained with anti-CCR7 antibody. Representative sections are shown. (**a**) synTxd6 (**b**) Txd6CyA (**c**) Txd28CyA and (**d**) Txd28CyAalt

cytotoxicity (CDC) (Fig. 10, $p = 0.03$ for Txd6CyA vs. Lewis Serum d0), while no cytotoxicity was observed after 28 days of daily or alternating CyA treatment, ($p = 0.03$ for Txd6CyA vs. Txd28CyAalt.), eventhough DSA were detected in this group by flow cytometry (Fig. 9b). These results are consistent with the pattern of C4d-staining in the different groups, which showed positive C4d staining at day 6 after allogeneic Tx, but not at day 28 after daily or intermittent immunosuppression (Fig. 1).

Discussion

Since non-adherence to immunosuppressive therapy is strongly associated with donor-specific antibodies and accelerated graft failure, our aim was to utilize a rat model of non-adherence in order to study the immunological mechanisms underlying chronic allograft injury.

In our model, MHC-mismatched rat strains were used for allogeneic renal transplantation. Acute humoral and cellular rejection was observed at day 6. As the animals were not pre-sensitized, the immunological risk was

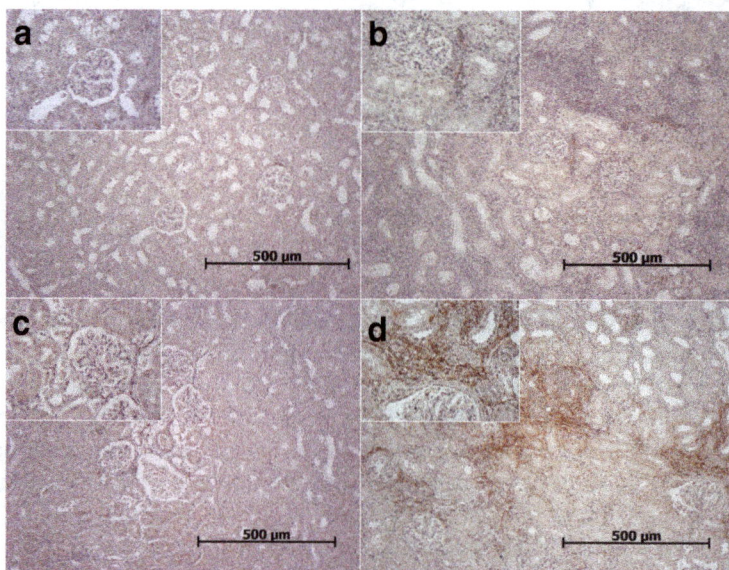

Fig. 7 a-d CCL21 expression in renal allografts. Two to three randomly selected sections per group were stained with anti-CCL21 antibody. Representative sections are shown. (**a**) synTxd6 (**b**) Txd6CyA (**c**) Txd28CyA and (**d**) Txd28CyAalt

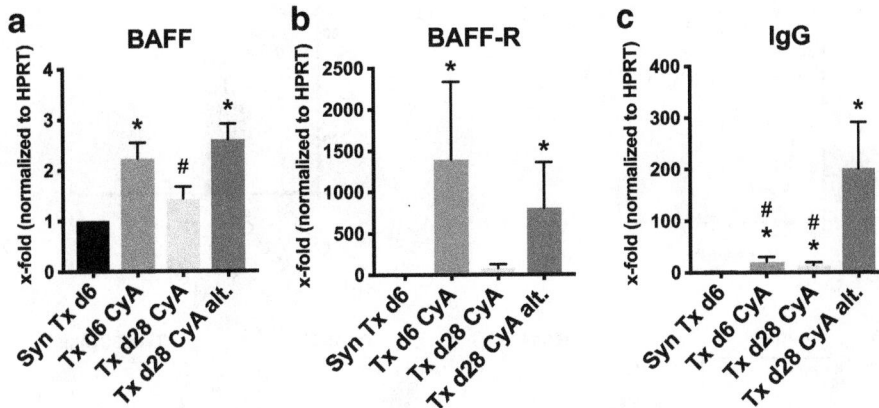

Fig. 8 a-c Quantitative RT-PCR analysis of BAFF, BAFF receptor and IgG expression from renal grafts after syngeneic or allogeneic transplantation treated with daily CyA for 6 or 28 days, or CyA on alternating days until d28. mRNA expression of target genes was normalized to the house-keeping gene HPRT and x-fold expression in comparison to syngeneic Tx d6 is shown. In (**a**) BAFF, (**b**) BAFF-Receptor, and (**c**) IgG. Data is shown as mean ± SEM. Groups consisted of at least 6 animals. Statistical analysis is shown (Mann-Whitney U Test). Significance is shown as * $p < 0.05$ compared to "SynTxd6", and # $p < 0.05$ compared to "Txd28CyAalt"

considered low, and no induction therapy was used. When immunosuppression was continued, rejection subsided in some animals, but not all, probably because the dose of cyclosporine used (5 mg/kg) was relatively low and no induction therapy or steroid was administered on top. Under daily cyclosporine administration, normal histology or mild cellular rejection was seen at day 28. In contrast, the non-adherence group suffered from a significant increase in the rate of cellular rejection with additional features of acute humoral rejection – illustrated by initiation of peritubular capillaritis. Our model intended to show mechanisms of early chronic parenchymal changes. Such changes were indeed induced in our model of non-adherence, as demonstrated by a significant increase in interstitial fibrosis.

While cellular infiltration was minimal after syngeneic transplantation, high numbers of inflammatory cells were seen early after allogeneic transplantation (day 6) with monocytes dominating the infiltrate. The numbers of monocytes, T cells and B cells declined when standard immunosuppression with daily CyA was continued. However, under conditions simulating non-adherence, T cell infiltration did not resolve as quickly as under daily immunosuppression. Meanwhile, B cell numbers remained elevated in comparison to syngeneic transplantation and monocyte numbers declined to a level similar to that after syngeneic transplantation. In line with these results, Hueso et al. previously showed that early interstitial fibrosis/tubular atrophy (IF/TA) and reduced graft survival are associated with increased

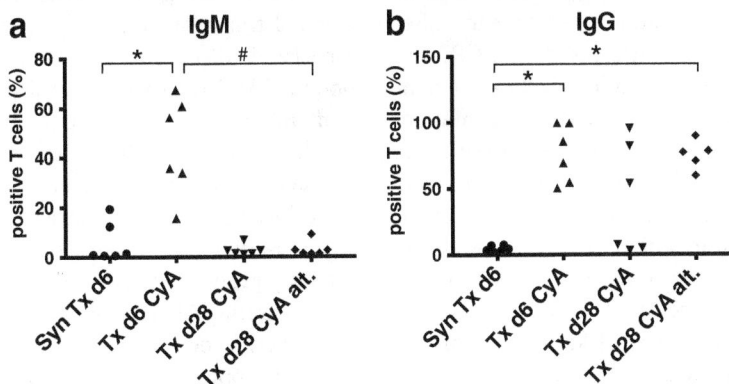

Fig. 9 a-b Detection of donor-specific antibodies from rats after syngeneic or allogeneic kidney transplantation treated with daily CyA for 6 or 28 days, or CyA on alternating days until d28. Donor splenocytes were incubated with recipient serum and then stained with (**a**) anti-rat IgM-antibody or (**b**) anti-rat IgG-antibody in duplicates and measured by flow cytometry. Percentages of IgG or IgM-positive cells are shown. Data is shown as single data points of each group on a scatter plot. Groups consisted of 5–6 animals. Statistical analysis is shown (Mann-Whitney U Test). Significance is shown as * $p < 0.05$ compared to "SynTxd6", # $p < 0.05$ compared to "Txd28CyAalt"

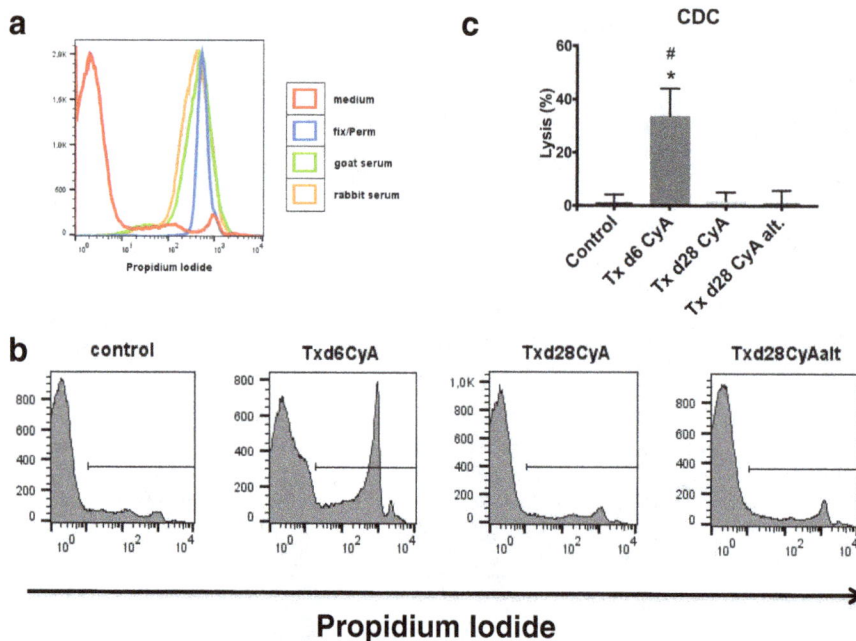

Fig. 10 Complement-dependent-cytotoxicity of donor-specific antibodies from rats after syngeneic or allogeneic kidney transplantation treated with daily CyA for 6 or 28 days, or CyA on alternating days until d28. Donor splenocytes were incubated with recipient serum and rabbit complement. Dead cells were stained with propidium iodide (PI) and measured by flow cytometry. (**a**) shows representative histograms of PI-staining for negative control (cell medium, shown in red) and positive controls (Fix/perm, shown in blue; goat serum shown in green; rabbit serum shown in orange). (**b**) shows representative histograms of PI-staining for control (Lew d0), Txd6CyA, Txd28CyA, and Txd28CyAalt. (**c**) shows quantitative analysis as percent lysis (n = 3–4 per group). Significance (Mann-Whitney U Test) is shown as * $p < 0.05$ compared to control (Lewis rat serum pre-Tx d0), # $p < 0.05$ compared to "Txd28CyAalt"

infiltration of T and B cells in human renal transplant biopsies [25].

The changes seen in the pattern of intra-renal chemokine transcription mirrored the changes in the composition of the cellular infiltrate, with chemokines attracting T and B lymphocytes, such as CCL19, CCL20, CCL21, CCL5 and lymphotoxin-β, increased in non-adherence.

Interestingly, CCL19, CCL20, and CCL21, were much more strongly induced in the setting of non-adherence than during the initial inflammatory reaction early after Tx (d6). CCL19, CCL21, and their receptor CCR7 are known to regulate homing and co-localization of dendritic cells and naïve T cells in lymphoid organs and are essential to T cell sensitization and the formation of an adaptive immune response [26]. However, they have also been implicated in the formation of tertiary lymphoid organs (TLO) in the context of chronic inflammation [24, 27, 28]. These structures have also been found in transplant organs and are associated with a poorer outcome [14, 29]. In a murine model of kidney transplantation, the fusion protein CCL19-IgG, which interferes with normal CCL19-CCR7 signaling, was found to strongly reduce graft rejection [30]. In our model of non-adherence, chemokines associated with TLO formation are strongly expressed, and this is accompanied with the formation of dense lymphocyte aggregates.

Another factor that has been associated with chronic inflammation and formation of B cell rich TLO is B cell activating factor (BAFF) [31]. BAFF is an activation, maturation and survival factor for B cells, expressed by lymph node stromal cells, neutrophils, macrophages, monocytes, dendritic cells and T cells [32]. A pathogenetic role for BAFF has been suggested for several autoimmune diseases, including Sjögren Syndrome, systemic lupus erythematosus, and multiple sclerosis [33–35]. In the context of renal transplantation, higher serum levels of BAFF are associated with donor-specific antibodies [36], blood cell-bound BAFF with worse renal graft function, and intra-graft BAFF expression is associated with ABMR and IF/TA [37]. We now show that BAFF transcription is increased within the graft during non-adherence. In line with this, IgG transcription levels are also increased during non-adherence. In fact, the non-adherence group was the only group that showed intra-renal IgG transcription, demonstrating that local intra-graft antibody formation exclusively occurred after prolonged suboptimal immunosuppression.

Although, fully developed TLO structures were not yet observed in our experimental setting at the analyzed time-points, the enhanced organization of B lymphocytes into dense clusters during our simulation of non-adherence together with the increased expression of

TLO-associated chemokines CCL19, CCL20, CCL21, and BAFF may be indicative of early steps in the formation of these highly organized structures. Furthermore, the appearance of intra-graft IgG transcription maybe linked to the development of an organized local adaptive immune response. Although our experiments cannot differentiate plasma cell infiltration from local differentiation from precursor cells, a possible explanation maybe that BAFF activates intra-renal B cells, which mature into antibody-secreting plasma cells within the graft. Similarly, our experiments cannot rule out that increased IgG transcription is due to turnover of local B cell populations in non-adherence, but evidence for local antibody production by plasma cells in chronic rejection has been provided by Thaunat et al. [14]. There is also evidence for clonal expansion of B cells inside grafts [38]. No conclusions can be drawn as to the specificity or diversity of the IgG produced in our non-adherence model, and further experiments will be needed to establish the source and specificity of intra-graft IgG production. Others have shown however, that locally and systemically produced antibodies differ in diversity and timing with more diverse HLA (human leukocyte antigen) specificities being generated from intra-graft antibody production [14, 39].

In our model, de novo DSA were detected in rat serum under conditions mimicking non-adherence to therapy. This corresponds to data from studies of renal transplant patients [3, 10, 11]. Antibodies were shown to be donor-specific, since binding of recipient Lewis rat splenocytes did not occur. Although our experiments could not specifically identify anti-MHC antibodies, endothelial non-MHC targets for these antibodies were unlikely since splenocytes were used in our assay. IgM and IgG DSA were detected early after transplantation (day 6), following a kinetic previously described for rat humoral responses after immunization [40, 41]. At the later timepoint, we saw a clear induction of a secondary humoral response, where IgM was no longer detected, while IgG levels remained elevated. We interpreted this as a sign that Ig class switching was completed, and that sensitization to donor antigens and initial DSA production takes place very early. Our results suggest that activated B cells and plasma cells are then armed and ready for antibody production, and are kept in check by appropriate immunosuppression with CNI. Analysis of CDC showed that DSA were cytotoxic early after Tx (d6), but not after non-adherence or daily CyA (d28), which was consistent with the pattern of C4d-staining observed in the different groups. Our experiments do not offer a specific mechanism to explain this phenomenon, but one possibility is that the different immunosuppressive treatments and

durations result in a switch in the IgG-subclass generated and thereby also determine the phenotype of ABMR, eg. C4d-positive vs. C4d-negative, in line with recently published observations of DSA IgG subclasses and rejection phenotypes in transplant patients [42]. In this study of renal transplant patients, chronic ABMR was associated with the non-complement activating IgG subclass IgG4 in humans, whereas acute ABMR was associated with the complement-fixing IgG3 [42].

Under-immunosuppression in a clinical setting may be due to non-adherence to therapy or to inter-individual variations in responsiveness to CNI, since CNI therapy is monitored using serum concentration, not functional tests. Considering this, even when optimal adherence to therapy is achieved, a group of patients may still effectively be "under-immunosuppressed" and at risk of chronic rejection.

While there is a lot of data showing the deleterious effects of DSA on graft outcome, there is an ongoing debate over which DSA are clinically relevant, or more precisely, what features of DSA, such as MFI (mean fluorescence intensity), complement-fixing capacity or IgG-subclass, are linked to deleterious outcomes and require treatment [42–44]. Our model offers an ideal framework for deciphering such critical issues.

Several animal models have been established in which preformed DSA are induced using pre-transplant immunization [45, 46]. Since in the majority of cases, DSA are de novo DSA and not DSA from pre-sensitization, our model - with reliable histological and serological entities of acute antibody mediated rejection during non-adherence - more closely resembles this highly prevalent group of patients.

Conclusion

In this study, we established and characterized a rat model of CNI under-immunosuppression in analogy to non-adherence to immunosuppressive therapy after allogeneic kidney transplantation. In this model, non-adherence led to mixed cellular and humoral rejections. This study shows that during prolonged under-immunosuppression, lymphocytic infiltrates take up an organized form within the graft. This is promoted by factors also associated with formation of secondary and tertiary lymphoid organs. Furthermore, intra-renal IgG mRNA synthesis was induced after prolonged under-immunosuppression. These intra-renal changes are accompanied by systemic production of donor-specific antibodies after non-adherence. The contribution of organized lymphocytic infiltrates to chronic allograft injury needs to be addressed in further studies.

Additional files

Additional file 1: *anti-CD20 and anti-CD3 immunofluorescence costaining of rat spleen follicles.* Anti-CD20-positive B cells are in the B cell zone of splenic follicles (yellow), and anti-CD3-positive T cells in the T cell zone of the splenic follicles (red), also shown are proliferating Ki67-positive cells in splenic follicles (green). (PDF 3198 kb)

Additional file 2: *anti-CD20, anti-CD3, and anti-CD68 immunofluorescence costaining of rat spleen follicle.* (A) shows anti-CD20-positive B cells in the B cell zone of a splenic follicle (green), anti-CD3-positive T cells in T cell zone of splenic follicle (red), and CD68-positive macrophages (yellow) in the splenic red pulp, also shown in (B) without costaining. (PDF 588 kb)

Additional file 3: *anti-CD11b/c and anti-CD68 FACS costain of rat spleno-cytes.* (A) shows unstained cells, (B) shows anti-CD11b/c-PE antibody only, and (C) shows anti-anti-CD11b/c-PE antibody and anti-CD68-APC antibody co-stain of rat splenocytes. (PDF 82 kb)

Additional file 4: *CXCR4 and CXCL12 expression.* This figure shows quantitative RT-PCR analysis of chemokine and chemokine receptor expression from renal grafts after syngeneic or allogeneic transplantation treated with CyA for 6 or 28 days, or CyA on alternating days until d28. mRNA expression of target genes was normalized to the house-keeping gene HPRT and x-fold expression in comparison to syngeneic Tx d6 is shown. (A) CXCR4 (B) CXCL12. Data is shown as mean ± SEM. Groups consisted of at least 6 animals. Statistical analysis is shown (Mann-Whitney U Test). Significance is shown as $*p < 0.05$ compared to "SynTxd6", and # $p < 0.05$ compared to "Txd28CyAalt". (PDF 24 kb)

Abbreviations
ABMR: Antibody-mediated rejection; BAFF: B cell activating factor belonging to the TNF family; BAFF-R: BAFF-receptor; BN: Brown Norway rat; CCL: CC chemokine ligand; CCR: CC chemokine receptor; CD: Cluster of differentiation; CDC: Complement dependent cytotoxicity; CNI: Calcineurin inhibitor; CXCL: CXC chemokine; CXCR: CXC chemokine receptor; CyA: Cyclosporine A; DSA: Donor-specific antibody; HLA: Human leukocyte antigen; IF/TA: Interstitial fibrosis and tubular atrophy; IgG: Immunoglobulin G; IgM: Immunoglobulin M; LEW: Lewis rat; MFI: Mean fluorescence intensity; MHC: Major histocompatibility complex; RT-PCR: Real-time polymerase chain reaction; SLE: Systemic lupus erythematosus; TLO: Tertiary lymphoid organ; Tx: Transplantation

Acknowledgements
We would like to thank Mrs. Stefanie Ellmann and Mrs. Alexandra Müller for their excellent technical assistance.

Funding
This work was supported by the Else Kröner-Fresenius-Stiftung to TB. The funding body Else-Kröner-Fresenius-Stiftung had no part in the design of the study, in the collection, analysis, and interpretation of data, or in writing the manuscript.

Authors' contributions
LK contributed to experimental design, performed data analysis and prepared the manuscript. BJ contributed to experimental design and data analysis. HP performed treatments and operations of animals. AS and SW helped with experimental design and data analysis. PR evaluated histopathology and immunohistochemistry, including Banff classification, and helped with manuscript writing. BB contributed to data analysis and manuscript writing as department head. TB contributed to experimental design, data analysis, manuscript writing and supervised the research project as group leader. All authors read and approved the final manuscript.

Competing interests
The authors declare that they have no competing interests.

Author details
[1]Department of Nephrology, University Hospital Regensburg, Franz-Josef-Strauß Allee 11, D-93053 Regensburg, Germany. [2]Department of Pathology, University Hospital Erlangen, Erlangen, Germany.

References
1. Gondos A, Dohler B, Brenner H, Opelz G. Kidney graft survival in Europe and the United States: strikingly different long-term outcomes. Transplantation. 2013;95(2):267–74.
2. Stegall MD, Gaston RS, Cosio FG, Matas A. Through a glass darkly: seeking clarity in preventing late kidney transplant failure. J Am Soc Nephrol. 2015; 26(1):20–9.
3. Wiebe C, Gibson IW, Blydt-Hansen TD, Karpinski M, Ho J, Storsley LJ, Goldberg A, Birk PE, Rush DN, Nickerson PW. Evolution and clinical pathologic correlations of de novo donor-specific HLA antibody post kidney transplant. Am J Transplant. 2012;12(5):1157–67.
4. Park WD, Griffin MD, Cornell LD, Cosio FG, Stegall MD. Fibrosis with inflammation at one year predicts transplant functional decline. J Am Soc Nephrol. 2010;21(11):1987–97.
5. Shishido S, Asanuma H, Nakai H, Mori Y, Satoh H, Kamimaki I, Hataya H, Ikeda M, Honda M, Hasegawa A. The impact of repeated subclinical acute rejection on the progression of chronic allograft nephropathy. J Am Soc Nephrol. 2003;14(4):1046–52.
6. Mannon RB, Matas AJ, Grande J, Leduc R, Connett J, Kasiske B, Cecka JM, Gaston RS, Cosio F, Gourishankar S, et al. Inflammation in areas of tubular atrophy in kidney allograft biopsies: a potent predictor of allograft failure. Am J Transplant. 2010;10(9):2066–73.
7. Sellares J, de Freitas DG, Mengel M, Reeve J, Einecke G, Sis B, Hidalgo LG, Famulski K, Matas A, Halloran PF. Understanding the causes of kidney transplant failure: the dominant role of antibody-mediated rejection and nonadherence. Am J Transplant. 2012;12(2):388–99.
8. Hidalgo LG, Campbell PM, Sis B, Einecke G, Mengel M, Chang J, Sellares J, Reeve J, Halloran PF. De novo donor-specific antibody at the time of kidney transplant biopsy associates with microvascular pathology and late graft failure. Am J Transplant. 2009;9(11):2532–41.
9. DeVos JM, Patel SJ, Burns KM, Dilioglou S, Gaber LW, Knight RJ, Gaber AO, Land GA. De novo donor specific antibodies and patient outcomes in renal transplantation. Clin Transpl. 2011;34:351–8.
10. Butler JA, Peveler RC, Roderick P, Horne R, Mason JC. Measuring compliance with drug regimens after renal transplantation: comparison of self-report and clinician rating with electronic monitoring. Transplantation. 2004;77(5):786–9.
11. Brown KL, El-Amm JM, Doshi MD, Singh A, Cincotta E, Morawski K, Losanoff JE, West MS, Gruber SA. Outcome predictors in African-American deceased-donor renal allograft recipients. Clin Transpl. 2009;23(4):454–61.
12. Vlaminck H, Maes B, Evers G, Verbeke G, Lerut E, Van Damme B, Vanrenterghem Y. Prospective study on late consequences of subclinical non-compliance with immunosuppressive therapy in renal transplant patients. Am J Transplant. 2004;4(9):1509–13.
13. Cosio FG, Gloor JM, Sethi S, Stegall MD. Transplant glomerulopathy. Am J Transplant. 2008;8(3):492–6.
14. Thaunat O, Patey N, Caligiuri G, Gautreau C, Mamani-Matsuda M, Mekki Y, Dieu-Nosjean MC, Eberl G, Ecochard R, Michel JB, et al. Chronic rejection triggers the development of an aggressive intragraft immune response through recapitulation of lymphoid organogenesis. J Immunol. 2010;185(1):717–28.
15. Sautenet B, Blancho G, Buchler M, Morelon E, Toupance O, Barrou B, Ducloux D, Chatelet V, Moulin B, Freguin C, et al. One-year results of the effects of Rituximab on acute antibody-mediated rejection in renal transplantation: RITUX ERAH, a multicenter double-blind randomized placebo-controlled trial. Transplantation. 2016;100(2):391–9.

16. Pontarini E, Fabris M, Quartuccio L, Cappelletti M, Calcaterra F, Roberto A, Curcio F, Mavilio D, Della Bella S, De Vita S. Treatment with belimumab restores B cell subsets and their expression of B cell activating factor receptor in patients with primary Sjogren's syndrome. Rheumatology (Oxford). 2015;54(8):1429–34.

17. Furie R, Petri M, Zamani O, Cervera R, Wallace DJ, Tegzova D, Sanchez-Guerrero J, Schwarting A, Merrill JT, Chatham WW, et al. A phase III, randomized, placebo-controlled study of belimumab, a monoclonal antibody that inhibits B lymphocyte stimulator, in patients with systemic lupus erythematosus. Arthritis Rheum. 2011;63(12):3918–30.

18. Hoffmann U, Bergler T, Jung B, Steege A, Pace C, Rummele P, Reinhold S, Kruger B, Kramer BK, Banas B. Comprehensive morphometric analysis of mononuclear cell infiltration during experimental renal allograft rejection. Transpl Immunol. 2013;28(1):24–31.

19. Bergler T, Hoffmann U, Bergler E, Jung B, Banas MC, Reinhold SW, Kramer BK, Banas B. Toll-like receptor 4 in experimental kidney transplantation: early mediator of endogenous danger signals. Nephron Exp Nephrol. 2012;121(3–4):e59–70.

20. Hoffmann U, Segerer S, Rummele P, Kruger B, Pietrzyk M, Hofstadter F, Banas B, Kramer BK. Expression of the chemokine receptor CXCR3 in human renal allografts–a prospective study. Nephrol Dial Transplant. 2006;21(5): 1373–81.

21. Sis B, Mengel M, Haas M, Colvin RB, Halloran PF, Racusen LC, Solez K, Baldwin WM 3rd, Bracamonte ER, Broecker V, et al. Banff '09 meeting report: antibody mediated graft deterioration and implementation of Banff working groups. Am J Transplant. 2010;10(3):464–71.

22. Zhou HL, Wang YT, Gao T, Wang WG, Wang YS. Distribution and expression of fibroblast-specific protein chemokine CCL21 and chemokine receptor CCR7 in renal allografts. Transplant Proc. 2013;45(2):538–45.

23. Aloisi F, Pujol-Borrell R. Lymphoid neogenesis in chronic inflammatory diseases. Nat Rev Immunol. 2006;6(3):205–17.

24. Luther SA, Bidgol A, Hargreaves DC, Schmidt A, Xu Y, Paniyadi J, Matloubian M, Cyster JG. Differing activities of homeostatic chemokines CCL19, CCL21, and CXCL12 in lymphocyte and dendritic cell recruitment and lymphoid neogenesis. J Immunol. 2002;169(1):424–33.

25. Hueso M, Navarro E, Moreso F, O'Valle F, Perez-Riba M, Del Moral RG, Grinyo JM, Seron D. Intragraft expression of the IL-10 gene is up-regulated in renal protocol biopsies with early interstitial fibrosis, tubular atrophy, and subclinical rejection. Am J Pathol. 2010;176(4):1696–704.

26. Comerford I, Harata-Lee Y, Bunting MD, Gregor C, Kara EE, McColl SR. A myriad of functions and complex regulation of the CCR7/CCL19/CCL21 chemokine axis in the adaptive immune system. Cytokine Growth Factor Rev. 2013;24(3):269–83.

27. Timmer TC, Baltus B, Vondenhoff M, Huizinga TW, Tak PP, Verweij CL, Mebius RE, van der Pouw Kraan TC. Inflammation and ectopic lymphoid structures in rheumatoid arthritis synovial tissues dissected by genomics technology: identification of the interleukin-7 signaling pathway in tissues with lymphoid neogenesis. Arthritis Rheum. 2007;56(8):2492–502.

28. Weninger W, Carlsen HS, Goodarzi M, Moazed F, Crowley MA, Baekkevold ES, Cavanagh LL, von Andrian UH. Naive T cell recruitment to nonlymphoid tissues: a role for endothelium-expressed CC chemokine ligand 21 in autoimmune disease and lymphoid neogenesis. J Immunol. 2003;170(9):4638–48.

29. Baddoura FK, Nasr IW, Wrobel B, Li Q, Ruddle NH, Lakkis FG. Lymphoid neogenesis in murine cardiac allografts undergoing chronic rejection. Am J Transplant. 2005;5(3):510–6.

30. Ziegler E, Gueler F, Rong S, Mengel M, Witzke O, Kribben A, Haller H, Kunzendorf U, Krautwald S. CCL19-IgG prevents allograft rejection by impairment of immune cell trafficking. J Am Soc Nephrol. 2006;17(9):2521–32.

31. Magliozzi R, Columba-Cabezas S, Serafini B, Aloisi F. Intracerebral expression of CXCL13 and BAFF is accompanied by formation of lymphoid follicle-like structures in the meninges of mice with relapsing experimental autoimmune encephalomyelitis. J Neuroimmunol. 2004;148(1–2):11–23.

32. Mackay F, Figgett WA, Saulep D, Lepage M, Hibbs ML. B-cell stage and context-dependent requirements for survival signals from BAFF and the B-cell receptor. Immunol Rev. 2010;237(1):205–25.

33. Mariette X, Roux S, Zhang J, Bengoufa D, Lavie F, Zhou T, Kimberly R. The level of BLyS (BAFF) correlates with the titre of autoantibodies in human Sjogren's syndrome. Ann Rheum Dis. 2003;62(2):168–71.

34. Gross JA, Johnston J, Mudri S, Enselman R, Dillon SR, Madden K, Xu W, Parrish-Novak J, Foster D, Lofton-Day C, et al. TACI and BCMA are receptors for a TNF homologue implicated in B-cell autoimmune disease. Nature. 2000;404(6781):995–9.

35. Thangarajh M, Gomes A, Masterman T, Hillert J, Hjelmstrom P. Expression of B-cell-activating factor of the TNF family (BAFF) and its receptors in multiple sclerosis. J Neuroimmunol. 2004;152(1–2):183–90.

36. Thibault-Espitia A, Foucher Y, Danger R, Migone T, Pallier A, Castagnet S, G-Gueguen C, Devys A, C-Gautier A, Giral M, et al. BAFF and BAFF-R levels are associated with risk of long-term kidney graft dysfunction and development of donor-specific antibodies. Am J Transplant. 2012;12(10):2754–62.

37. Xu H, He X, Liu Q, Shi D, Chen Y, Zhu Y, Zhang X. Abnormal high expression of B-cell activating factor belonging to the TNF superfamily (BAFF) associated with long-term outcome in kidney transplant recipients. Transplant Proc. 2009;41(5):1552–6.

38. Cheng J, Torkamani A, Grover RK, Jones TM, Ruiz DI, Schork NJ, Quigley MM, Hall FW, Salomon DR, Lerner RA. Ectopic B-cell clusters that infiltrate transplanted human kidneys are clonal. Proc Natl Acad Sci U S A. 2011; 108(14):5560–5.

39. Zarkhin V, Kambham N, Li L, Kwok S, Hsieh SC, Salvatierra O, Sarwal MM. Characterization of intra-graft B cells during renal allograft rejection. Kidney Int. 2008;74(5):664–73.

40. Antoine JC, Petit C, Avrameas S. Development of immunoglobulin and antibody-synthesizing cells after immunization with different doses of antigen. Immunology. 1976;31(6):921–30.

41. Temple L, Kawabata TT, Munson AE, White KL Jr. Comparison of ELISA and plaque-forming cell assays for measuring the humoral immune response to SRBC in rats and mice treated with benzo[a]pyrene or cyclophosphamide. Fundam Appl Toxicol. 1993;21(4):412–9.

42. Lefaucheur C, Loupy A, Hill GS, Andrade J, Nochy D, Antoine C, Gautreau C, Charron D, Glotz D, Suberbielle-Boissel C. Preexisting donor-specific HLA antibodies predict outcome in kidney transplantation. J Am Soc Nephrol. 2010;21(8):1398–406.

43. Guidicelli G, Guerville F, Lepreux S, Wiebe C, Thaunat O, Dubois V, Visentin J, Bachelet T, Morelon E, Nickerson P, et al. Non-complement-binding de novo donor-specific anti-HLA antibodies and kidney allograft survival. J Am Soc Nephrol. 2016;27(2):615–25.

44. Jordan SC. Donor-specific HLA antibody IgG subclasses are associated with phenotypes of antibody-mediated rejection in sensitized renal allograft recipients. J Am Soc Nephrol. 2016;27(1):6–8.

45. Huang G, Wilson NA, Reese SR, Jacobson LM, Zhong W, Djamali A. Characterization of transfusion-elicited acute antibody-mediated rejection in a rat model of kidney transplantation. Am J Transplant. 2014;14(5):1061–72.

46. Reese SR, Wilson NA, Huang G, Redfield RR 3rd, Zhong W, Djamali A. Calcineurin inhibitor minimization with Ixazomib, an investigational Proteasome inhibitor, for the prevention of antibody mediated rejection in a preclinical model. Transplantation. 2015;99(9):1785–95.

14

Characteristics of the specific humoral response in patients with advanced solid tumors after active immunotherapy with a VEGF vaccine, at different antigen doses and using two distinct adjuvants

Javier Sánchez Ramírez[1][*][†], Yanelys Morera Díaz[1][†], Mónica Bequet-Romero[1], Francisco Hernández-Bernal[2], Katty-Hind Selman-Housein Bernal[3], Ana de la Torre Santos[4], Eduardo Rafael Santiesteban Álvarez[5], Yenima Martín Bauta[2], Cimara H. Bermúdez Badell[2], Josué de la Torre Pupo[3], Jorge V. Gavilondo[1], CENTAURO-2 Team of Investigators and Marta Ayala Avila[1]

Abstract

Background: CIGB-247, a VSSP-adjuvanted VEGF-based vaccine, was evaluated in a phase I clinical trial in patients with advanced solid tumors (CENTAURO). Vaccination with the maximum dose of antigen showed an excellent safety profile, exhibited the highest immunogenicity and was the only one showing a reduction on platelet VEGF bioavailability. However, this antigen dose level did not achieve a complete seroconversion rate in vaccinated patients. These clinical results led us to the question whether a "reserve" of untapped immune response potential against VEGF could exist in cancer patients. To address this matter, CENTAURO-2 clinical trial was conducted where antigen and VSSP dose scale up were studied, and also incorporated the exploration of aluminum phosphate as adjuvant. These changes were made with the aim to increase immune response against VEGF.

Results: The present study reports the characterization of the humoral response elicited by CIGB-247 from the combining of different antigen doses and adjuvants. Cancer patients were immunologically monitored for approximately 1 year. Vaccination with different CIGB-247 formulations exhibited a very positive safety profile. Cancer patients developed IgM, IgG or IgA antibodies specific to VEGF. Elicited polyclonal antibodies had the ability to block the interaction between VEGF and its receptors, VEGFR1 and VEGFR2. The highest humoral response was detected in patients immunized with 800 μg of antigen + 200 μg of VSSP. Off-protocol long-term vaccination did not produce negative changes in humoral response.

Conclusions: Vaccination with a human VEGF variant molecule as antigen in combination with VSSP or aluminum phosphate is immunogenic. The results of this study could contribute to the investigation of this vaccine therapy in an adequately powered efficacy trial.

Trial registration: Trial registration number: RPCEC00000155. Cuban Public Clinical Trial Registry. Date of registration: June 06, 2013. Available from: http://registroclinico.sld.cu/.

Keywords: CIGB-247, VEGF, Cancer vaccine, Humoral response, Clinical trial

* Correspondence: javier.sanchez@cigb.edu.cu
[†]Equal contributors
[1]Department of Pharmaceuticals, Center for Genetic Engineering and Biotechnology (CIGB), P.O. Box 6162, Playa Cubanacán, Havana 10600, Cuba
Full list of author information is available at the end of the article

Background

Over the last decade promising results on cancer vaccines have been achieved in clinical trials and the field is rapidly expanding [1]. An attractive approach is the development of vaccines against molecular markers expressed in the tumor vasculature or directly against one of the most prominent molecular angiogenic players: the vascular endothelial growth factor (VEGF). This type of strategy, known as specific active immunotherapy, has been mostly developed in the oncological arena. VEGF is one of the most important growth factors with a relevant role on tumor angiogenesis, and it has become an attractive target for cancer immunotherapy [2]. Within this research line, our group has developed CIGB-247, a VEGF-based vaccine, that uses a recombinant human VEGF variant molecule as antigen [3] in combination with VSSP, a bacterial-derived adjuvant [4].

CIGB-247 has previously shown anti-tumor and anti-metastatic effects in mice, stimulating the development of VEGF-blocking antibodies and specific T cell responses [3, 5, 6]. After extensive preclinical studies [5, 7], this vaccine candidate was evaluated between 2011 and 2012 in a Phase I clinical trial (code name CENTAURO), where safety, tolerance, and immunogenicity were studied in 30 patients with advanced solid tumors [8].

The CENTAURO study was a first-in-human phase 1 trial to evaluate a cancer therapeutic vaccine based on human VEGF. This clinical trial included three antigen levels (50, 100 and 400 µg), all in combination with 200 µg of VSSP, delivered subcutaneously once a week for 8 weeks, with a booster re-immunization on week 12. CIGB-247 showed an excellent safety and tolerance profile, and was immunogenic at the three studied antigen doses. Results suggested an antigen dose effect on immunogenicity. The immunogenicity increased with higher antigen doses, in terms of the number of patients with anti-VEGF IgG antibodies, the ability of serum to block VEGF/VEGF receptor 2 (VEGFR2) interactions, and positivity in specific gamma-IFNγ ELISPOT tests. Patients with higher accumulated survival times were positive to all these immune response tests. The higher antigen dose patient cohort (400 µg of antigen + 200 µg of VSSP) was the only one showing a reduction on platelet VEGF bioavailability, indicating a functionality of induced antibodies. However, this group did not achieve a complete seroconversion rate [8].

Clinical results of the CENTAURO study led us to the question whether a "reserve" of untapped immune response potential against VEGF could exist in cancer patients, which could be further manipulated by increasing the amount of antigen. As experimental basis for this matter, our group achieved satisfactory results in non-human primates by increasing the amount of antigen in combination with VSSP as adjuvant and using a weekly vaccination scheme [7]. VSSP has shown immunopotentiating properties on the humoral and cellular responses [9–11], however, it has not yet been explored whether increasing the amount of VSSP in the vaccine lead to higher antibody titers specific to VEGF.

An alternative strategy to enhance the vaccine immunogenicity is changing adjuvant composition in the CIGB-247 vaccine formulation. Up to date, aluminum salts are considered as the gold standard because of their effectiveness at enhancing antibody responses and their strong safety records among human adjuvants [12]. Hence, we developed a variant of CIGB-247 that incorporates aluminum phosphate as adjuvant. VEGF antigen formulated in aluminum was found to be safe in two mouse strains and in non-human primates; in mice, it inhibits tumor growth and metastases, and elicits anti-VEGF blocking antibodies and cell-mediated direct cytotoxic responses [13]. However, it has not been tested whether VEGF formulated in aluminum produces or not higher specific IgG antibody titers and VEGF/VEGFR2 blocking activities with respect to the same antigen dose per injection and VSSP as adjuvant.

Based on the unanswered questions, we firstly tested in pre-clinical animal models all of the above mentioned changes in the vaccine formulation. Then, these changes were explored in a second phase I (b) clinical trial (code name CENTAURO-2) that involved CIGB-247 vaccine candidate. This clinical trial was done in patients with advanced solid tumors. Different antigen doses and adjuvants were evaluated in terms of safety and immunogenicity, taking as reference 400 µg of antigen + 200 µg of VSSP, previously evaluated in the CENTAURO study. Because of the importance of anti-VEGF antibodies in the vaccine's potential anti-tumor effects, the present paper is mainly devoted to the description and discussion of the humoral response results of the trial, and of those obtained during the follow up of surviving patients that continued to be vaccinated off-trial.

Methods

Investigational product

The antigen used in this study is a recombinant fusion protein, representative of human VEGF isoform 121 [3]. The lyophilized antigen was produced under GMP conditions in vials of 400 µg (lots VED 12403/0 and VEN 13401/0) by the Development Unit of Center for Genetic Engineering and Biotechnology (CIGB, Havana, Cuba).

The adjuvants used were aluminum phosphate (lots VAN 1301/0 and VAN 1303/0) and VSSP (lot 711301). VSSP are very small sized particles obtained from the *Neisseria meningitides* outer membrane, supplied by the Center for Molecular Immunology of Havana, Cuba. Both adjuvants were produced under GMP conditions.

At the moment of vaccination, one or two antigen vials were dissolved in pre-calculated amounts of injection water, and the required amount was mixed with the established quantity of VSSP or aluminum phosphate, up to a final volume never exceeding 0.25 mL (mice) or 1 mL (rabbits, non-human primates and patients) per injection dose.

Animals

Female C57BL/6 and Balb/c mice, 7–9 weeks of age housed under pathogen-free conditions, were maintained at five animals per cage in contained areas. Female New Zealand rabbits weighting 1.5–2 kg (7–8 weeks of age) and healthy adult green monkeys (Chlorocebus-formerly Cercopithecus-aethiops sabaeus) weighting 3–7 kg, were caged individually in special tasked areas. All animals were purchased from the National Center for Animal Breeding (CENPALAB, Havana, Cuba), and maintained in the animal facility of the Center for Genetic Engineering and Biotechnology in accordance with the Cuban guidelines for the care and use of laboratory animals. All studies were approved by the Institute's Animal Care and Use Committee.

Pre-clinical study for the evaluation of VEGF-specific antibody response elicited at different VSSP doses and using two distinct adjuvants

Immunization was done subcutaneously in mice, rabbits and non-human primates. The immunization scheme with VSSP as adjuvant comprised eight weekly vaccinations, meanwhile using aluminum phosphate, the schedule included four bi-weekly administrations.

Humoral response was followed using an ELISA test for specific anti-human VEGF antibody titer and a competitive ELISA test for serum blockade on VEGF/VEGFR2 interaction, as previously described [3, 5, 7].

Design of the Centauro-2 trial and immunization protocol

The CENTAURO-2 clinical trial was a phase Ib, multicenter, open, non-controlled study of the CIGB-247 cancer vaccine, where different antigen doses and adjuvants were evaluated in fifty patients with advanced solid tumors. Written informed consent was obtained for all patients. The protocol and patient informed consent forms were approved by the hospitals institutional review boards and ethics committees, and by the Cuban Regulatory Authority (CECMED). This study was conducted in accordance with the ethical guidelines of the Declaration of Helsinki.

Patients were enrolled by the CIMEQ (Havana, Cuba), Celestino Hernández Robau (Santa Clara, Cuba) and José Ramón López Tabranes (Matanzas, Cuba) hospitals. Inclusion and exclusion criteria were similar to those applied for CENTAURO study [8]. However, patients with brain metastases were excluded of this trial.

Fifty patients were randomly allocated in each of the five vaccination cohorts (10 individuals per group), corresponding to: (a) 400 µg of antigen + 200 µg of VSSP referred herein as Ag + V or reference group (maximum dose previously evaluated in CENTAURO study); (b) 400 µg of antigen + 400 µg of VSSP referred herein as Ag + 2 V; (c) 800 µg of antigen + 200 µg of VSSP referred herein as 2Ag + V; (d) 200 µg of antigen + 0.7 mg Al^{3+} referred herein as ½Ag + Al; (e) 400 µg of antigen + 0.7 mg Al^{3+} referred herein as Ag + Al. All vaccinations were administered subcutaneously as a single site dose. Figure 1a details the immunization protocol for groups Ag + V, Ag + 2 V and 2Ag + V, and Fig. 1b for the ½Ag + Al and Ag + Al cohorts.

At week sixteen, data from each patient were gathered and processed for the final report to be submitted to CECMED. Individuals surviving the trial period were eligible under medical supervision to start off-trial voluntary re-immunizations. Re-immunizations started on week sixteen, once every four weeks, until death, intolerance, marked disease progression or patient's withdrawal of consent.

Human blood samples

Venous blood samples were collected using a blood collection set with pre-attached holder (Becton Dickinson 367355) and taken into an EDTA tube or into a serum separator tube for plasma and serum analyses respectively. Serum and plasma samples were immediately stored at -70 °C until use.

Blood samples were taken during the trial period at weeks 0 (pre-vaccination), 5 or 6, 9, 13 (one week after the end of trial vaccinations) and 16 (end of trial period and start of off-trial re-immunizations). For investigations conducted during the off-trial re-immunizations, blood samples were taken at different time points, depending on patient availability.

ELISAs reagents

GST-fused human VEGF isoform 121 (GST-hVEGF) was produced in E. coli as previously described [14]. Human VEGF isoform 121 (rhVEGF) was produced in CHO cells [15]. Skim milk powder (A0830) and Tween 20 (A1389) were supplied by AppliChem. HRP-conjugated sheep anti-mouse IgG antibody (Sigma A6782) or HRP-conjugated goat anti-rabbit IgG antibody (Sigma A0545) were used for detecting mouse or rabbit serum IgG respectively. HRP-conjugated goat anti-human IgG (Fc γ fragment specific) antibody (Jackson Immunoresearch Laboratories, 109-035-098) was used for detecting human or monkey serum IgG at 80 ng/mL. Biotinylated antibodies specific for human IgM (3840-6-250), human IgA (3860-6-250) and human IgE (3810-8-250) were supplied by Mabtech. Biotinylated mouse monoclonal

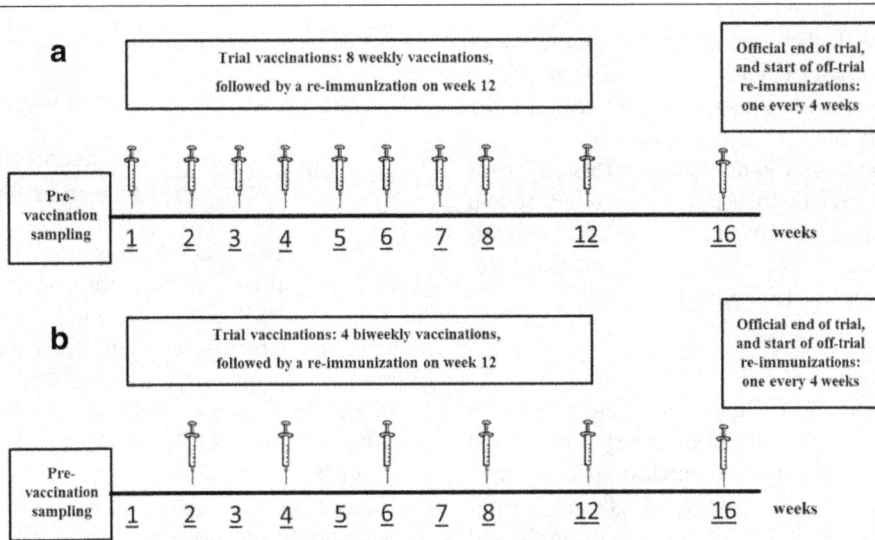

Fig. 1 Vaccination schedules. CIGB-247 combinations using VSSP or aluminum phosphate as adjuvants were administered weekly (**a**) or bi-weekly (**b**), respectively. Pre-vaccination sampling included sera and plasma. After the end of the trial period (week 16), a re-immunization was done once every 4 weeks until death, intolerance, marked disease progression or patient's withdrawal of consent

antibodies specific for human IgG1 (ab9975), IgG2 (ab99785), IgG3 (ab99830) and IgG4 (ab99824) were purchased from Abcam. Recombinant human VEGF receptor 2/Fcγ chimera (Sigma, V6758) and recombinant human VEGF receptor 1/Fcγ chimera (Sigma, V1385) were used in competitive ELISAs as described below. Bevacizumab, a commercially available monoclonal antibody specific to human VEGF (Roche, Switzerland) was used as a positive control for VEGF/VEGFR2 and VEGF/VEGFR1 blockade. In the competitive ELISAs, biotinylated goat antibodies specific for human VEGFR2 (BAF357) or human VEGFR1 (BAF321) were supplied by R&D Systems for detecting VEGF/VEGFR2 or VEGF/VEGFR1 bindings respectively, and used at 0.1 μg/mL. Streptavidin-peroxidase conjugate (Sigma, S5512), was used at 1/30,000 dilution.

ELISA for specific anti-human VEGF IgG, IgM, IgA and IgE antibodies

The levels of human IgG, IgM, IgA and IgE antibodies against rhVEGF were measured by a conventional isotype-specific indirect ELISA. Wells were coated with rhVEGF (2.5 μg/mL) during overnight incubation at 4 °C (100 μL/well). Following blocking step (250 μL/well), the wells were incubated with serum samples (100 μL/well, 1 h at 37 °C) and IgG, IgM, IgA or IgE antibodies were detected with HRP-conjugated goat anti-human IgG antibody, biotinylated goat anti-human IgM antibody (specific for Fc5μ), biotinylated anti-human IgA monoclonal antibody (specific for Fc part) and biotinylated anti-human IgE monoclonal antibodies respectively. For biotinylated conjugates the detection system consisted of a 1:30,000 dilution of streptavidin-conjugated HRP

(100 μL/well, 45 min at 37 °C). Plates were developed by using H_2O_2 as substrate and OPD or TMB as chromogen (100 μL/well). After 15 min, the reaction was stopped by the addition of 2.0 N H_2SO_4 (50 μl/well), and the absorbance was measured at 492 or 450 nm, respectively.

For IgG assay, the wells were blocked with 2.5% goat serum, 2% skim milk, 0.05% Tween20. Serum samples were diluted with blocking buffer. Secondary antibody was diluted with 2% skim milk, 0.05% Tween20. IgG anti-VEGF ELISA has been previously described in details by Sánchez et al. [15]. ELISAs for detecting IgM, IgA and IgE antibodies specific to VEGF used as blocking reagent the following buffer: 2.5% goat serum, 2% BSA, 0.05% Tween20. Serum samples were diluted with RD6 (R&D Systems, diluent of kit SVE00). Biotinylated conjugates and streptavidin-conjugated HRP were diluted in 1% BSA.

IgG antibody titer was estimated as previously described [15]. The procedure was similar for IgM, IgA and IgE with the difference that the interpolated value on "x" axis was determined by adding five standard deviations to the duplicated mean of the blank optical density.

Titer ratio and "VEGF-specific antibody titer" were calculated as follow:

$$\text{Titer ratio} = \frac{\text{Post vaccination titer}}{\text{Pre vaccination titer}} \quad (A)$$

Specific antibody titer = Post vaccination titer-Pre vaccination titer (B)

To declare a given serum sample taken during vaccination to be positive for VEGF-specific IgG, IgM, IgA, or

IgE antibodies, the obtained "titer ratio" must be ≥2 (formula A). In the particular case of IgG antibodies, additionally to the criterion depicted above, for a sample to be considered positive, it has also to comply with a value of "specific antibody titer" ≥1/100 (formula B).

The term seroconversion is only used in this paper for IgG antibodies and refers to a patient that has shown two or more samples positive for VEGF-specific antibodies during trial vaccinations or off-trial re-immunizations (seroconverted patient) [8].

IgG subclasses assays

Antigen-specific IgG1, IgG2, IgG3, and IgG4 antibodies were determined by indirect ELISA using biotinylated mouse monoclonal anti-human subclass-specific antibodies (IgG1, IgG2, IgG3 and IgG4). Briefly, microtiter plates were coated with rhVEGF (2.5 µg/mL) and blocked with 4% BSA. Sera were diluted with 0.4% BSA and incubated during 1 h at 37 °C. The subsequent steps of the reaction were developed as described above.

To declare a given serum sample taken during vaccination as "non-detectable" for VEGF-specific IgG1, IgG2, IgG3, or IgG4 antibodies, "specific antibody titer" must be < 1/10. Values ≥ 1/10 make samples to be classified as "detectable". For each patient, the IgG subclass classified as "detectable" with the highest "specific antibody titer" was declared as "predominant".

Competitive ELISA for serum blockade of VEGF/VEGFR2 and VEGF/VEGFR1 interactions

Competitive ELISA has been previously described in details by Sánchez et al. [15]. Briefly, plates were coated overnight at 4 °C with rhVEGF. After three washes with 0.1% Tween 20 in PBS, the plates were blocked with 4% BSA for 1 h at 37 °C, followed by new washes. Serial dilutions of test sera (1/50, 1/100, 1/200, 1/400), Bevacizumab (1 µg/mL) or dilution buffer were added (100 µL/well) and incubated for 1 h at 37 °C. Then, 100 µL of 25 ng/mL of VEGFR2-Fc or 125 ng/mL of VEGFR1-Fc were added to the wells (12.5 and 62.5 ng/mL final concentration respectively) and additionally incubated for 45 min at 37 °C. After washes, wells were incubated with biotinylated anti-human VEGFR2 or VEGFR1 antibodies, the latter followed by streptavidin-peroxidase conjugate. The subsequent steps of the reaction were developed as described in previous sub-sections.

Maximum bindings of VEGFR2 or VEGFR1 were obtained from wells incubated with dilution buffer (instead of serum sample) and VEGF receptors/Fcγ chimeras (VEGFR2-Fc or VEGFR1-Fc). The inhibition caused by a given sample (sera or positive control) on VEGF/VEGFR2 or VEGF/VEGFR1 interactions was expressed as percentage, according to the following formula:

$$\% \text{ inhibition} = 100\% - \left[\left(\frac{\text{absorbance of test sample}}{\text{absorbance of "Maximum Binding"}}\right) * 100\right] \text{ (C)}$$

Inhibition levels were expressed as a % ratio:

$$\text{inhibition levels} = \frac{\text{Post vaccination inhibition }(\%)}{\text{Pre vaccination inhibition }(\%)} \text{ (D)}$$

A given serum sample was considered positive for neutralizing anti-VEGF antibodies when the value resulting from this ratio was ≥2 (formula D). Patients showing at least one serum sample with neutralizing anti-VEGF antibodies during trial vaccinations or off-trial re-immunizations were considered with a positive blocking activity on the VEGF/VEGFR1 or VEGF/VEGFR2 bindings [8].

Results from competitive ELISA tests were accepted if the assay shows a variability below 10% (assay criterion). The effect of re-immunization on VEGF/VEGFR2 blockade was studied during off-trial re-immunizations. In this phase, sample "A" (before re-immunization) and sample "B" (7–10 days after re-immunization) were analyzed, where certain levels of anti-VEGF blocking antibodies could be circulating as result of monthly vaccinations. Based on assay criterion and a work published by other authors [16], a value of 10% was established as the cut off to consider an increase or not in anti-VEGF blocking activity between samples "A" and "B".

Measurements of platelet VEGF and sVEGFR-2 in plasma

VEGF and soluble VEGFR2 (sVEGFR-2) concentrations in serum and/or plasma samples were measured with commercially available sandwich enzyme-linked immunosorbent assay kits from R&D Systems (SVE00 and SVR200 respectively). All standard reagents and solutions, supplied by kits, were used in accordance with the manufacturer's instructions.

VEGF released per platelet was calculated using the following formula [17]:

$$\text{Platelet VEGF} = \frac{(\text{Serum VEGF-plasma VEGF}) \, x \, (1 - \text{haematocrit})}{\text{platelet counts}}$$

Platelet VEGF was expressed in picograms of VEGF per million platelets. Levels of platelet VEGF and plasma sVEGFR-2 were measured at baseline (pre-vaccination), at the end of trial vaccinations (week 13) and thereafter during re-immunizations.

In the re-immunization phase, the number of available patients decreased and therefore statistical tests were not used. For each individual, platelet VEGF and sVEGFR-2 were determined in a sample taken 7–10 days after a given re-immunization. The variation of both parameters (denominated ΔVEGF or ΔsVEGFR-2) was expressed in percentage and was calculated using the following formula:

$$\Delta VEGF \text{ or } \Delta sVEGFR\text{-}2 = \left[\left(\frac{\text{levels after re-immunization}}{\text{pre-vaccination levels}} \right) * 100 \right] - 100\%$$

Based on criteria established by other authors [18], $\Delta \leq -30\%$ was considered a decrease; $\Delta \geq 30\%$ was considered an increase; $-30\% < \Delta < 30\%$ indicated a stability.

Statistical analysis

All experiments included at least duplicated measurements. Data, graphs and statistic were analyzed with Graphpad Prism software version 5.0 (Graphpad Software Inc., La Jolla, CA). Differences in anti-VEGF antibodies or blocking activity were evaluated using unpaired t-test in pre-clinical settings. In patients, matched comparisons of platelet VEGF and plasma sVEGFR-2 from weeks 0 and 13 per treatment group, were done using paired t test (data that were normally distributed or after log transformation). Spearman correlation test was used to measure the correlation between one non-parametric variable with one parametric variable. Statistical significance was considered as $p < 0.05$.

Results

Pre-clinical research to explore the influence of dose and different adjuvants on VEGF-specific IgG antibodies and VEGF/VEGFR2 blocking activities

In order to investigate the effects on VEGF-specific antibody response of higher doses of VSSP in the VEGF vaccine formulation or the antigen combination with aluminum phosphate, we performed a pre-clinical study. This pre-clinical study was based on immunogenicity experiments done in mice, rabbits and non-human primates.

In mice when the amount of VSSP was doubled in the vaccine formulation (¼Ag + V), anti-VEGF antibody titers were significantly higher than those found in the group ¼Ag + ½ V (unpaired t-test, $p = 0.0180$) (Fig. 2a). At the same antigen dose level, the combination with aluminum phosphate elicited VEGF-specific antibody titers and VEGF/VEGFR2 blocking activities with values significantly higher than the combination with VSSP (unpaired t-test, $p = 0.0009$ and $p = 0.0010$ respectively) (Fig. 2b and c).

Rabbits immunized with Ag + Al showed antibody titers and blocking activities seven and three times higher than the group of rabbits vaccinated with Ag + V (Fig. 2d and e). As shown in Fig. 2 f, monkeys vaccinated with Ag + Al developed anti-VEGF antibody titers four times higher than the antibody titers seen in the group immunized with Ag + V. Only in this animal species, a similar level of blocking activity in serum was detected between both groups (Fig. 2g).

All these experimental evidences indicated that the increase of the VSSP dose or the change of adjuvant towards aluminum phosphate induce a positive effect on the humoral response specific to VEGF. For that reason, we decided to evaluate such new vaccine formulations in the framework of a clinical trial in cancer patients (CENTAURO-2).

Patients characteristics and immunization compliance

Table 1 depicts the basic characteristics of patients included in the CENTAURO-2 clinical study. Of the fifty patients, 33 were females and 17 males (Table 1). Subjects had a variety of malignancies at original diagnosis, being the most common breast (n = 11 for a 22%), colon (n = 8 for a 16%), lung and ovary (for each one n = 7 for a 14%). At the moment of inclusion in the CENTAURO-2 trial, 96% of the patients had metastatic disease and 74% were classified as progressive disease, according the RECIST criteria. Eastern Cooperative Oncology Group performance status (ECOG) was 1 or 2 for 84% of the enrolled patients.

Forty-one patients completed the trial immunization scheme (82%). Of the nine non-evaluated patients, two abandoned voluntarily, other five died; one abandoned due to disease progression and one patient was excluded of the study due to the early development of brain metastasis (exclusion criteria).

Safety

In order to investigate the safety of the different vaccine formulations, medical evaluations were done before and after each vaccination. Injection site grade I events accounted for 87.74% of all adverse events seen during the trial period (up to week 16) that could be classified as probably or definitively related to the vaccine (Additional file 1). With VSSP as adjuvant, other thirty general adverse events were also recorded, most of them grade I, exception made of one event of grade II, and two events of grade III. With aluminum as adjuvant, the majority of the adverse events were local, exception made of one case of asthenia, and all grade I. Hence, a majority of the documented adverse effects attributable to vaccination were low grade injection site events. Because of the strong bacterial contents of VSSP, the individuals immunized with VSSP vaccine formulations showed a higher amount of low grade local adverse events than when aluminum was used as adjuvant. All these events were controlled, and patients with adverse events were treated either with pharmacological or non-pharmacological therapies. All documented events happened in 29 patients (58%) of the 50 recruited individuals (Additional file 1). All deaths during trial period or re-immunization phase were attributable to the progression of their base disease.

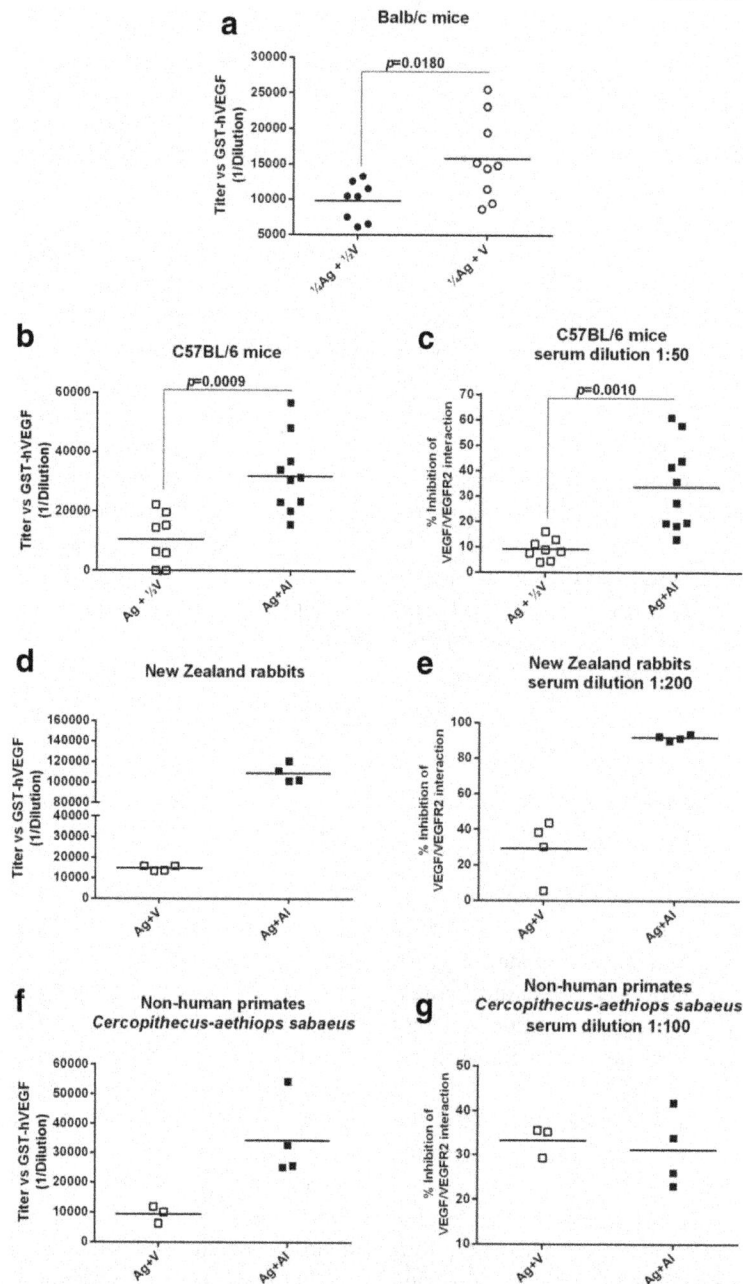

Fig. 2 Humoral response in pre-clinical models. Specific IgG antibodies were detected by ELISA using GST-hVEGF as coating antigen (**a**, **b**, **d** and **f**). The ability of animal sera antibodies to block VEGF/VEGFR2 interaction was determined using a competitive ELISA, where a soluble VEGFR2 competes with diluted serum in plates coated with GST-hVEGF (**c**, **e** and **g**). CIGB-247 combinations using VSSP or aluminum phosphate as adjuvants were administered weekly (eight vaccinations) or bi-weekly (four vaccinations) respectively. Horizontal bars represent the mean values of antibody titer or blocking activity, which are shown for each group. *p*-Values were calculated according to unpaired *t*-test. Reference dose (A + V): 400 µg of antigen + 200 µg of VSSP; (¼Ag + ½ V): 100 µg of antigen + 100 µg of VSSP; (¼Ag + V): 100 µg of antigen + 200 µg of VSSP; (Ag + Al): 400 µg of antigen + aluminum phosphate

Antibody classes responses specific to VEGF after completion the trial vaccination scheme

To study in depth the vaccine-induced polyclonal humoral immune response, four classes of human immunoglobulins were determined by ELISAs. Of the 41 patients that finished all programmed immunizations,

serum samples from 39 individuals were available for antibody tests on week 13 (one week after completion the trial vaccination scheme).

Figure 3a–c display specific antibody titers against VEGF for IgG, IgM, and IgA respectively, for patients of all cohorts. Each patient is represented as an empty

Table 1 Patients enrolled in the CENTAURO-2 phase Ib clinical trial

Characteristic	n	Percent
Age		
≥ 50	38	76%
< 50	12	24%
Sex		
Female	33	66%
Male	17	34%
Primary tumor site[a]		
Breast	11	22%
Colon	8	16%
Lung	7	14%
Ovary	7	14%
Kidney	3	6%
Uterus	3	6%
Soft tissues	3	6%
Anal canal	2	4%
Rectum	2	4%
Others	4	8%
Metastasis[b]		
Liver	13	27%
Lung	8	16%
Bone	6	12%
Lymph nodes	6	12%
Suprarenal glands	4	8%
Soft tissue	2	4%
Others	9	16%
Without metastasis	2	4%
Status[c]		
PD	37	74%
SD	13	26%
ECOG PS		
0	8	16%
1	34	68%
2	8	16%
Trial vaccinations		
Completed[d]	41	82%
No completed	9	18%

Patients were eligible for enrollment after having received available therapy and were no longer responding. ECOG PS, Eastern Cooperative Oncology Group performance status; PD, progressive disease; SD, stable disease. [a]at the time of initial diagnosis; [b]at the time of trial inclusion; [c]RECIST classification at the time of trial inclusion; [d]39 patients of the 41 were available for antibody tests and sVEGFR-2 at week thirteen; 38 patients were available for platelet VEGF

symbol (serum sample positive for antibody at week 13) or filled symbol (serum sample negative for antibody at week 13). It can be seen that of the 39 evaluated

patients, 26 individuals (66.7%) had positive samples to VEGF-specific IgG antibodies, 11 (28.2%) for IgA, and 7 (18%) for IgM. No patient had detectable levels of specific IgE (Additional file 2).

At week 13, the group 2Ag + V exhibited the highest number of samples positive for IgG or IgM or IgA antibodies specific to VEGF (Fig. 3). At this moment, there were patients with triple-positive samples (IgG/IgM/IgA). Individuals with IgG/IgA or IgG/IgM double-positive samples were detected, however, the combination IgM/IgA was not observed. All cases with single-positive samples were IgG but neither IgM nor IgA (Additional file 3).

Specific antibody titers values showed the following trend: IgG > IgM > IgA, excluding the groups Ag + 2 V and ½ Ag + Al, in which IgM antibodies specific to VEGF were higher than IgG antibodies (Fig. 3). Irrespective of the used adjuvant, VSSP or aluminum phosphate, CIGB-247 induces anti-VEGF IgG antibodies as principal class of immunoglobulins. For that reason, it was the class of immunoglobulin under study at different time points during trial vaccinations (weeks 5 or 6, 9 and 13). Vaccination increased specific IgG titers in at least one serum sample, in 43 of the 47 evaluable patients, with values as low as 1/10 and as high as 1/93981 (Additional file 4).

Specific anti-VEGF IgG seroconversion in patients that completed the trial vaccination scheme

In order to evaluate the seroconversion, the principal immunoglobulin class specific to VEGF was chosen for this analysis. Figures 4a depicts the results of IgG seroconversion (patient that has shown two or more samples positive for VEGF-specific antibodies) for those patients that completed the trial vaccination scheme. The reference group (Ag + V) showed six seroconverted patients out of the eight evaluable individuals (75%) (Fig. 4a). When the antigen dose was increased to 800 μg (group 2Ag + V), the proportion of seroconverted patients increased (8/8 for a 100%). The opposite effect was observed when the adjuvant VSSP was increased to 400 μg: in the Ag + 2 V group, the proportion of seroconverted patients decreased (5/8 for a 62.5%). With the same antigen dose (400 μg) and aluminum phosphate as adjuvant (group Ag + Al), the proportion of seroconverted patients was similar (6/8 for a 75%) to that of the reference group. The lowest proportion of seroconverted patients was found in the cohort vaccinated with 200 μg of antigen and aluminum phosphate as adjuvant (group ½Ag + Al) with only one patient of nine for a 11% (Fig. 4a). The percentage of seroconverted patients per cohort, showed the following order: 2Ag + V > Ag + V = Ag + Al > Ag + 2 V > ½ Ag + Al (Fig. 4a).

Early seroconversion occurs when a seroconverted patient has a positive serum sample at week 5 (VSSP-

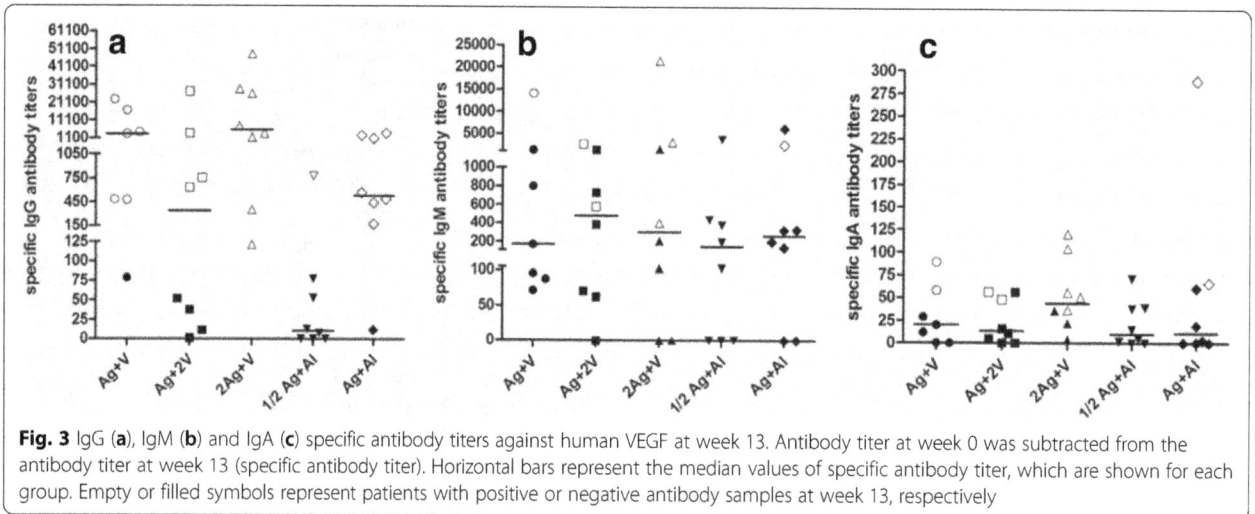

Fig. 3 IgG (**a**), IgM (**b**) and IgA (**c**) specific antibody titers against human VEGF at week 13. Antibody titer at week 0 was subtracted from the antibody titer at week 13 (specific antibody titer). Horizontal bars represent the median values of specific antibody titer, which are shown for each group. Empty or filled symbols represent patients with positive or negative antibody samples at week 13, respectively

adjuvanted cohorts) or week 6 (aluminum-adjuvanted cohorts). Figure 4b shows that early seroconversion responses were preferably found in VSSP-adjuvanted cohorts. The number of early seroconverted patients for the groups 2Ag + V, Ag + 2 V and Ag + V were 5/8, 4/8, and 3/8, respectively, compared to 1/8 and 0/8 in the Ag + Al and ½Ag + Al cohorts.

VEGF/VEGFR2 and VEGF/VEGFR1 blocking activities in patients that completed the trial vaccination scheme

VEGF and its receptors VEGFR1 and VEGFR2 play major roles in tumor angiogenesis [19]. In order to assess the ability of serum antibodies from a vaccinated patient to block the binding of VEGF to its receptors, a competitive ELISA was performed.

Figure 5a shows the number of patients with positive blocking activity on the VEGF/VEGFR2 binding. Individuals showing at least one serum sample with neutralizing anti-VEGF antibodies were considered positive for blocking activity. In the reference group, five out of eight patients (62.5%) had a positive blocking activity on the VEGF/VEGFR2 binding, similar to the group 2Ag + V. A slightly lower number of positive patients were observed for the aluminum-adjuvanted cohorts: ½Ag + Al (5/9 for a 55.6%) and Ag + Al (4/8 for a 50%). The lowest number of positive patients was found in the Ag + 2 V group (2/8 for a 25%).

Figure 5b depicts a similar analysis for the VEGF/VEGFR1 blocking activity test. The reference group (Ag + V) exhibited the lowest number of positive patients (3/8 for a 37.5%). When the amount of antigen or VSSP were doubled as compared to the reference group, the proportion of positive patients increased in both groups, (6/8 for a 75%) and (5/7 for a 71.4%), respectively. In the aluminum- adjuvanted cohorts, the rates were 6 out of 8 patients for the Ag + Al group (75%), and 5 out of 9 patients for the ½Ag + Al group (56%).

All results shown above demonstrated that using of aluminum as adjuvant, a higher humoral response was obtained at the antigen dose level of 400 μg. Of all antigen doses and adjuvant combinations, the most immunogenic dose was 800 μg of antigen in combination with 200 μg of VSSP.

IgG seroconversion and VEGF/VEGFR2 blocking activity in patients that received off-trial re-immunizations

One of the features of this study is the relatively long period over which the patients were immunologically evaluated (up to week 60), receiving up to eleven re-immunizations (Additional file 5). Re-immunizations were administered every four weeks. Patients belonging to groups Ag + V and 2Ag + V conserved their original vaccine formulation in this phase of the study. Patients from the Ag + 2 V, ½Ag + Al and Ag + Al cohorts kept their original vaccine formulation for re-immunization, until the approval of the final trial report by CECMED. At this point, taking into consideration the results of safety and humoral response, these three cohorts switched to 800 μg of antigen + 200 μg of VSSP, always under medical supervision. For each patient, the time point of dose change is shown in Additional file 5. Because of their distinct recruitment moment, the exact time point of the switch was different between individuals, even in a same cohort.

Of the thirty-two patients that were eligible for off-trial re-immunizations, twenty-two individuals had at least two serum samples after week sixteen (Additional file 5). In these patients, studies involving seroconversion and VEGF/VEGFR2 blocking activity were done. VEGF/VEGFR1 blockade was not studied.

Of these 22 patients, 16 seroconverted individuals (72.7%) during trial vaccinations conserved their status during re-immunization phase. Three patients (13.6%) with no evidence of seroconversion turned to seroconverted status

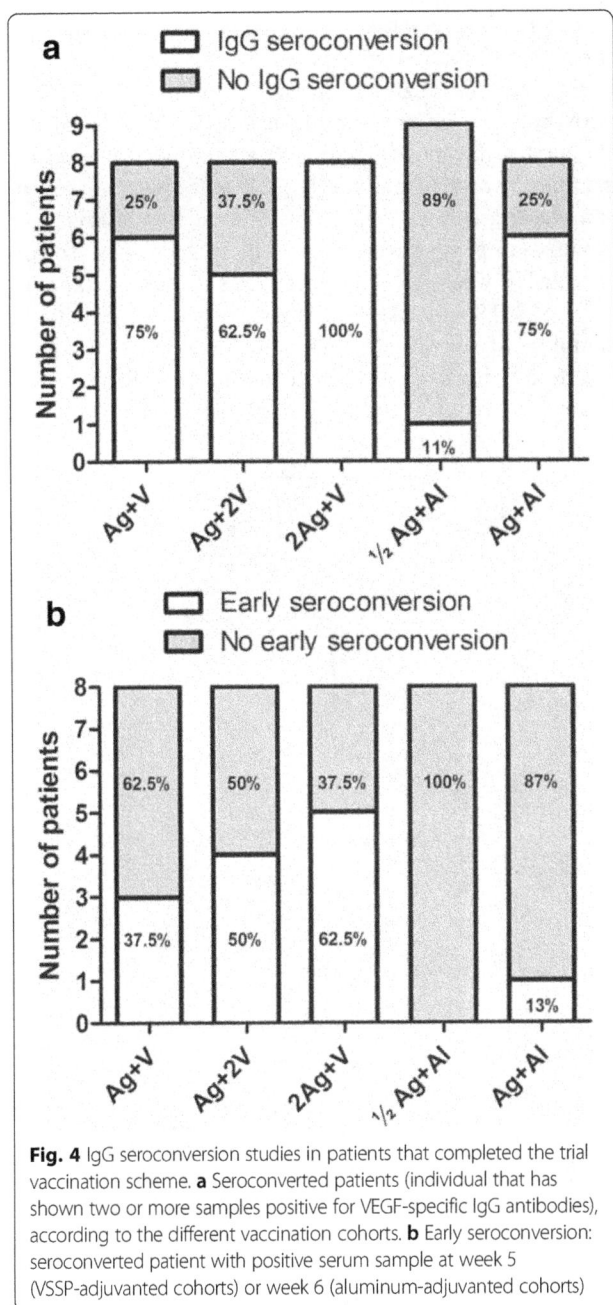

Fig. 4 IgG seroconversion studies in patients that completed the trial vaccination scheme. **a** Seroconverted patients (individual that has shown two or more samples positive for VEGF-specific IgG antibodies), according to the different vaccination cohorts. **b** Early seroconversion: seroconverted patient with positive serum sample at week 5 (VSSP-adjuvanted cohorts) or week 6 (aluminum-adjuvanted cohorts)

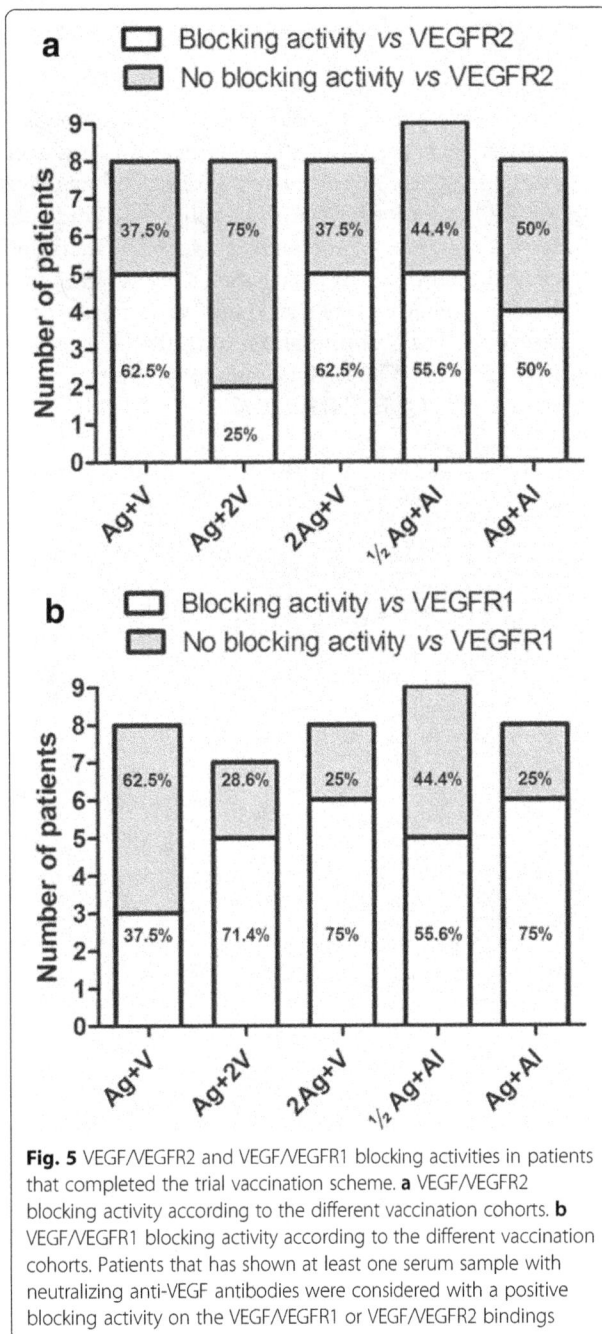

Fig. 5 VEGF/VEGFR2 and VEGF/VEGFR1 blocking activities in patients that completed the trial vaccination scheme. **a** VEGF/VEGFR2 blocking activity according to the different vaccination cohorts. **b** VEGF/VEGFR1 blocking activity according to the different vaccination cohorts. Patients that has shown at least one serum sample with neutralizing anti-VEGF antibodies were considered with a positive blocking activity on the VEGF/VEGFR1 or VEGF/VEGFR2 bindings

after off-trial re-immunizations. Two individuals (9.1%) remained negative in both phases and one patient (4.5%) lost his seroconverted status. In the case of VEGF/VEGFR2 blocking activity, eleven individuals (50%) with positive blocking activity during trial vaccinations conserved their status during re-immunization phase. Five patients (22.7%) with no documented blocking activity turned to positive status after off-trial re-immunizations. Three individuals (13.6%) remained negative in both phases and another three patients lost their positive blocking activity during re-immunization phase.

Evolution of VEGF-specific IgG antibodies and VEGF/VEGFR2 blockade in twelve patients submitted to long-term re-immunizations

Twelve of the thirteen patients submitted to long-term re-immunizations with an overall survival longer than 45 weeks (approximately 1 year) were studied. In these patients, evolution of VEGF-specific IgG antibodies and VEGF/VEGFR2 blockade were studied in more detail, including their pre-vaccination values (week 0) and values at week 13 (one week after the last immunization of the trial vaccinations). All these patients were individually followed in Fig. 6.

For most patients, serum samples obtained during re-immunization phase had VEGF-specific IgG antibodies titers higher than pre-vaccination, regardless of the fact that samples could be considered positive or negative (Fig. 6). Only in patient JL42, IgG antibodies gradually decreased to pre-vaccination levels at week 50. Taking as reference the end of trial vaccinations (week 13), anti-VEGF IgG antibody titers presented an increase or a decrease during the re-immunization phase. Regarding positivity of anti-VEGF IgG antibody titers, eight patients (JL12, CQ13, CH19, CH27, JL29, CH33, CH45 and JL49) had positive serum sample at week 13 and then maintained their positivity in samples taken during re-immunization period. One subject (CH20), with negative serum sample at week 13, showed for the first time, positivity for three consecutive serum samples. Another patient (JL30), with positive serum sample at week 13, lost this status in five consecutive serum samples. Patient JL42 had a positive serum sample at week 13, conserved this status in samples of weeks 18 and 28, and then lost his positivity in samples of weeks 36, 44 and 49. Finally, patient CH08 did not exhibit positivity in any of the times when the serum sampling was made.

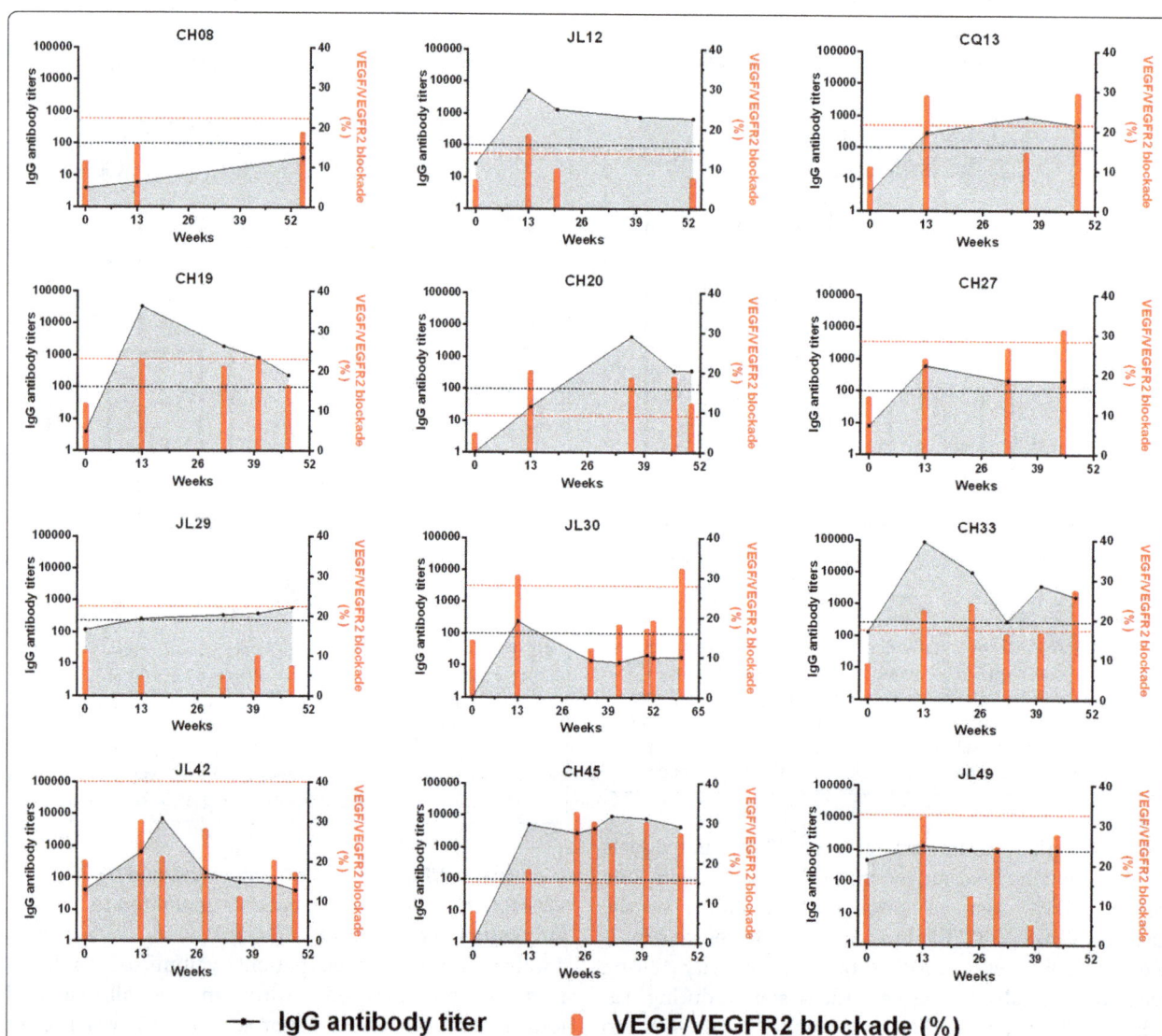

Fig. 6 Evolution of VEGF-specific IgG antibodies and VEGF/VEGFR2 blockade in patients submitted to long-term re-immunizations. Samples, taken at different time points, came from twelve patients (depicted by their trial code name) with an overall survival longer than 45 weeks (approximately 1 year). Antibody titers and VEGF/VEGFR2 blockade percentages are shown as *black dots* and *red bars*, respectively. Week 0 is pre-vaccination and week 13 is one week after finishing the trial vaccinations. Cut-off values that define the positivity for IgG antibodies (*black discontinued line*) and VEGF/VEGFR2 blockade (*red discontinued line*) are shown for each patient

The VEGF/VEGFR2 blockade, expressed in percentage, is characterized by a very fluctuating behavior during the course of sustained immunization (Fig. 6). Concerning positivity for VEGF/VEGFR2 blockade, Fig. 6 shows that one patient (CH27) with negative serum sample at week 13, increased the percentage values at week 32, being positive at week 45. Two individuals (CH45 and CH20) had a positive serum sample at week 13, and all serum samples taken during off-trial re-immunization maintained their positivity. Three patients (CQ13, JL30 and CH33) were positive at week 13, and during the re-immunization phase these patients restored their positive status after having lost it. In two other patients (JL12 and CH19), samples taken during the re-immunization phase did not show the positive status that have been present in week 13. Finally, serum samples for four patients (CH08, JL29, JL42 y JL49) never reached values above cut-off and remained negative.

Re-immunizations effects on VEGF-specific antibodies and VEGF/VEGFR2 blockade in twelve patients submitted to long-term re-immunizations

All these aforementioned findings could be influenced by the moment in which the sample was taken. The samples available during off-trial re-immunizations were mostly acquired at the moment of a new vaccination, i.e., approximately four weeks after a previous re-immunization. However, it is well known that the earliest time at which serum antibody peaks following vaccination is at about 7–14 days. To better study the effect of re-immunization on anti-VEGF antibody levels and VEGF/VEGFR2 blockade, blood samples from 12 patients submitted to long-term vaccinations were taken just before the re-immunization (sample A) and then, these patients were summoned 7 to 10 days after this re-immunization for additional blood sampling (sample B). Table 2 shows the study results for IgG, IgM and IgA antibodies specific to VEGF, as well as VEGF/VEGFR2 blockade in these serum samples. Re-immunization was considered effective if: i) sample "B" conserves or gains positivity or ii) value in sample "B" is higher than value obtained in sample "A" (*antibody titer: sample "B" - sample "A" ≥ 1/100 or VEGF/VEGFR2 blockade: sample "B" - sample "A" ≥ 10%*).

Regarding positivity of anti-VEGF IgG antibody titers, nine of the twelve patients (JL12, CQ13, CH19, CH20, CH27, JL29, CH33, CH45 and JL49) with the re-immunization conserved their positivity for the test. Samples "A" and "B" were positive in all cases (Table 2). For IgM, the re-immunization was effective in four patients (JL12, CH33, CH45 and JL49). In the case of patient JL12, had a negative sample "A", after the re-immunization, he gained positivity in sample "B". For

IgA, only patient CH33 conserved positivity (both samples "A" and "B" were positive). Concerning VEGF/VEGFR2 blockade, the re-immunization was effective in eight of the twelve patients. Of these eight patients, five individuals (CQ13, CH20, CH27, CH33 and CH45) had positive results both in sample acquired at re-immunization time (sample "A"), and 7–10 days afterwards (sample "B"). The remaining three individuals (JL12, CH19 and JL49) had sample "A" classified as negative, and they changed to positive in the sample taken later (sample "B") (Table 2).

The effect of re-immunization on antibody levels was studied in the same cohort of patients underwent long-term vaccinations. In general, the re-immunization had a limited effect on specific-IgG or IgA antibody levels. For IgG, only two individuals increased their IgG antibody titers, from 1/589 (sample "A") to 1/795 (sample "B") in patient JL29 and from 1/947 to 1/1110 in patient JL49. For IgA, no increments were detected. A different scenario was seen for IgM, with seven patients (CQ13, CH19, CH27, JL29, CH33, JL42 and CH45) showing IgM antibody titers in sample "B" higher than the values obtained in sample "A" (Table 2). In the case of VEGF/VEGFR2 blockade, in three patients (CH19, JL29 and JL42), inhibition percentages were found to be higher in sample "B" than the values obtained in sample"A".

IgG subclasses

As was demonstrated previously, anti-VEGF IgG antibodies were the principal class of immunoglobulins. In order to study the contribution of each one of the four VEGF-specific IgG subclasses, indirect ELISA was performed using human VEGF as coating antigen. Figure 7 shows IgG subclasses analysis without regarding antigen doses or vaccination schedules. The study was made for three different vaccination periods or stages: weeks 5–16 (trial period), weeks 20–36 (early off-trial re-immunizations) and weeks 46–56 (long-term re-immunizations). In each of these stages, and for the available patients, serum samples with the highest anti-VEGF IgG antibody titers were chosen for these measurements.

IgG1, IgG2 and IgG4 subclasses specific to VEGF were found in all periods. Only IgG3 was not detected during long-term re-immunizations (Fig. 7). The predominant subclass in all periods was IgG1, accounting for 50% of patients in the first two stages, and 38.5% in the third and last. Both, IgG2 and IgG3, were the second most important immunoglobulins during trial period with 13.6% of the patients. IgG2 was conserved over time as "detectable" or as "predominant" subclass. IgG3 had a tendency to disappear. Finally, IgG4 increased over time as "predominant" subclass from 0% in trial period to 30.8% of the patients during long-term re-immunizations, being the second most relevant IgG subclass during this latter period.

Table 2 Effect of the re-immunization on VEGF-specific IgG, IgA and IgM antibodies or VEGF/VEGFR2 blockade

Patient code	IgG antibody titer			IgA antibody titer			IgM antibody titer			VEGF/VEGFR2 blockade (%)		
	Pre-vaccination	Re-immunization phase		Pre-vaccination	Re-immunization phase		Pre-vaccination	Re-immunization phase		Pre-vaccination	Re-immunization phase	
	Week 0	Sample A	Sample B	Week 0	Sample A	Sample B	Week 0	Sample A	Sample B	Week 0	Sample A	Sample B
CH08	4	36	31	49	70	71	1183	1035	1101	11.2	18.7	11.9
JL12	26	700*	770*	49	93	56	298	528	604*	6.92	7.5	15.2*
CQ13	4	505*	582*	335	286	305	1655	2090	2198†	10.8	29.4*	24.5*
CH19	4	232*	244*	49	59	68	1180	1462	1978†	11.5	16.1	31.5*,#
CH20	1	374*	339*	110	94	62	963	629	675	4.6	12.1*	16.7
CH27	8	207*	236*	268	472*	319*	1947	3422	3732†	14.2	31.1*	29.9*
JL29	118	589*	795*,†	87	124	144	707	438	557†	11.2	7.2	20.8#
JL30	1	17	17	69	72	75	886	663	688	14	19	18
CH33	133	1655*	1697*	111	676*	530*	2591	341140*	3859811*,†	8.7	27.2*	28.9*
JL42	41	40	56	70	73	96	1788	1374	2426†	20	17	27#
CH45	0	4474*	3825*	48	80	84	543	4108*	4995*,†	7.6	27.4*	23*
JL49	463	947*	1110*,†	70	155*	125	509	1114*	1027*	16.3	27.5	34.1*

Sample "A": is the value for the sample taken just before the re-immunization; Sample "B": is the value for the sample acquired 7–10 days after the taking of the sample "A". [*]: sample meets the positivity criteria for specific-IgG (using formulas A and B), IgA or IgM antibodies (using formula A) or VEGF/VEGFR2 blockade (using formula D). (†): sample meets the criterion of increase for antibody titer: sample "B" - sample "A" ≥ 1/100. (#): sample meets the criterion of increase for VEGF/VEGFR2 blockade: sample "B" - sample "A" ≥ 10%. Patients: CH08 (sample A taken at week 55; sample B taken at week 56); JL12 (sample A taken at week 53; sample B taken at week 54); CQ13 (sample A taken at week 48; sample B taken at week 49); CH19 (sample A taken at week 47; sample B taken at week 48); CH20 (sample A taken at week 50; sample B taken at week 51); CH27 (sample A taken at week 45; sample B taken at week 46); JL29 (sample A taken at week 48; sample B taken at week 49); JL30 (sample A taken at week 52; sample B taken at week 53); CH33 (sample A taken at week 48; sample B taken at week 49); JL42 (sample A taken at week 49; sample B taken at week 50); CH45 (sample A taken at week 48; sample B taken at week 49); JL49 (sample A taken at week 44; sample B taken at week 45)

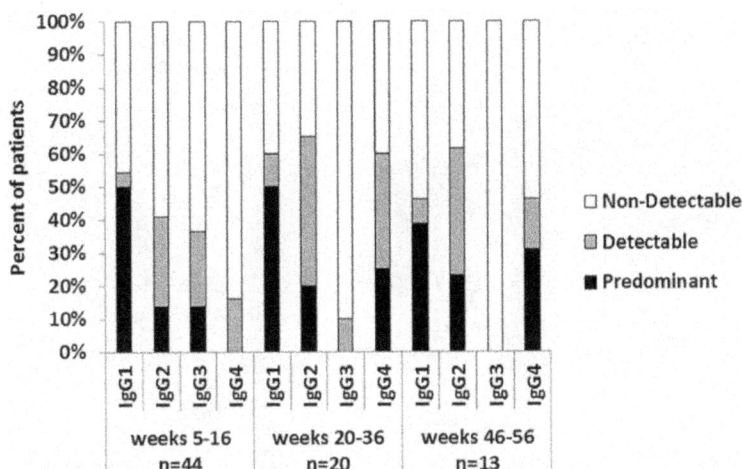

Fig. 7 Percentages of patients with different VEGF-specific IgG subclasses in the weeks 5–16, 20–36 and 46–56. In each of these stages, and for the available patients, the study was made in the sample with the highest specific IgG antibody titer. "n" represents the number of evaluated patients. Terms "non-detectable", "detectable" and "predominant" are detailed in Methods

Platelet VEGF and plasma levels of sVEGFR-2

VEGF and sVEGFR-2 have been extensively studied in several anti-cancer or anti-angiogenesis treatment strategies [20–23]. In order to evaluate the dynamic changes on platelet VEGF and sVEGFR-2 during vaccination with CIGB-247, we measured the baseline levels (week 0 or pre-vaccination), at the end of the trial vaccinations (week 13) and approximately 1 year after initial immunization.

Table 3 shows that a statistically significant reduction on platelet VEGF values with vaccination only occurred in the groups 2Ag + V ($p = 0.0244$) and Ag + Al ($p = 0.0086$). No change was observed on plasma levels of sVEGFR-2 for any of the immunization groups.

The relationship between the variation of platelet VEGF (ΔVEGF), and specific IgG antibodies titers (week 13 – week 0), was studied in 38 patients disregarding the vaccine dose and scheme. An inverse and statistically significant correlation was observed (Spearman correlation coefficient, $r = -0.5888$, $p < 0.0001$) indicating that patients with higher specific IgG antibody titers decreased their platelet VEGF levels. However, there were not statistically significant correlations between ΔVEGF and IgA antibody titers ($r = -0.1979$, $p = 0.2337$) or ΔVEGF and IgM antibody titers ($r = -0.2145$, $p = 0.1960$).

Twelve of the thirteen patients submitted to long-term re-immunizations with an overall survival longer than 45 weeks (approximately 1 year) provided blood samples. (Figure 6). Serum and plasma samples were collected, 7-10 days after a given re-immunization time point (time point for the taking of sample "B", see Fig. 8 for specific week). These patients were checked for platelet VEGF (Fig. 8a) and sVEGFR-2 (Fig. 8b). Most patients (10/12 for an 83%) had platelet VEGF levels lower than baseline (ΔVEGF ≤ -30%, decrease of platelet VEGF). The

remaining two patients (2/12 for a 17%), showed stability in platelet VEGF (-30% < ΔVEGF >30%). For sVEGFR-2, most patients (11/12 for a 92%) had no change and only one individual (1/12 for an 8%) had levels of sVEGFR-2 lower than baseline.

Discussion

So far CENTAURO and CENTAURO-2 clinical trials show the only available results worldwide for a VEGF active immunization procedure in humans. The novelty of our VEGF-based vaccine makes difficult to find comparable settings in the clinical practice. A similar therapeutic vaccine that uses a VEGF peptide in combination with the adjuvant RFASE is being investigated in a phase I clinical trial (NCT02237638), but this study is still recruiting patients and no results are available yet. Thus, we focus our comparisons in the results found in this trial (CENTAURO-2) and the previous one (CENTAURO) [8]. We also discuss some pre-clinical experiments to bridge the gap between the two clinical trials. Additionally, we compare our results with cancer vaccines directed to other self-antigens.

The excellent safety results of the CIGB-247 vaccine candidate (using VSSP as adjuvant), together with its ability to induce specific anti-VEGF antibodies able to block the interaction between VEGF and VEGFR2, were among the main hallmarks of the CENTAURO trial [8]. The CENTAURO-2 phase Ib clinical trial was designed to test new vaccine compositions, incorporating higher antigen doses in combination with the adjuvants VSSP or aluminum phosphate.

Evidences gathered in a majority of the enrolled patients showed that vaccination with different CIGB-247 formulations exhibited a very positive safety profile. This

Table 3 Comparison of platelet VEGF and plasma sVEGFR-2 per treatment groups in the CENTAURO-2 trial

Groups	pg of VEGF/10^6platelets Mean (range) [n]		pg/mL of sVEGFR-2 Mean (range) [n]	
	Week 0	Week 13	Week 0	Week 13
Ag + V	1.21 (0.30–2.20) [7]	0.61 (0.10–1.43) [7] ns	9736 (6939–11724) [7]	9792 (7427–11162) [7] ns
Ag + 2 V	0.93 (0.55–1.46) [7]	1.01 (0.08–3.29) [7] ns	10455 (8116–12653) [8]	10423 (7262–12882) [8] ns
2Ag + V	2.07 (0.11–8.19) [8]	0.57 (0.22–2.05) [8] $p = 0.0244$*	9736 (7078–12637) [8]	9948 (9125–11098) [8] ns
½Ag + Al	1.90 (0.90–3.64) [8]	1.98 (0.63–3.54) [8] ns	10228 (7555–12735) [8]	9567 (7820–13372) [8] ns
Ag + Al	1.58 (0.72–3.19) [8]	1.06 (0.15–2.91) [8] $p = 0.0086$**	10131 (8491–12223) [8]	10296 (8611–13294) [8] ns

The table summarizes the data per vaccine dose cohorts and the results of paired t-test (ns: non-significant; *$p < 0.05$; **$p < 0.01$). (n) number of patients

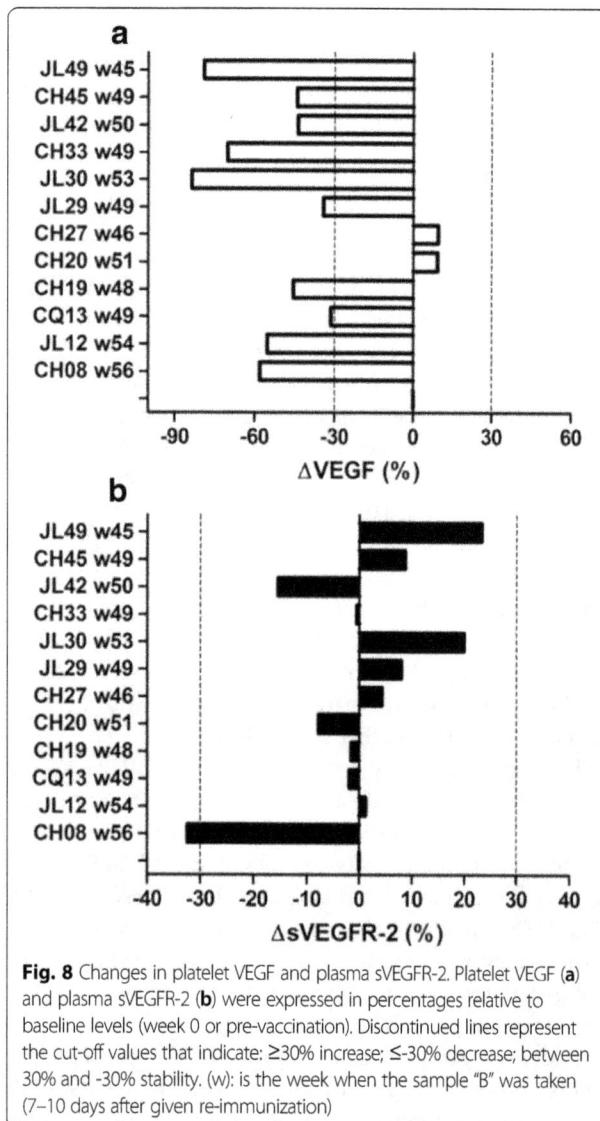

Fig. 8 Changes in platelet VEGF and plasma sVEGFR-2. Platelet VEGF (**a**) and plasma sVEGFR-2 (**b**) were expressed in percentages relative to baseline levels (week 0 or pre-vaccination). Discontinued lines represent the cut-off values that indicate: ≥30% increase; ≤-30% decrease; between 30% and -30% stability. (w): is the week when the sample "B" was taken (7–10 days after given re-immunization)

is in line with the fact that it is generally recognized that many cancer vaccines have few adverse reactions [24].

Some clinical studies on cancer vaccines have revealed a relationship between the high levels of elicited antibodies and an improved survival; and even have been able to elucidate the specific immunoglobulin class associated with overall survival [25–27]. Although these types of correlations are not applicable to phase I clinical trials, there is no doubt about the importance of studying in depth the humoral response in early evaluations of cancer vaccines in humans [24]. A special emphasis was done in this paper in the characterization of the vaccine-induced humoral response in terms of quantity, quality, kinetic, dynamic and composition.

An important goal of this study (CENTAURO-2) was to determine if CIGB-247 antigen in different settings of adjuvants and higher doses of antigen or adjuvant is capable to elicit a specific humoral response against human VEGF higher than the response seen in CENTAURO clinical trial [8].

The reference Ag + V group and the Ag + Al cohort had similar seroconversion rates, but unexpectedly, the former showed faster (earlier) seroconversion and also developed higher titers of specific IgG antibodies. An explanation to this difference has to consider first the use of different adjuvants. While aluminum has been employed by others in cancer patient vaccination [28, 29], the bacterially-derived VSSP has previously shown to be a very strong stimulator of specific humoral responses in cancer patients [30, 31], and its use in our case may favor the speed and intensity of the response against VEGF. The second aspect that could explain these differences is the total amount of antigen administered, which is much lower in the aluminum cohort due to the bi-weekly vaccination scheme. If this is true, the results differ substantially from those of our pre-clinical studies done in mice, rabbits, and non-human primates, where using bi-weekly immunization schedules with the VEGF antigen formulated in aluminum produced higher specific IgG antibody titers or VEGF/VEGFR2 blocking activities, with respect to control groups immunized weekly with the same antigen dose per injection, and VSSP as adjuvant. Irrespectively of the fact that we do not have at present a mechanistic explanation for these differences in the behavior of pre-clinical models and human cancer patients, our findings illustrate how carefully extrapolations between them should be done.

Another dissimilar result between pre-clinical models and cancer patients was found when the amount of VSSP was doubled in the vaccine formulation. Although in mice a doubled dose of VSSP led to an increase in anti-VEGF antibody titers, in cancer patients, a lower amount of IgG seroconverted individuals was observed in the Ag + 2 V cohort as compared with the Ag + V group. This result could be due to the high dose of VSSP, which has a negative effect on humoral response only in humans. The amount of powerful bacterial antigens present in this dose of VSSP could be competing against VEGF for a humoral response, a phenomenon known as antigenic competition. In fact, VSSP is known to induce high levels of anti-VSSP antibodies in cancer patients [30, 31]. Although the actual mechanisms of antigenic competition are still not fully understood, it is well established that the degree of competition increases as the dose of the competing antigen is increased [32, 33].

The results of CENTAURO-2 study show that vaccinating with VEGF, combined either with VSSP or aluminum phosphate, leads to the production of specific anti-VEGF IgG, IgM, and IgA antibodies. These three types of immunoglobulins elicited in patients by using other cancer vaccines based on defined specific tumor antigens have demonstrated complement dependent cytotoxicity (CDC) and antibody dependent cellular cytotoxicity (ADCC) activities [27, 34, 35]. However, these effector mechanisms of antibodies are typical when their respective antigens are membrane surface proteins. In our case, VEGF is a soluble protein, and together with IgG, we can now add a possible role of IgM and IgA to the potential of the antibody response elicited by CIGB-247 in blocking the interactions of VEGF and VEGF receptors. Additional to ligand depletion, FcγR–mediated enhancement of antigen presentation is another mechanism contributing to tumor immunity [36]. It has been reported that immune complexes, formed as a consequence of IgG antibody binding to its antigen, can enhance in dendritic cells antigen uptake and upregulate antigen presentation, both to MHC class II-restricted CD4$^+$ T cells and to CD8+ T cells [37, 38]. It is being increasingly recognized that IgG immunoglobulin are potent integrators of innate and cellular immunity or a link between humoral and cellular immunity, resulting in increased immune responses [39]. Similar

mechanisms have been described for IgM and IgA antibodies via Fcα/μR (Fc receptor for IgM and IgA immunoglobulins) or FcαRI [40, 41].

For a vaccine candidate targeting a growth factor relevant for tumor growth is imperative to test not only the specific antibody response elicited against VEGF but also the ability of such antibodies to block the binding of VEGF to VEGFR2 or VEGFR1. Because of the aforementioned, VEGFR2 and VEGFR1 blocking activities documented in serum samples from CENTAURO-2 patients deserve special attention. In particular, the blockade of VEGF/VEGFR1 interaction had not been studied before with our vaccine candidate, and these results add another possible mechanism to others involved in the final anti-tumor potential of CIGB-247. The humoral response induced by CIGB-247 vaccine, could be able to impair VEGF/VEGFRs axis that mediates important processes for tumor development including tumoral angiogenesis and tumor-induced immunosuppression [19, 42].

The second part of this discussion will be devoted to the analysis of the humoral response results in patients from the CENTAURO-2 trial that received off-trial monthly re-immunizations. In the field of cancer therapeutic vaccines, chronic vaccination is regarded as essential, especially when the vaccines involve self-antigens [43]. Immunizations may boost pre-vaccination anti-VEGF antibodies detected in some patients, improving it in terms of quantity and quality. This particular effect could be more relevant for patients who already naturally have anti-VEGF blocking antibodies.

Regarding the assessment of boost vaccination effect in patients with longer survival and baseline anti-VEGF blocking antibodies, an ideal situation could be the one where the antibody assessment during off-trial monthly re-immunizations could be controlled by the inclusion a non-vaccinated patients in order to determine whether this is specific to the vaccination administered or whether this post-vaccination blocking activity is found naturally in these patients. It is not feasible to obtain control samples from non-treated patients in this clinical trial because of three major reasons: (a) patients of CENTAURO-2 trial had a variety of malignancies, for that reason the non-vaccinated patients should be representative of this heterogeneity; (b) most of the patients of CENTAURO-2 trial had metastatic disease and were classified as progressive disease according the RECIST criteria. The non-vaccinated patients should be representative of this advanced illness, where a survival greater than 1 year is a big challenge; (c) patients were eligible for enrollment in this clinical trial after having received available therapy and were no longer responding. Thus, it is not ethically correct that a group of patients without treatment options were not eligible for the vaccine candidate, even more, when in our hands we have data about patients with advanced illness and immunized with the vaccine candidate able to show objective clinical benefits [8, 44]. Additionally, it is well studied that patients in frank progression have a strong tumor-induced immunosuppression [45, 46]. This immunosuppression has a negative impact on the cellular and humoral responses. In this context, the probability of increasing a basal blocking activity over time is quite low. Therefore, the increase of the basal blocking activity over time observed in these longer survival patients can only be explained by the monthly re-immunizations.

Despite the limitations imposed from the switch of patients from their original vaccine formulation to that of 800 µg of antigen + 200 µg of VSSP during off-trial re-immunizations, with respect the scope of the conclusions to be drawn, the off-trial vaccination phase and patient follow up allowed us to document that re-immunization was safe. Additionally, re-immunization was relevant for a number of patients, in terms of helping to maintain positive specific IgG antibody titers and/or VEGF/VEGFR2 blocking ability, or eventually achieving a seroconversion or VEGF/VEGFR2 blocking status, not documented during the trial period, or lost thereafter. These results are in line with our findings in the preceding CENTAURO clinical study [8], and other follow up studies about the vaccine candidate in combination with VSSP [44, 47].

Continued vaccination was also important to produce a gradual shift in the anti-VEGF IgG response from IgG1 to IgG4. IgG1/IgG4 subclass switching has been previously reported using a CEA-based vaccine in colorectal cancer patients [48]. IgG4 antibodies are prominent only after prolonged immunization with protein antigens, and have been associated with the affinity maturation process [49]. They are considered the highest affinity antibodies that could lead to more efficient antigen neutralization [50]. The potential generation of VEGF-specific antibodies of much greater affinity relative to those obtained during the trial vaccination scheme is highly relevant because of the high affinity of the interaction between VEGF and VEGFR2 (Kd = 37×10^{-12} M) [51]. The presence of these high-affinity antibodies requires further investigation by surface plasmon resonance.

We found that re-immunizations during off-trial vaccinations increased specific anti-VEGF IgM antibody titer. While IgM is commonly associated with a primary immune response after initial exposure to an antigen, Seifert et al. have also found IgM memory B cells that are generated in T cell-dependent immune responses, with similar features of class-switched memory B cells: enhanced antigen response, proliferation, increased metabolic turnover, a propensity to plasmablast differentiation and a higher and faster reactivity [52]. This experimental evidence could explain the presence of specific IgM antibodies during long-term vaccination with CIGB-247.

VEGF is a soluble factor and platelets are considered one of the most important physiological transporters of VEGF [53]. Blood platelets have an active role on tumor angiogenesis and metastasis formation [54]. All these elements suggest that VEGF content within platelets may be a meaningful interesting potential biomarker for studying the effect of VEGF-based immunotherapies.

In the preceding CENTAURO clinical trial, we have documented that only the cohort that received the highest antigen dose (400 µg antigen + 200 µg VSSP) showed statistically significant reduced levels of platelet VEGF, with respect to pre-vaccination values [8]. However, in CENTAURO-2 study this drop in platelet VEGF was not observed in the group with the same dose and schedule (reference group). These apparently contradictory results in the two trials could be related to differences in the types of tumors, localization and stages. Another element to always consider is the relatively low number of individuals per group, which limits the scope of the results and the extension of them from one study to another. Our findings strongly support that elicited antibodies specific to VEGF in different adjuvants settings do not only block the interaction with its receptors but also reduce in vivo platelet VEGF bioavailability. Such results shed some light on the mechanism of CIGB-247 anti-tumoral effects by adding antigen sequestration capabilities to the already described specific neutralization of the ligand interaction with the receptor.

In this work, we found a statistically significant correlation between IgG response and the variation of platelet VEGF when pooling all trial patients. Not many cancer therapeutic vaccines have been developed using soluble growth factors as target antigens, but a result that is in line with our findings is that reported by Rodríguez et al. in a phase III study of CIMAvax-EGF, a therapeutic vaccine for the treatment of patients with non-small cell lung cancer, where EGF is the antigen. These authors also found a significant inverse correlation between the anti-EGF antibody titers and serum EGF concentration [55].

Modulation of the soluble version of membrane VEGFR2 (sVEGFR-2) has been extensively studied after treatment with tyrosine kinase inhibitors (TKIs) or with single-agent Bevacizumab, a humanized monoclonal antibody specific to human VEGF. Patients treated with TKIs have decreased levels of sVEGFR-2 [20, 21, 56, 57]; however Bevacizumab induces the opposite effect (i.e., an increase in sVEGFR-2 levels) [22, 23, 58]. A different modulation profile regarding sVEGFR-2 has been ascribed to receptor blockade with TKIs or direct ligand depletion with Bevacizumab.

The sVEGFR-2 levels were not studied in the CEN-TAURO trial. In the CENTAURO-2 clinical trial the majority of the patients, both during the trial, and off-trial, did not show any significant changes with respect to pre-vaccination levels. Bevacizumab and antibodies elicited by CIGB-247 possibly share VEGF neutralizing antibodies as part of their potential anti-tumor mechanisms; however they did not produce the same effect. In fact, specific immunoglobulin concentrations in blood after therapy onset are dissimilar for these two different therapeutic strategies (active immunotherapy *versus* passive immunotherapy).

In order to explain this difference, we will be based on the theory presented by Loupakis et al., which indicates that the increase of sVEGFR-2 levels on Bevacizumab-containing therapies may be related to the switch on of activated endothelial cells or progenitors of the tumor's microenvironment [59]. This possible tumor and host-driven resistance mechanism could be caused by induced stress due to the high dose of Bevacizumab administered during infusion. However, in the context of vaccination with CIGB-247, levels of vaccine-induced antibodies are not so extremely high as to cause this phenomenon. This type of strategy could be seen as a sort of metronomic therapy with low levels of elicited antibodies as compare with intravenous administration of Bevacizumab. At these lower specific antibody levels, both toxicity for normal tissues and the induction of sVEGFR-2 increase are most probably not favored.

Taking into account the results of all ELISA tests described here, with aluminum as adjuvant, a further increase in antigen dose over 400 µg is foreseen in order to achieve a higher specific humoral response. The best results of humoral response seen at the dose level of 800 µg of antigen indicate the potential use of this dose in combination with either VSSP or aluminum phosphate as adjuvants.

Conclusions

The present study shows that vaccination with CIGB-247 at different antigen doses and in combination with different adjuvants, is safe, and induces predominantly IgG, but also IgM, and IgA antibodies specific to human VEGF. Elicited antibodies also block the interaction between VEGF and its receptors VEGFR1 and VEGFR2. Vaccination with CIGB-247 is associated with a depletion of platelet VEGF. All these properties are preserved with monthly immunizations up to 1 year. Particularly, as immunizations number increases, anti-VEGF IgG response shifts gradually from IgG1 to IgG4, being the former the predominant subclass. Both strategies using either VSSP or aluminum phosphate as adjuvants combined with the highest dose of antigen (800 µg) deserve further evaluations in phase II clinical trials.

Additional files

Additional file 1: Reported adverse events which were probably or definitively related to the vaccine during trial period. (PDF 113 kb)

Additional file 2: IgE antibody titers specific to human VEGF. (XLSX 13 kb)

Additional file 3: Detection of specific-IgG, IgM or IgA immunoglobulin classes at the end of trial vaccinations (week 13). (PDF 100 kb)

Additional file 4: Anti-VEGF IgG antibody titers prior and after vaccination during trial vaccinations. (XLS 41 kb)

Additional file 5: Off-trial re-immunizations. (PDF 97 kb)

Acknowledgments
The present study had a collaboration group named as "CENTAURO-2 Team of Investigators". The names of the individual members are: Mariela Pérez de la Iglesia, Sheila Padrón Morales, Lian Trimiño Lorenzo, Gerardo R. Hernández González, Yasmiana Muñoz Pozo, Eduardo Ibañez Carrillo, Rodolfo A. Morales Yera, Jesús Piñero Molinér and Kirenia Camacho Sosa.

Funding
This work was supported by Heber Biotec and Chemo. They were involved in all stages of the study conduct and analysis. The costs associated with the development and publishing of the manuscript were also covered by Heber Biotec.

Authors' contributions
JS and YM performed the immunological determinations and took part in the trial design, data management, interpretation of the results and paper writing. MB took part in the trial design, data management, interpretation of the results and paper reviewer. FH designed the trial, was its main coordinator, and took part in data management, analyses and interpretation of the results. KH, AT, ES and JT were the clinical investigators that recruited and treated the patients, participated in the trial design and data collection. YM and CB took part in the trial coordination, monitoring, and data acquisition and management; JG and MA were project managers and took part in the trial design, data management and interpretation of the results; CENTAURO-2 Team of Investigators were supplier of CIGB-247 antigen, coating antigen for ELISAs or were responsible for the care and welfare of the patients, as well as data acquisition. All authors read and approved the final manuscript.

Authors' information
Not applicable.

Competing interests
The authors declare that they have no competing interests.

Author details

[1]Department of Pharmaceuticals, Center for Genetic Engineering and Biotechnology (CIGB), P.O. Box 6162, Playa Cubanacán, Havana 10600, Cuba. [2]Department of Clinical Research, CIGB, P.O. Box 6162, Playa Cubanacán, Havana 10600, Cuba. [3]Center of Medical and Surgical Research (CIMEQ), Playa, Siboney, Havana 12100, Cuba. [4]"Celestino Hernández Robau" Hospital, Santa Clara 50100, Cuba. [5]"José Ramón López Tabranes" Hospital, Matanzas 40100, Cuba.

References

1. Wentink MQ, Huijbers EJ, de Gruijl TD, Verheul HM, Olsson AK, Griffioen AW. Vaccination approach to anti-angiogenic treatment of cancer. Biochim Biophys Acta. 2015;1855(2):155–71.

2. Ferrara N. VEGF as a therapeutic target in cancer. Oncology. 2005;69 Suppl 3:11–6.

3. Morera Y, Bequet M, Ayala M, Lamdán H, Agger EM, Andersen P, Gavilondo JV. Anti-tumoral effect of active immunotherapy in C57BL/6 mice using a recombinant human VEGF protein as antigen and three chemically unrelated adjuvants. Angiogenesis. 2008;11(4):381–93.

4. Estévez F, Carr A, Solorzano L, Valiente O, Mesa C, Barroso O, Sierra GV, Fernández LE. Enhancement of the immune response to poorly immunogenic gangliosides after incorporation into very small size proteoliposomes (VSSP). Vaccine. 1999;18(1-2):190–7.

5. Morera Y, Bequet M, Ayala M, Velazco JC, Pérez PP, Alba JS, Ancízar J, Rodríguez M, Cosme K, Gavilondo JV. Immunogenicity and some safety features of a VEGF-based cancer therapeutic vaccine in rats, rabbits and non-human primates. Vaccine. 2010;28(19):3453–61.

6. Bequet M, Morera Y, Ayala M, Ancízar J, Soria Y, Blanco A, Suárez-Alba J, Gavilondo JV. CIGB-247: a VEGF-based therapeutic vaccine that reduces experimental and spontaneous lung metastasis of C57Bl/6 and BALB/c mouse tumors. Vaccine. 2012;30(10):1790–9.

7. Morera Y, Bequet M, Ayala M, Pérez PP, Castro J, Sánchez J, Alba JS, Ancízar J, Cosme K, Gavilondo JV. Antigen dose escalation study of a VEGF-based therapeutic cancer vaccine in non human primates. Vaccine. 2012;30(2):368–77.

8. Gavilondo JV, Hernández F, Ayala M, de la Torre AV, de la Torre J, Morera Y, Bequet M, Sánchez J, Valenzuela CM, Martin Y, et al. Specific active immunotherapy with a VEGF vaccine in patients with advanced solid tumors. results of the CENTAURO antigen dose escalation phase I clinical trial. Vaccine. 2014;32(19):2241–50.

9. Mesa C, De Leon J, Rigley K, Fernandez LE. Very small size proteoliposomes derived from Neisseria meningitidis: an effective adjuvant for Th1 induction and dendritic cell activation. Vaccine. 2004;22(23-24):3045–52.

10. Fernandez A, Mesa C, Marigo I, Dolcetti L, Clavell A, Oliver L, Fernandez LE, Bronte V. Inhibition of tumor-induced myeloid-derived suppressor cell function by a nanoparticulated adjuvant. J Immunol. 2011;186(1):264–74.

11. Oliver L, Fernandez A, Raymond J, Lopez-Requena A, Fernandez LE, Mesa C. Very small size proteoliposomes derived from Neisseria meningitidis: an effective adjuvant for antigen-specific cytotoxic T lymphocyte response stimulation under leukopenic conditions. Vaccine. 2012;30(19):2963–72.

12. Petrovsky N. Comparative safety of vaccine adjuvants: a summary of current evidence and future needs. Drug Saf. 2015;38(11):1059–74.

13. Pérez Sánchez L, Morera Diaz Y, Bequet-Romero M, Ramses Hernández G, Rodríguez Y, Castro Velazco J, Puente Pérez P, Ayala Avila M, Gavilondo JV. Experimental studies of a vaccine formulation of recombinant human VEGF antigen with aluminum phosphate. Hum Vaccin Immunother. 2015;11(8):2030–7.

14. Morera Y, Lamdán H, Bequet M, Ayala M, Rojas G, Muñoz Y, Gavilondo JV. Biologically active vascular endothelial growth factor as a bacterial recombinant glutathione S-transferase fusion protein. Biotechnol Appl Biochem. 2006;44(Pt 1):45–53.

15. Sánchez Ramírez J, Morera Díaz Y, Musacchio Lasa A, Bequet-Romero M, Muñoz Pozo Y, Pérez Sánchez L, Hernández-Bernal F, Mendoza Fuentes O, Selman-Housein KH, Gavilondo Cowley JV, et al. Indirect and competitive enzyme-linked immunosorbent assays for monitoring the humoral response against human VEGF. J Immunoassay Immunochem. 2016;37(6):636–58.

16. Danziger-Isakov L, Cherkassky L, Siegel H, McManamon M, Kramer K, Budev M, Sawinski D, Augustine JJ, Hricik DE, Fairchild R, et al. Effects of influenza immunization on humoral and cellular alloreactivity in humans. Transplantation. 2010;89(7):838–44.

17. Adams J, Carder PJ, Downey S, Forbes MA, MacLennan K, Allgar V, Kaufman S, Hallam S, Bicknell R, Walker JJ, et al. Vascular endothelial growth factor (VEGF) in breast cancer: comparison of plasma, serum, and tissue VEGF and microvessel density and effects of tamoxifen. Cancer Res. 2000;60(11):2898–905.

18. Recchia F, Candeloro G, Necozione S, Bisegna R, Bratta M, Rea S. Immunotherapy in patients with less than complete response to chemotherapy. Anticancer Res. 2009;29(2):567–72.

19. Zhang Z, Neiva KG, Lingen MW, Ellis LM, Nor JE. VEGF-dependent tumor angiogenesis requires inverse and reciprocal regulation of VEGFR1 and VEGFR2. Cell Death Differ. 2010;17(3):499–512.

20. Shah MA, Wainberg ZA, Catenacci DV, Hochster HS, Ford J, Kunz P, Lee FC, Kallender H, Cecchi F, Rabe DC, et al. Phase II study evaluating 2 dosing schedules of oral foretinib (GSK1363089), cMET/VEGFR2 inhibitor, in patients with metastatic gastric cancer. PLoS One. 2013;8(3):e54014.

21. Zhu AX, Sahani DV, Duda DG, di Tomaso E, Ancukiewicz M, Catalano OA, Sindhwani V, Blaszkowsky LS, Yoon SS, Lahdenranta J, et al. Efficacy, safety, and potential biomarkers of sunitinib monotherapy in advanced hepatocellular carcinoma: a phase II study. J Clin Oncol. 2009;27(18):3027–35.

22. Boige V, Malka D, Bourredjem A, Dromain C, Baey C, Jacques N, Pignon JP, Vimond N, Bouvet-Forteau N, De Baere T, et al. Efficacy, safety, and biomarkers of single-agent bevacizumab therapy in patients with advanced hepatocellular carcinoma. Oncologist. 2012;17(8):1063–72.

23. Willett CG, Duda DG, di Tomaso E, Boucher Y, Ancukiewicz M, Sahani DV, Lahdenranta J, Chung DC, Fischman AJ, Lauwers GY, et al. Efficacy, safety, and biomarkers of neoadjuvant bevacizumab, radiation therapy, and fluorouracil in rectal cancer: a multidisciplinary phase II study. J Clin Oncol. 2009;27(18):3020–6.

24. Guidance Development Review C, Working Group for Clinical Studies of Cancer I, Working Group for Effector Cell T, Working Group for CMCNcS, Working Group for Cancer V, Adjuvants, Working Group for Anti-immune Checkpoint T, Comprehensive Cancer I, Biostatistics S, Arato T, et al. Guidance on cancer immunotherapy development in early-phase clinical studies. Cancer Sci. 2015;106(12):1761–71.

25. Gonzalez G, Crombet T, Neninger E, Viada C, Lage A. Therapeutic vaccination with epidermal growth factor (EGF) in advanced lung cancer: analysis of pooled data from three clinical trials. Hum Vaccin. 2007;3(1):8–13.

26. Ullenhag GJ, Frodin JE, Jeddi-Tehrani M, Strigard K, Eriksson E, Samanci A, Choudhury A, Nilsson B, Rossmann ED, Mosolits S, et al. Durable carcinoembryonic antigen (CEA)-specific humoral and cellular immune responses in colorectal carcinoma patients vaccinated with recombinant CEA and granulocyte/macrophage colony-stimulating factor. Clin Cancer Res. 2004;10(10):3273–81.

27. Staff C, Magnusson CG, Hojjat-Farsangi M, Mosolits S, Liljefors M, Frodin JE, Wahren B, Mellstedt H, Ullenhag GJ. Induction of IgM, IgA and IgE antibodies in colorectal cancer patients vaccinated with a recombinant CEA protein. J Clin Immunol. 2012;32(4):855–65.

28. Gonzalez G, Crombet T, Catala M, Mirabal V, Hernandez JC, Gonzalez Y, Marinello P, Guillen G, Lage A. A novel cancer vaccine composed of human-recombinant epidermal growth factor linked to a carrier protein: report of a pilot clinical trial. Ann Oncol. 1998;9(4):431–5.

29. Alfonso S, Valdés-Zayas A, Santiesteban ER, Flores YI, Areces F, Hernández M, Viada CE, Mendoza IC, Guerra PP, García E, et al. A randomized, multicenter, placebo-controlled clinical trial of racotumomab-alum vaccine as switch maintenance therapy in advanced non-small cell lung cancer patients. Clin Cancer Res. 2014;20(14):3660–71.

30. Osorio M, Gracia E, Reigosa E, Hernandez J, de la Torre A, Saurez G, Perez K, Viada C, Cepeda M, Carr A, et al. Effect of vaccination with N-glycolyl GM3/VSSP vaccine by subcutaneous injection in patients with advanced cutaneous melanoma. Cancer Manage Res. 2012;4:341–5.

31. de la Torre A, Hernandez J, Ortiz R, Cepeda M, Perez K, Car A, Viada C, Toledo D, Guerra PP, Garcia E, et al. NGlycolylGM3/VSSP Vaccine in Metastatic Breast Cancer Patients: Results of Phase I/IIa Clinical Trial. Breast Cancer: Basic Clin Res. 2012;6:151–7.

32. Kim YT, Merrifield N, Zarchy T, Brody NI, Siskind GW. Studies on antigenic competition. 3. Effect on antigenic competition on antibody affinity. Immunology. 1974;26(5):943–55.

33. Dagan R, Eskola J, Leclerc C, Leroy O. Reduced response to multiple vaccines sharing common protein epitopes that are administered simultaneously to infants. Infect Immun. 1998;66(5):2093–8.

34. Ragupathi G, Liu NX, Musselli C, Powell S, Lloyd K, Livingston PO. Antibodies against tumor cell glycolipids and proteins, but not mucins, mediate complement-dependent cytotoxicity. J Immunol. 2005;174(9):5706–12.

35. Snijdewint FG, von Mensdorff-Pouilly S, Karuntu-Wanamarta AH, Verstraeten AA, Livingston PO, Hilgers J, Kenemans P. Antibody-dependent cell-mediated cytotoxicity can be induced by MUC1 peptide vaccination of breast cancer patients. Int J Cancer. 2001;93(1):97–106.

36. Wen YM, Mu L, Shi Y. Immunoregulatory functions of immune complexes in vaccine and therapy. 2016;8(10):1120-1133.

37. de Jong JM, Schuurhuis DH, Ioan-Facsinay A, Welling MM, Camps MG, van der Voort EI, Huizinga TW, Ossendorp F, Verbeek JS, Toes RE. Dendritic cells, but not macrophages or B cells, activate major histocompatibility complex class II-restricted CD4+ T cells upon immune-complex uptake in vivo. Immunology. 2006;119(4):499–506.

38. den Haan JM, Bevan MJ. Constitutive versus activation-dependent cross-presentation of immune complexes by CD8(+) and CD8(-) dendritic cells in vivo. J Exp Med. 2002;196(6):817–27.

39. Hamano Y, Arase H, Saisho H, Saito T. Immune complex and Fc receptor-mediated augmentation of antigen presentation for in vivo Th cell responses. J Immunol. 2000;164(12):6113–9.

40. Shen L, van Egmond M, Siemasko K, Gao H, Wade T, Lang ML, Clark M, van De Winkel JG, Wade WF. Presentation of ovalbumin internalized via the immunoglobulin-A Fc receptor is enhanced through Fc receptor gamma-chain signaling. Blood. 2001;97(1):205–13.

41. Shibuya A, Honda S. Molecular and functional characteristics of the Fcalpha/muR, a novel Fc receptor for IgM and IgA. Springer Semin Immunopathol. 2006;28(4):377–82.

42. Voron T, Marcheteau E, Pernot S, Colussi O, Tartour E, Taieb J, Terme M. Control of the immune response by pro-angiogenic factors. Front Oncol. 2014;4:70.

43. González G, Crombet T, Lage A. Chronic vaccination with a therapeutic EGF-based cancer vaccine: a review of patients receiving long lasting treatment. Curr Cancer Drug Targets. 2011;11(1):103–10.

44. Selman-Housein KH, de la Torre A, Hernández-Bernal F, Martin Y, Garabito A, Piñero J, Morera Diaz Y, Sánchez Ramírez J, Bequet-Romero M, Bermúdez C, et al. Clinical benefits in patients with advanced solid tumors after long-term immunization with a VEGF therapeutic vaccine. Open J Clin Med Case Rep. 2017, 3(2).

45. Almand B, Clark JI, Nikitina E, van Beynen J, English NR, Knight SC, Carbone DP, Gabrilovich DI. Increased production of immature myeloid cells in cancer patients: a mechanism of immunosuppression in cancer. J Immunol. 2001;166(1):678–89.

46. Gross S, Walden P. Immunosuppressive mechanisms in human tumors: why we still cannot cure cancer. Immunol Lett. 2008;116(1):7–14.

47. Morera Y, Sánchez J, Bequet-Romero M, Selman-Housein KH, de la Torre A, Hernández-Bernal F, Martin Y, Garabito A, Pinero J, Bermúdez C, et al. Specific humoral and cellular immune responses in cancer patients undergoing chronic immunization with a VEGF-based therapeutic vaccine. Vaccine. 2017;35(28):3582–90.

48. Ullenhag GJ, Frodin JE, Strigard K, Mellstedt H, Magnusson CG. Induction of IgG subclass responses in colorectal carcinoma patients vaccinated with recombinant carcinoembryonic antigen. Cancer Res. 2002;62(5):1364–9.

49. Collins AM, Jackson KJ. A Temporal Model of Human IgE and IgG Antibody Function. Front Immunol. 2013;4:235.

50. Prechl J. A generalized quantitative antibody homeostasis model: antigen saturation, natural antibodies and a quantitative antibody network. bioRxiv. 2016.

51. Cunningham SA, Tran TM, Arrate MP, Brock TA. Characterization of vascular endothelial cell growth factor interactions with the kinase insert domain-containing receptor tyrosine kinase. A real time kinetic study. J Biol Chem. 1999;274(26):18421–7.

52. Seifert M, Przekopowitz M, Taudien S, Lollies A, Ronge V, Drees B, Lindemann M, Hillen U, Engler H, Singer BB, et al. Functional capacities of human IgM memory B cells in early inflammatory responses and secondary germinal center reactions. Proc Natl Acad Sci U S A. 2015;112(6):E546–555.

53. Banks RE, Forbes MA, Kinsey SE, Stanley A, Ingham E, Walters C, Selby PJ. Release of the angiogenic cytokine vascular endothelial growth factor (VEGF) from platelets: significance for VEGF measurements and cancer biology. Br J Cancer. 1998;77(6):956–64.

54. Sabrkhany S, Griffioen AW, Oude Egbrink MG. The role of blood platelets in tumor angiogenesis. Biochim Biophys Acta. 2011;1815(2):189–96.

55. Rodríguez PC, Popa X, Martínez O, Mendoza S, Santiesteban E, Crespo T, Amador RM, Fleytas R, Acosta SC, Otero Y, et al. A Phase III Clinical Trial of the Epidermal Growth Factor Vaccine CIMAvax-EGF as Switch Maintenance Therapy in Advanced Non-Small Cell Lung Cancer Patients. Clin Cancer Res. 2016.

56. Dror Michaelson M, Regan MM, Oh WK, Kaufman DS, Olivier K, Michaelson SZ, Spicer B, Gurski C, Kantoff PW, Smith MR. Phase II study of sunitinib in men with advanced prostate cancer. Ann Oncol. 2009;20(5):913–20.

57. Sleijfer S, Gorlia T, Lamers C, Burger H, Blay JY, Le Cesne A, Scurr M, Collin F, Pandite L, Marreaud S, et al. Cytokine and angiogenic factors associated with efficacy and toxicity of pazopanib in advanced soft-tissue sarcoma: an EORTC-STBSG study. Br J Cancer. 2012;107(4):639–45.

58. Kopetz S, Hoff PM, Morris JS, Wolff RA, Eng C, Glover KY, Adinin R, Overman MJ, Valero V, Wen S, et al. Phase II trial of infusional fluorouracil, irinotecan, and bevacizumab for metastatic colorectal cancer: efficacy and circulating angiogenic biomarkers associated with therapeutic resistance. J Clin Oncol. 2010;28(3):453–9.

59. Loupakis F, Cremolini C, Fioravanti A, Orlandi P, Salvatore L, Masi G, Di Desidero T, Canu B, Schirripa M, Frumento P, et al. Pharmacodynamic and pharmacogenetic angiogenesis-related markers of first-line FOLFOXIRI plus bevacizumab schedule in metastatic colorectal cancer. Br J Cancer. 2011; 104(8):1262–9.

15

Low HLA binding of diabetes-associated CD8+ T-cell epitopes is increased by post translational modifications

John Sidney[1]*, Jose Luis Vela[2], Dave Friedrich[2], Ravi Kolla[1], Matthias von Herrath[2], Johnna D. Wesley[2] and Alessandro Sette[1]

Abstract

Background: Type 1 diabetes (T1D) is thought to be an autoimmune disease driven by anti-islet antigen responses and mediated by T-cells. Recent published data suggests that T-cell reactivity to modified peptides, effectively neoantigens, may promote T1D. These findings have given more credence to the concept that T1D may not be solely an error of immune recognition but may be propagated by errors in protein processing or in modifications to endogenous peptides occurring as result of hyperglycemia, endoplasmic reticulum (ER) stress, or general beta cell dysfunction. In the current study, we hypothesized that diabetes-associated epitopes bound human leukocyte antigen (HLA) class I poorly and that post-translational modifications (PTM) to key sequences within the insulin-B chain enhanced peptide binding to HLA class I, conferring the CD8+ T-cell reactivity associated with T1D.

Results: We first identified, through the Immune Epitope Database (IEDB; www.iedb.org), 138 published HLA class I-restricted diabetes-associated epitopes reported to elicit positive T-cell responses in humans. The peptide binding affinity for their respective restricting allele(s) was evaluated in vitro. Overall, 75% of the epitopes bound with a half maximal inhibitory concentration (IC50) of 8250 nM or better, establishing a reference affinity threshold for HLA class I-restricted diabetes epitopes. These studies demonstrated that epitopes from diabetes-associated antigens bound HLA with a lower affinity than those of microbial origin (binding threshold of 500 nM for 85% of the epitopes). Further predictions suggested that diabetes epitopes also bind HLA class I with lower affinity than epitopes associated with other autoimmune diseases. Therefore, we measured the effect of common PTM (citrullination, chlorination, deamidation, and oxidation) on HLA-A*02:01 binding of insulin-B-derived peptides, compared to native peptides. We found that these modifications increased binding for 44% of the insulin-B epitopes, but only 15% of the control peptides.

Conclusions: These results demonstrate that insulin-derived epitopes, commonly associated with T1D, generally bind HLA class I poorly, but can be subject to PTM that improve their binding capacity and may, in part, be responsible for T-cell activation in T1D and subsequent beta cell death.

Keywords: Diabetes, Insulin, T cell epitopes, Class I MHC, HLA-peptide binding affinity

* Correspondence: jsidney@lji.org
[1]La Jolla Institute for Allergy and Immunology, La Jolla, CA 92130, USA
Full list of author information is available at the end of the article

Background

Type 1 diabetes (T1D) is characterized by the presence of autoantibodies and islet beta cell loss leading to metabolic dysfunction and hyperglycemia. Beta cell loss is, in part, mediated by T-cells that are reactive to insulin-derived epitopes [1]. Recent studies have indicated that processing defects in proinsulin may lead to antigen processing errors or altered expression of proinsulin-derived epitopes. Additionally, the distinctive inflammation in the pancreas may trigger increased expression of enzymes, such as tissue transglutimase (tTG), or other mechanisms leading to post-translational modifications (PTMs) of native epitopes, generating peptides with greater binding affinity to HLA, and enhancing T-cell recognition and activation and increased beta cell death [2]. Responding T-cells would have appropriately passed through negative selection in the thymus by recognizing weakly immunogenic native epitopes and migrated into the periphery. Then, in the periphery, in T1D-susceptible individuals, PTM of epitopes during antigen processing leads to a higher affinity to HLA, allowing T-cells to recognize the peptide-HLA (pHLA) complex and undergo activation and expansion, rather than anergy. This then leads to pancreatic inflammation and beta cell death.

The polymorphisms of HLA class II genes are major risk factors for T1D and CD4 T-cells are widely studied and continue to be of high interest. Human CD4 T-cells recognizing a modified epitope from the insulin-A chain were first described in the context of HLA DR4 [3]. Another study demonstrated activation of CD4 T-cells from a recent-onset T1D patient in response to a modified preproinsulin-derived epitope [4]. Additionally, in a recent study from DeLong et al. [5], CD4 T-cells reactive to epitopes from fused peptides were found in insulitic lesions in T1D. Though cytolytic CD8 T-cells (CTLs) have been seen in the pancreatic infiltrate and diabetes antigen-specific cells can be detected in the periphery, HLA class I and CD8 T-cell-pHLA interactions have not been as broadly investigated in T1D [6].

We hypothesized that CTLs recognizing diabetes epitopes could escape negative selection in the thymus by having only weak HLA class I binding capacity. The present study was designed to systematically address the issue of HLA binding affinity of human class I-restricted epitopes derived from diabetes-associated antigens. Accordingly, we experimentally determined the HLA class I binding capacity of epitopes from diabetes-associated proteins that were reported to illicit positive CTL responses in humans with T1D. Further, utilizing bioinformatic predictions, we compared the class I binding patterns of diabetes epitopes with those of non-diabetes autoimmune disease and viral epitopes. Finally, we experimentally tested whether PTM modification by citrullination, chlorination, deamidation, and oxidation of insulin epitopes could increase peptide binding to HLA-A*02:01, the HLA class I allele most commonly studied in the context of T1D is HLA-A*02:01, and thereby potentially leading to a stronger in vivo T-cell response.

Results

Diabetes-associated CTL epitopes in the published literature

To identify diabetes-associated CTL epitopes from the published literature, we employed a bioinformatics tool recently developed in the Sette laboratory [7]. This tool automatically extracts relevant data from the Immune Epitope Database (IEDB; www.iedb.org) and generates reference sets of validated epitopes from various disease indications. Here, the tool was applied to epitopes in the IEDB that are derived from a set of human proteins associated with diabetes [8], further modified to take advantage of the IEDB's search interface that allows for identification of epitope records directly associated with studies related to a specific disease and/or auto-immune context.

Accordingly, using the IEDB disease finder, the query was configured to include epitopes derived from antigens associated with T1D, pre-diabetes, and diabetes mellitus studies (Additional file 1). The query was also structured for epitopes reported to elicit positive T-cell responses in human hosts as determined using multimer/tetramer staining assays or readouts based on intracellular cytokine staining (ICS), enzyme-linked immunospot (ELISPOT), or ^{51}Cr-release assays. Responses induced following either in vitro or ex vivo stimulation were allowed. Finally, only epitopes between 8 and 11 residues in length were considered, agreeing with the most canonical peptide sizes bound by class I molecules. This generated a set of 138 epitopes (Additional file 2). Notably, 114 of the 138 epitopes (83%) were restricted by HLA-A*02:01 or A2 serological specificities. As A*02 alleles are the most common in almost all major ethnic/geographic populations worldwide [9, 10] and, as a result, have been the most extensively studied, it is unlikely that this bias is related to diabetes incidence.

HLA class I binding capacity of T1D-associated CTL epitopes

The 138 peptides were tested for their capacity to bind their respective HLA class I restricting allele(s) in classical competition assays based on the inhibition of the binding of high affinity radiolabeled ligands to purified major histocompatibility (MHC) molecules, as described in the Methods. In instances where the precise restriction was not available, binding to the most common representative subtype from the same allele family was assayed (e.g., A*02:01 for A02; B*07:02 for B7; A*03:01 for A03, etc.). The affinity of each epitope to its reported

HLA restricting allele(s) is shown in Table 1. For epitopes reported to be restricted by multiple alleles, each restriction is shown separately. The different alleles assayed, a tally of the number of corresponding peptides tested, and the number that were considered high or intermediate binders, are provided in Table 2.

In total, 56 (48.7%) of the 115 A*02:01-restricted epitopes bound with high affinity (IC50 < 500 nM); another 34 (29.6%) bound with intermediate affinity (IC50 in the 500–5000 nM range). Of the 38 non-A*02 restrictions, only 3 (7.9%) were associated with an affinity of 500 nM or better and another 10 (26.3%) bound with only intermediate affinity. Thus, overall, 103 of 153 (67.3%) of the HLA/epitope combinations were associated with binding at the 5000 nM, or better, level; that is, 59 (38.6%) were associated with high affinity, and another 44 (28.8%) with intermediate affinity.

In terms of thresholds, 75% of the epitopes bound with an IC50 of 8250 nM or better, and 90% of the epitopes bound with an IC50 of 48,000 nM (Fig. 1). These results established a reference threshold for binding affinities of HLA class I-restricted diabetes epitopes, and confirmed that the majority of diabetes epitopes bound with detectable affinity to HLA, consistent with HLA binding being a necessary (albeit not sufficient) requisite for HLA class I-specific immunogenicity.

Comparative HLA class I binding capacity of diabetes-associated CTL epitopes

The binding threshold identified above is notable in that it is somewhat higher (i.e., associated with lower affinity) than the binding threshold (500 nM) previously found to be associated with the vast majority (> 80%) of HLA class I-restricted T-cell epitopes derived from various pathogens [11–13]. To more directly compare diabetes-associated epitopes to those of pathogenic origin, we next utilized a bioinformatic approach used previously [13] and generated predicted binding affinities for each diabetes-associated epitope to its restricting allele(s) utilizing the SMM algorithm hosted by the IEDB analysis resource. Predictions were also generated for a large panel of over 2200 virus-derived epitopes identified in the IEDB. The cumulative predicted affinity of the two epitope sets were then compared (Fig. 2). As shown, the virus-derived epitopes were predicted to bind at a higher rate than the diabetes-associated epitopes, where a predicted binding threshold of 500 nM captured about 70% of the virus epitopes, but only 60% of the diabetes epitopes. Similarly, 75% of the virus epitopes were expected to bind at 750 nM or better, in comparison to 1260 nM for the diabetes epitopes. The results for the viral epitopes were consistent with previous reports where a binding threshold of 500 nM was associated with approximately 85% of epitopes [11, 12]. These findings indicate that the overall binding affinity is lower for diabetes-associated T-cell epitopes when compared to virus-derived peptides.

These observations were not entirely surprising, as it has been hypothesized that self-epitopes might bind with reduced affinity, and that this is likely characteristic of autoimmunity in general (see, e.g., [2, 14]). However, when we evaluated the predicted binding affinity of 53 non-diabetes autoimmune epitopes retrieved from the IEDB using identical methodology, we found that these epitopes were not only predicted to bind better than diabetes-associated peptides, but even better than the viral epitopes. In fact, a 500 nM threshold identifies 80% of the selected non-diabetes autoimmune-associated epitopes, with 75% of them predicted to bind at the 355 nM level or better (Fig. 2).

Selection of post-translationally modified peptides

The measured and predicted lower affinity of diabetes epitopes could be explained if the epitopes recognized by diabetes-associated T-cells are often PTM products, and the modification is associated with increased HLA binding. To test this hypothesis, which was also previously suggested by McGinty and James [15], we analyzed the binding affinity of diabetes-associated epitopes, specifically from the insulin-B 30-mer, and control non-epitopes, modified by common PTMs, including citrullination, oxidation, deamidation, and chlorination. In each case, as described following, sets of all possible overlapping 9- or 10-mer sequences incorporating the various modifications were synthesized.

In terms of oxidation, Strollo et al. [16] using sodium dodecyl sulfate polyacrylamide gel electrophoresis (SDS-PAGE), three-dimensional fluorescence, and mass spectrometry (MS) demonstrated that histidine (His5), cysteine (Cys7), and L-phenylalanine (Phe24) residues could be oxidized in insulin-B (corresponding to positions 29, 31, and 49, respectively, in the full unspliced insulin sequence). To address the impact of oxidation of these residues on pHLA binding, 66 peptides were synthesized (see Additional file 3), comprising 14 peptides with oxidized Cys7; 14 with oxidized Phe24; and 38 with all residues oxidized (i.e., pan oxidation; see Methods).

Strollo et al. also reported that the tyrosines (Tyr) in positions 16 and 26 in the insulin B-chain (positions 40 and 50 in the unspliced sequence) were chlorinated. Therefore, another 29 peptides were synthesized to evaluate chlorination of both tyrosine residues.

Further, deamination of asparagine (Asn) and glutamine (Gln) residues have been described [4]. Deamination of Asn or Gln leads to and aspartic acid (Asp) or glutamic acid (Glu), respectively, or isoaspartic and isoglutamic acid, respectively. To evaluate the impact of Asn or Gln deamination of insulin B-chain eptipes, we synthesized another 16 peptides.

Table 1 HLA class I binding of CTL epitopes associated with previously defined diabetes-associated proteins

Source protein	Epitope sequence	Target assay	IC50 nM
AN1-type zinc finger protein 5	SASVQRADTSL	B*07:02	11
Bruton agammaglobulinemia tyrosine kinase	CLCLLNPQGT	A*02:01	–
	HLASEKVYAI	A*02:01	4064
	KLANIQCLCL	A*02:01	97
	KLANIQCPCL	A*02:01	121
	LASEKVYAI	A*02:01	6926
	SLTAISTTL	A*02:01	242
	SLTTISTTL	A*02:01	237
	YIPSCTVVGM	A*02:01	9506
Fms-related tyrosine kinase 3	KVLHELFGMDI	A*02:01	11
	VLHELFGMDI	A*02:01	287
Fms-related tyrosine kinase 3 ligand	ALARGAGTVPL	A*02:01	29
	SMPQGTFPV	A*02:01	631
Glial fibrillary acidic protein isoform 2	NLAQDLATV	A*02:01	67
	QLARQQVHV	A*02:01	–
	SLEEEIRFL	A*02:01	472
Glutamate decarboxylase 2	RFKMFPEVK	A*11:01	18,296
	MFPEVKEKG	A*11:01	–
	SPGSGFWSF	B*07:02	1173
	TSEHSHFSL	B*35:01	–
	ELAEYLYNI	A*02:01	637
	FLQDVMNIL	A*02:01	70
	ILMHCQTTL	A*02:01	478
	LLQEYNWEL	A*02:01	35
	RMMEYGTTMV	A*02:01	709
	VMNILLQYV	A*02:01	2024
	VMNILLQYVV	A*02:01	2308
	ACDGERPTL	B*07:02	28,719
	AHVDKCLEL	B*07:02	–
	APVIKARMM	B*07:02	18,197
	HPRYFNQLST	B*07:02	1252
	IPSDLERRIL	B*07:02	3858
Heat shock 70 kDa protein 1	LLDVAPLSL	A*02:01	51
	LLLLDVAPL	A*02:01	10
	LMGDKSENV	A*02:01	7374
Heat shock 70 kDa protein 6	FIQVYEVERA	A*02:01	7024
	FMTSSWWGA	A*02:01	378
	FMTSSWWRA	A*02:01	101
	FMTSSWWRAPL	A*02:01	84
	GIPPAPHGV	A*02:01	219
	GLLQVHHSCPL	A*02:01	5.8
	GVFIQVYEV	A*02:01	460
	KCQEVLAWL	A*02:01	–

Table 1 HLA class I binding of CTL epitopes associated with previously defined diabetes-associated proteins *(Continued)*

Source protein	Epitope sequence	Target assay	IC50 nM
	LLGRFELIGI	A*02:01	233
	LLHVHHSCPL	A*02:01	7839
	LLQVHHSCPL	A*02:01	3087
	NLLGRFELI	A*02:01	764
	NLLGRFELIGI	A*02:01	1.8
	SLASLLPHV	A*02:01	9.1
	SMCRFSPLTL	A*02:01	1149
	SVASLLPHV	A*02:01	1758
	VLNSLASLL	A*02:01	4968
	VLNSVASLL	A*02:01	1143
	VLVEGSTRI	A*02:01	17,161
Heat shock 70 kDa protein 6 variant	SLFEGVDFYT	A*02:01	51
Heat shock 70 kDa protein 1A variant	GIPPAPRGV	A*02:01	1226
	LIFDLGGGT	A*02:01	5416
Heat shock protein HSP 90-beta	ILDKKVEKV	A*02:01	11,237
Insulin	WGPDPAAA	A*02:01	–
	GIVEQCCTSI	A*02:01	7446
	LCGSHLVEAL	A*02:01	–
	SHLVEALYLV	A*02:01	2153
	ALWGPDPAAA	A*02:01	1008
	HLVEALYLV	A*02:01	134
	SLYQLENYC	A*02:01	16,923
	RLLPLLALL	A*02:01	145
		A*24:02	10,212
	VCGERGFFYT	A*01:01	–
		A*02:01	–
		B*08:01	–
		B*18:01	626
	ALWMRLLPLL	A*02:01	190
		A*24:02	6181
		B*08:01	33
	ALWMRLLPL	A*02:01	218
		B*08:01	107
	GSHLVEALY	A*01:01	30,269
	LVCGERGFFY	A*01:01	–
		A*03:01	27,363
		A*11:01	27,207
	GERGFFYT	A*01:01	–
		B*08:01	1377
	LALWGPDPAA	A*02:01	30,300
	RLLPLLALLAL	A*02:01	109

Table 1 HLA class I binding of CTL epitopes associated with previously defined diabetes-associated proteins (Continued)

Source protein	Epitope sequence	Target assay	IC50 nM
	HLCGSHLVEA	A*02:01	7536
	SLQKRGIVEQ	A*02:01	–
	LYLVCGERGF	A*24:02	5255
	LWMRLLPLL	A*24:02	545
	ALWGPDPAAAF	A*01:01	–
		A*24:02	15,101
	ERGFFYTPK	A*03:01	–
	PLALEGSLQK	A*03:01	–
	PLLALLALWG	A*03:01	–
	ALYLVCGER	A*03:01	2793
		A*11:01	28,341
	SLQPLALEG	A*02:01	–
		A*03:01	–
	LPLLALLAL	B*07:02	610
		B*35:01	12,300
		B*51:01	1164
	WMRLLPLLAL	B*07:02	2359
	FYTPKTRRE	B*08:01	13,033
Islet amyloid polypeptide precursor	FLIVLSVAL	A*02:01	26
	KLQVFLIVL	A*02:01	1372
Islet-specific glucose-6-phosphatase	FLWSVFMLI	A*02:01	26
Islet-specific glucose-6-phosphatase isoform 1	FLWSVFWLI	A*02:01	55
	RLLCALTSL	A*02:01	91
	LNIDLLWSV	A*02:01	684
	VLFGLGFAI	A*02:01	149
	NLFLFLFAV	A*02:01	1228
	YLLLRVLNI	A*02:01	57
	FLFAVGFYL	A*02:01	1.1
Protein tyrosine phosphatase	LLPPLLEHL	A*02:01	444
	SLAAGVKLL	A*02:01	3686
	SLSPLQAEL	A*02:01	101
	ALTAVAEEV	A*02:01	1306
	SLYHVYEVNL	A*02:01	209
	TIADFWQMV	A*02:01	4693
	VIVMLTPLV	A*02:01	2117
	MVWESGCTV	A*02:01	126
Tyrosine-protein kinase BTK	LASEKVYTI	A*02:01	1254
Tyrosine-protein kinase Lyn isoform B	LMFWSPSHSCA	A*02:01	143
	RLQREWHTL	A*02:01	1230
Tyrosine-protein phosphatase non-receptor type 11	RLGPVARTRV	A*02:01	581
	STVASRLGPV	A*02:01	25,069
	STVASWLGPV	A*02:01	9227

Table 1 HLA class I binding of CTL epitopes associated with previously defined diabetes-associated proteins (Continued)

Source protein	Epitope sequence	Target assay	IC50 nM
	TLSSRVCCRT	A*02:01	2784
	TVASRLGPV	A*02:01	7695
Zinc finger protein 36, C3H1 type-like 2	GLPAGAAAQA	A*02:01	530
	HLSYHRLLPL	A*02:01	4259
	HLSYHWLLPL	A*02:01	3817
	RLLPLWAAL	A*02:01	52
	RLLPLWAALPL	A*02:01	5.4
	RLRPLCCTA	A*02:01	8234
	WLLPLWAAL	A*02:01	4.2
	WLLPLWAALPL	A*02:01	3.2
Zinc transporter 8 isoform a	ALGDLFQSI	A*02:01	76
	AVAANIVLTV	A*02:01	575
	FLLSLFSLWL	A*02:01	16
	HIAGSLAVV	A*02:01	216
	ILAVDGVLSV	A*02:01	2.2
	ILKDFSILL	A*02:01	39
	ILVLASTITI	A*02:01	675
	IQATVMIIV	A*02:01	9043
	KMYAFTLES	A*02:01	880
	RLLYPDYQI	A*02:01	124
	SISVLISAL	A*02:01	1555
	TMHSLTIQM	A*02:01	104
	VAANIVLTV	A*02:01	320
	VTGVLVYL	A*02:01	9.0
	LLIDLTSFL	A*02:01	8.1
	LLSILCIVV	A*02:01	734
	LLSLFSLWL	A*02:01	152

A dash indicates IC50 >40,000 nM

In addition to the various published PTMs of the B-chain, we also investigated the effect of citrullination throughout the entire unspliced insulin sequence, which required the synthesis of 70 peptides. Collectively, a total of 276 peptides were synthesized, comprising 181 modified peptides and the corresponding 95 unmodified 9- and 10-mers. All peptides were evaluated for binding to HLA-A*02:01, as described in the Methods. The HLA-A*02:01 binding of each modified peptide is listed, along with its cognate unmodified (i.e., wild type, WT) peptide, in Additional file 3. The location of the various residues subjected to modification in the full-length insulin sequence is shown in Additional file 4.

HLA-A*02:01 binding of PTM insulin-derived peptides

We next evaluated the impact of these PTMs on the HLA-A*02:01 binding capacity of insulin-derived peptides,

Table 2 HLA class I tested, and epitope binding rates

Target assay	n	High affinity	% high	Int. affinity	% int.	Total binders	% binders
A*01:01	5	0	0.0	0	0.0	0	0.0
A*02:01	115	56	48.7	34	29.6	90	78.3
A*03:01	6	0	0.0	1	16.7	1	16.7
A*11:01	4	0	0.0	0	0.0	0	0.0
A*24:02	5	0	0.0	1	20.0	1	20.0
B*07:02	9	1	11.1	5	55.6	6	66.7
B*08:01	5	2	40.0	1	20.0	3	60.0
B*18:01	1	0	0.0	1	100.0	1	100.0
B*35:01	2	0	0.0	0	0.0	0	0.0
B*51:01	1	0	0.0	1	100.0	1	100.0
Total	153	59	38.6	44	28.8	103	67.3

including nine that were previously reported as A*02:01 restricted T cell epitopes (see Additional file 3). Of the nine previously reported epitopes, four (44%) were associated with a PTM-dependent improvement of affinity of at least two-fold (average = 3.76 +/− 2.73-fold) compared to the WT peptide (Table 3, top 4 epitopes). These improved peptides include the leader sequence 2–10 9-mer and 2–11 10-mer epitopes; here, modification of the arginine (Arg) in position 6 by citrullination improved binding of the 9-mer and 10-mer 7.83- and 2.76-fold, respectively. Two peptides (one 9- and one 10-mer) from the 33–42 region of the beta chain with chlorination of Tyr40 bound 2- to 2.5-fold better than the corresponding WT sequences. Overall, because in several cases multiple modifications of each epitope were tested, 26.7% (4/15) of the total modifications to known insulin-derived A*02:01-restricted T-cell epitopes resulted in a peptide with increased binding.

In addition to these previously published PTM epitopes, another 13 peptides (Table 3, bottom 13, below line) were found to be associated with improved binding as a result of PTM, compared to the unmodified counterpart. (For the 9-mer B-chain sequence, YLVCGERGF, 2 different modifications led to increased binding). However, only one of the 14 modified peptides — a citrullinated leader sequence peptide —bound with an affinity < 100 nM. By comparison, three of the four modified known HLA-A*02:01 restricted epitopes bound with affinities < 100 nM. The difference in the rate of improvement seen between these two peptide sets is significant ($p = 0.0147$).

Additional analyses evaluated the effect of 166 modifications of 86 control non-epitopes (or epitopes restricted by non-A*02 alleles). For these control peptides, improved binding (i.e., > 2-fold increase in affinity) was found for only 14 of the 166 modifications (8.4%); this

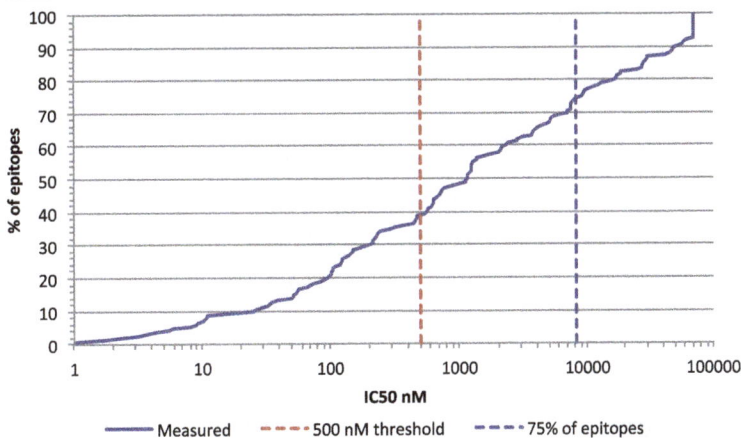

Fig. 1 HLA class I binding capacity of diabetes-associated CTL epitopes: A cumulative percentage of diabetes associated epitopes is plotted as a function of the binding capacity of the epitopes assayed for their corresponding HLA class I restricting allele. As shown, about 40% of the epitopes bound with an affinity of 500 nM (red dashed line), or better, and 75% bound at the 8250 nM level (blue dashed line)

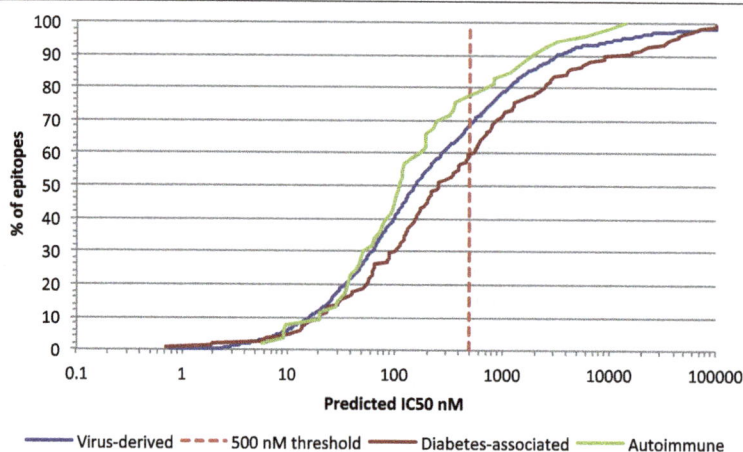

Fig. 2 Binding capacity of various types of class I epitopes: The predicted binding affinity of diabetes-associated epitopes (red line) is compared with the predicted binding capacity of virus derived epitopes (blue line), and epitopes associated with other autoimmune diseases (green line). The 500 nM threshold (dashed red line) identifies 60%, 70%, and 78% of the respective epitopes

corresponded to only 13/86 (15%) unique control peptides acquiring higher affinity following modification. The difference in rate of improvement, compared to the A*02-restricted insulin-B-derived epitope set, was significant ($p = 0.05$).

The effects of specific modifications on the binding of A*02 epitopes, non-epitopes, and in total, are summarized in Table 4. With respect to the epitopes, 2/3 (67%)

sequences subjected to chlorination, and 2/5 (40%) modified by citrullination, resulted in improved binding. Oxidation did not result in improved binding in any of the seven cases examined. Taken together, however, it should be noted that the number of events probed here are not sufficient to make statements regarding statistical significance of differences between the different modifications. Further, because Asn or Gln residues were not present in

Table 3 Insulin-derived epitope-HLA-A*02 binding was improved by PTMs

Set	Start	Segment	Len	Sequence WT	Modified	Modification	A*02:01 binding WT	Modified	Fold increase
Improved A*02 epitopes	2	Leader	9	ALWMRLLPL	ALWMULLPL	Citrullination	218	28	7.83
			10	ALWMRLLPLL	ALWMULLPLL	Citrullination	190	69	2.76
	33	B chain	10	SHLVEALYLV	SHLVEALJLV	Chlorination	2153	1066	2.02
	34	B chain	9	HLVEALYLV	HLVEALJLV	Chlorination	134	55	2.43
Other improved peptides	1	Leader	9	MALWMRLLP	MALWMULLP	Citrullination	4539	2117	2.14
	1	Leader	10	MALWMRLLPL	MALWMULLPL	Citrullination	1255	262	4.79
	3	Leader	10	LWMRLLPLLA	LWMULLPLLA	Citrullination	406	61	6.62
	4	Leader	10	WMRLLPLLAL	WMULLPLLAL	Citrullination	654	310	2.11
	28	B chain	9	QHLCGSHLV	EHLCGSHLV	Deamidation	–	7237	> 5
	31	B chain	10	CGSHLVEALY	BGSHLVEALY	Oxidation of C	33,691	8043	4.19
	37	B chain	10	EALYLVCGER	EALYLVCGEU	Citrullination	10,069	3100	3.25
	38	B chain	10	ALYLVCGERG	ALJLVCGERG	Chlorination	8784	2734	3.21
	39	B chain	9	LYLVCGERG	LYLVCGEUG	Citrullination	28,006	12,493	2.24
	40	B chain	9	YLVCGERGF	JLVCGERGF	Chlorination	6742	3163	2.13
					YLVBGERGY	Pan oxidation	6742	3244	2.08
	45	B chain	10	ERGFFYTPKT	ERGYYYTPKT	Pan oxidation	–	5730	> 7
	46	B chain	9	RGFFYTPKT	RGYYYTPKT	Pan oxidation	–	8805	> 4
	80	C peptide	10	LALEGSLQKR	LALEGSLQKU	Citrullination	–	16,354	> 2

A dash indicates IC50 > 40,000 nM

Table 4 Summary of effects of specific PTMs on HLA A*02:01 binding capacity

	Epitopes		Non-epitopes		Total	
Modification	n	% improved	n	% improved	n	% improved
Chlorination	3	66.7	26	7.7	29	13.8
Citrullination	5	40.0	65	10.8	70	12.9
Deamidation	0	–	16	6.3	16	6.3
Oxidation	7	0.0	59	6.8	66	6.1
Total	15	26.7	166	8.4	181	9.9

the respective epitopes, none of the corresponding peptide sequences were subject to deamidation.

Discussion

The role of T-cells in T1D has been demonstrated in mouse models and supported by the presence of CD4+ and CD8+ T-cells in human pancreata. Further, with the use of multimer technology and functional assays, inflammatory T-cells responsive to pancreas-derived antigens can be detected in peripheral blood samples from T1D subjects. Notably, these autoreactive T-cells have also been found in healthy, non-diabetic individuals, suggesting that such T-cells commonly make it through thymic selection and enter the peripheral tissue with little consequence to the individual. Peripheral modifications (PTM, mutation, processing defects) of native epitopes that are weakly to non-immunogenic in the thymus could induce unanticipated T-cell activation in the periphery. This would imply that T1D is less an error of the immune system and more the result of peripheral tissue dysfunction. Recent publications demonstrating the presence of hybrid and modified peptides, as well as reactive T-cells, in T1D+ subjects provides additional evidence to support this idea [17].

The present analyses assessed the capacity of 138 diabetes-associated CTL epitopes identified in the published literature to bind their reported HLA class I restricting allele(s). The data generated established a binding affinity reference threshold of 8250 nM that captures 75% of HLA class I-restricted diabetes epitopes, representing an affinity threshold somewhat lower than observed for pathogen-derived epitopes and predicted for epitopes from non-T1D autoimmune diseases. Notably, only 38.6% (59/138) of the diabetes epitopes studied bound at least one of its reported restriction elements with high affinity (IC50 < 500 nM) and another 28.8% (44/138) bound at least one allele with intermediate affinity (IC50 in the 500–5000 nM range). A generally lower rate of binding was associated with non-A2 alleles, possibly related to the fact these alleles have been less studied, and therefore the dataset might be inherently less representative and associated with reduced accuracy in terms of HLA restriction determination. It is

also possible, as reported in a previous study [13], that different HLA alleles might be associated with epitope repertoires of differing breadth. Abreu and colleagues have similarly found that preproinsulin epitopes tend to be associated with low HLA class I (A02) binding affinity [2].

Intriguingly, from our data it appears that the lower overall affinity of diabetes-associated epitopes might be unique to this indication, as lower binding affinity thresholds do not extend to other autoimmune epitopes. The reasons for these apparent differences are not clear, but might be related to inherent differences in the immune response associated with T1D progression compared to multiple sclerosis and rheumatoid arthritis, the two indications from which the other autoimmune epitopes evaluated in the current study were derived.

To evaluate the potential impact of common PTMs on the HLA class I binding capacity, we synthesized a large set of insulin-derived A*02:01-restricted T-cell epitopes, and also control peptides derived from human insulin but not associated with T1D, incorporating various modifications, including citrullination, chlorination, deamidation, and oxidation. We found that these modifications increased binding for 44% of the known T-cell epitopes, but only 15% of the control peptides. This data supports the hypothesis that the epitopes recognized by diabetes-associated T-cells are often PTM products, and these modified epitopes are associated with increased HLA binding in peripheral tissue. Further study is required to understand the exact contribution of PTMs in T1D disease onset and to ascertain if they initiate disease, are a by-product of disease, or play a role in progression, and also to evaluate if they can be developed diagnostically to identify pathogenic T cells or clinically as a therapeutic.

It will be important for future studies to establish the generality of these findings by testing epitopes restricted by other HLA molecules. Query of the IEDB revealed that at least a dozen insulin-derived epitopes are restricted by other, non-A*02, alleles. The analyses could also be expanded to include HLA class II molecules, since posttranslational modifications (and citrullination in particular) have been discussed as a potential factor in modulating autoreactivity in rheumatoid arthritis and other autoimmune pathologies. Further, the present study provides a model to extend a similar analysis towards other antigens associated with T1D, such as GAD, HSP-70, IA-2, and IGRP.

It will also be crucial to test the modified epitopes associated with increased binding for recognition using PBMCs from at-risk, diabetic, and non-diabetic individuals. We have herein identified modified peptides that are high affinity A*02:01 binders, and could represent novel epitopes. It is of obvious interest to include these potential new epitopes in experiments using HLA-A*02:01+ PBMC from healthy, at-risk, and T1D+ donors for functional assessments, including T-cell proliferation and cytokine production. Parallel experiments could address similar analyses of insulin peptides, both native and post-translationally modified, that bind the K^d and D^b class I expressed by NOD mice to allow for a detailed in vivo evaluation of disease relevance. Further experiments could also start to address whether similar findings can be extended to insulin peptides that bind HLA class II, and in particular utilizing the diabetes associated DQ8 molecule.

Clearly, our understanding of the functional role of T-cells and HLA in T1D development and progression is continually evolving. Overall, these findings provide further evidence that human T1D is not solely the result of autoimmunity and may be driven by immune responses to neoantigens, generated from protein processing defects and metabolic dysregulation leading to cell stress.

Conclusions

The present study experimentally and bioinformatically assessed the MHC binding capacity of HLA class I restricted T cell epitopes to demonstrate that T1D-associated may have lower overall affinity than epitopes associated with other pathological indications. These observations lend credence to the hypothesis that T1D-associated epitopes may be products of posttranslational modification, and that these modified epitopes are associated with increased HLA binding in peripheral tissue. Indeed, assessment of the binding capacity of PTM versions of known HLA A*02:01 restricted T1D-associated epitopes found increased binding capacity for 44% of the known T-cell epitopes, but only 15% of control peptides. Overall, these findings provide further evidence that human T1D is not solely the result of autoimmunity and may be driven by immune responses to neoantigens, generated from protein processing defects and metabolic dysregulation leading to cell stress.

Methods

HLA-peptide binding assays

Peptide-MHC affinities were measured using classical competition assays based on the inhibition of binding of a high affinity radiolabeled ligand to purified HLA class I molecules, as previously described [18]. Briefly, 0.1–1 nM of radiolabeled peptide is co-incubated at room temperature with purified MHC in the presence of a cocktail of protease inhibitors. Following a two-day incubation, MHC bound radioactivity is determined by capturing MHC/peptide complexes on W6/32 (anti-HLA class I) mAb coated Lumitrac 600 plates (Greiner Bio-one, Frickenhausen, Germany), and bound cpm measured using the TopCount (Packard Instrument Co., Meriden, CT) microscintillation counter. The concentration of peptide yielding 50% inhibition of binding of the radiolabeled peptide is calculated. Under the conditions utilized, where [label] < [MHC]

and IC50 ≥ [MHC], measured IC50 values are reasonable approximations of true K_d. Each competitor peptide is tested at six different concentrations covering a 100,000-fold range, and in three or more independent experiments. As a positive control, the unlabeled version of the radiolabeled probe is also tested in each experiment. Utilizing a previously defined threshold [11, 12], peptides with an affinity of 500 nM or better for their restricting allele were defined as high affinity binders; peptides with affinities in the 500–5000 nM range were defined as intermediate binders.

HLA-peptide binding predictions

Binding predictions were performed using the command-line version of the SMM prediction tool available on the Immune Epitope Database website (http://www.iedb.org) [19, 20]. Besides strong performance in predicting A*02:01 binding capacity, SMM also consistently performs as one of the best prediction tools across a wide array of alleles, and also provides predicted IC50 nM values for all of the alleles considered here. In addition to predicted affinity (IC_{50}), the SMM algorithm provides a percentile score expressing the relative capacity of each peptide to bind each specific allele, compared to a universe of potential sequences of the same size.

Peptide synthesis

Peptides were synthesized by A and A (San Diego) as crude material on a 1 mg scale, or purified (> 95%) by reverse phase HPLC. PTM of individual residues, including deamidation, citrullination, chlorination and oxidation of cysteine was performed as part of the standard Fmoc synthesis. Because of the unavailability of Fmoc-Oxo-His, oxidation of histidine was performed post-synthesis. As a result, histidine cannot be individually oxidized, and in all corresponding peptides all other oxidizable residues (e.g., Cys and Met) are similarly oxidized. Throughout, in the corresponding peptide sequences, the respective PTMs are identified as follows. B: Cysteic acid; J: chloryl tyrosine; O: iso-aspartic acid; Z: iso-glutamic acid; U: citrulline. The human insulin sequence utilized was UniProt accession number P01308.

Additional files

Additional file 1: Diabetes-associated proteins. Table (Word; .docx) listing antigens associated with T1D, pre-diabetes, and diabetes mellitus studies. (DOCX 56 kb)

Additional file 2: CTL epitopes associated with previously defined diabetes-associated proteins. Table (Word; .docx) listing identified following IEDB query structured as described in the text. (DOCX 131 kb)

Additional file 3: Measured binding affinities. Table (Word; .docx) listing the modified and native peptides studied and their measured HLA A*02:01 binding capacity. (DOCX 135 kb)

Additional file 4: Location of modified residues in full length insulin sequence. Figure (.pdf) highlighting specific insulin residues targeted for modification, as described in the text. (DOCX 103 kb)

Abbreviations
CTLs: Cytolytic CD8 T-cells; ELISPOT: Enzyme-linked immunospot assay; ER: Endoplasmic reticulum; HLA: Human leukocyte antigen; IC50: Half maximal inhibitory concentration; ICS: Intracellular cytokine staining; IEDB: Immune Epitope Database; MHC: Major histocompatibility; MS: Mass spectrometry; PTM: Post-translational modification; SDS-PAGE: Sodium dodecyl sulfate polyacrylamide gel electrophoresis; T1D: Type 1 diabetes; tTG: Tissue transglutimase; WT: Wild type; amino acids have been abbreviated using standard 3-letter codes.

Acknowledgements
Erin Moore, Mikaela Lindvall, and Eugene Moore are acknowledged for contributing their efforts and technical expertise towards the performance of all MHC-peptide binding assays. The late Jalāl ad-Dīn Muhammad Rūmī (Balkhī) is thanked for inspiration and invaluable advice.

Funding
Not applicable.

Authors' contributions
JS performed and/or supervised the performance of all experimental procedures, designed, analyzed and interpreted the MHC-peptide binding studies, and participated in writing the manuscript. JLV, DF, RK, MvH, JDW contributed to the study design, data interpretation, and writing the manuscript. AS oversaw all aspects of the study, to include design, logistics, data analysis and interpretation, and writing of the manuscript. All authors read and approved the final manuscript.

Competing interests
Matthias von Herrath is a member of the editorial board (Associate Editor) of BMC Immunology. Otherwise, all authors declare that they have no competing interests.

Author details
[1]La Jolla Institute for Allergy and Immunology, La Jolla, CA 92130, USA. [2]Novo Nordisk Research Center Seattle, Inc., 530 Fairview Ave N, Seattle, WA 98109, USA.

References
1. Pugliese A. Autoreactive T cells in type 1 diabetes. J Clin Invest. 2017;127(8):2881–91.
2. Abreu JR, Martina S, Verrijn Stuart AA, Fillie YE, Franken KL, Drijfhout JW, Roep BO. CD8 T cell autoreactivity to preproinsulin epitopes with very low human leucocyte antigen class I binding affinity. Clin Exp Immunol. 2012;170(1):57–65.
3. Mannering SI, Harrison LC, Williamson NA, Morris JS, Thearle DJ, Jensen KP, Kay TW, Rossjohn J, Falk BA, Nepom GT, et al. The insulin A-chain epitope recognized by human T cells is posttranslationally modified. J Exp Med. 2005;202(9):1191–7.
4. van Lummel M, Duinkerken G, van Veelen PA, de Ru A, Cordfunke R, Zaldumbide A, Gomez-Tourino I, Arif S, Peakman M, Drijfhout JW, et al. Posttranslational modification of HLA-DQ binding islet autoantigens in type 1 diabetes. Diabetes. 2014;63(1):237–47.
5. Delong T, Wiles TA, Baker RL, Bradley B, Barbour G, Reisdorph R, Armstrong M, Powell RL, Reisdorph N, Kumar N, et al. Pathogenic CD4 T cells in type 1 diabetes recognize epitopes formed by peptide fusion. Science. 2016;351(6274):711–4.
6. Coppieters KT, Dotta F, Amirian N, Campbell PD, Kay TW, Atkinson MA, Roep BO, von Herrath MG. Demonstration of islet-autoreactive CD8 T cells in insulitic lesions from recent onset and long-term type 1 diabetes patients. J Exp Med. 2012;209(1):51–60.
7. Carrasco Pro S, Sidney J, Paul S, Lindestam Arlehamn C, Weiskopf D, Peters B, Sette A. Automatic Generation of Validated Specific Epitope Sets. J Immunol Res. 2015;2015:763461.
8. Seymour E, Damle R, Sette A, Peters B. Cost sensitive hierarchical document classification to triage PubMed abstracts for manual curation. BMC bioinformatics. 2011;12:482.
9. Middleton D, Menhaca L, Rood H, Komerofsky R. New allele frequency database http://www.allelefrequencies.net. Tissue Antigens. 2003;61(5):403–7.
10. Meyer D, Singe R, Mack S, Lancaster A, Nelson M, Erlich H, Frenandez-Vina M, Thomson G: Single Locus Polymorphism of Classical HLA Genes. Immunobiology of the Human MHC: Proceedings of the 13th International Histocompatibility Workshop and Conference; Seattle: IHWG Press. 2007: 653–704.
11. Sette A, Vitiello A, Reherman B, Fowler P, Nayersina R, Kast WM, Melief CJ, Oseroff C, Yuan L, Ruppert J, et al. The relationship between class I binding affinity and immunogenicity of potential cytotoxic T cell epitopes. J Immunol. 1994;153(12):5586–92.
12. Assarsson E, Sidney J, Oseroff C, Pasquetto V, Bui HH, Frahm N, Brander C, Peters B, Grey H, Sette A. A quantitative analysis of the variables affecting the repertoire of T cell specificities recognized after vaccinia virus infection. J Immunol. 2007;178(12):7890–901.
13. Paul S, Weiskopf D, Angelo MA, Sidney J, Peters B, Sette A. HLA class I alleles are associated with peptide-binding repertoires of different size, affinity, and immunogenicity. J Immunol. 2013;191(12):5831–9.
14. Ferlin WG, Mougneau E, Hugues S, Appel H, Jang MH, Cazareth J, Beaudoin L, Schricke C, Lehuen A, Wucherpfennig KW, et al. Self-peptides that bind with low affinity to the diabetes-associated I-A(g7) molecule readily induce T cell tolerance in non-obese diabetic mice. Eur J Immunol. 2004;34(10):2656–63.
15. McGinty JW, Marre ML, Bajzik V, Piganelli JD, James EA. T cell epitopes and post-translationally modified epitopes in type 1 diabetes. Curr Diab Rep. 2015;15(11):90.
16. Strollo R, Vinci C, Arshad MH, Perrett D, Tiberti C, Chiarelli F, Napoli N, Pozzilli P, Nissim A. Antibodies to post-translationally modified insulin in type 1 diabetes. Diabetologia. 2015;58(12):2851–60.
17. Kent SC, Babon JA. Narrowing in on the anti-beta cell-specific T cells: looking 'where the action is'. Curr Opin Endocrinol Diabetes Obes. 2017;24(2):98–102.
18. Sidney J, Southwood S, Moore C, Oseroff C, Pinilla C, Grey HM, Sette A: Measurement of MHC/peptide interactions by gel filtration or monoclonal antibody capture. Curr Protoc Immunol 2013, Chapter 18:Unit 18 13.
19. Kim Y, Ponomarenko J, Zhu Z, Tamang D, Wang P, Greenbaum J, Lundegaard C, Sette A, Lund O, Bourne PE, et al. Immune epitope database analysis resource. Nucleic Acids Res. 2012;40(Web Server issue):W525–30.
20. Vita R, Overton JA, Greenbaum JA, Ponomarenko J, Clark JD, Cantrell JR, Wheeler DK, Gabbard JL, Hix D, Sette A, et al. The immune epitope database (IEDB) 3.0. Nucleic Acids Res. 2015;43(Database issue):D405–12.

16

Blocking IL-10 signalling at the time of immunization does not increase unwanted side effects in mice

Guoying Ni[1], Zaowen Liao[2], Shu Chen[2], Tianfang Wang[3], Jianwei Yuan[4], Xuan Pan[4], Kate Mounsey[3], Shelley Cavezza[3], Xiaosong Liu[2,3,4*] and Ming Q. Wei[1]

Abstract

Background: Cancer therapeutic vaccine induced cytotoxic T cell (CTL) responses are pivotal for the killing of tumour cells. Blocking interleukin 10 (IL-10) signalling at the time of immunization increases vaccine induced CTL responses and improves prevention of tumour growth in animal models compared to immunization without an IL-10 signalling blockade. Therefore, this immunization strategy may have potential to curtail cancer in a clinical setting. However, IL-10 deficiency leads to autoimmune disease in the gut. Blocking IL-10 at the time of immunization may result in unwanted side effects, especially immune-pathological diseases in the intestine.

Methods: We investigated whether blocking IL-10 at the time of immunization results in intestinal inflammation responses in a mouse TC-1 tumour model and in a NOD autoimmune disease prone mouse model.

Results: We now show that blocking IL-10 at the time of immunization increases IL-10 production by CD4+ T cells in the spleen and draining lymph nodes, and does not result in blood cell infiltration to the intestines leading to intestinal pathological changes. Moreover, immunization with papillomavirus like particles combined with simultaneously blocking IL-10 signalling does not increase the incidence of autoimmune disease in Non-obese diabetic (NOD) mice.

Conclusions: Our results indicate that immunization with an IL-10 inhibitor may facilitate the generation of safe, effective therapeutic vaccines against chronic viral infection and cancer.

Keywords: Il-10, CD4+ T cells, Intestine, Inflammation, Immunotherapy

Background

Cervical cancer is the second most common cancer in women worldwide [1, 2]. Chronic infection of human papillomavirus (HPV), especially HPV subtype 16 and 18, leads to the development of cervical cancer [3–6]. Although a prophylactic vaccine against HPV infection has been introduced, treatment of patients with chronic HPV infection and cervical cancer, remains a big challenge [7, 8].

Therapeutic vaccine targeting viral infected or cancer cells without hurting normal tissues or organs, is a potential therapeutic for the treatment of chronic HPV infection and HPV infection related cancers, by stimulating cytotoxic T cells (CTLs) against viral/tumour antigens [9]. The HPV early proteins E6 and E7 are expressed in HPV-associated cancers and are ideal targets for a therapeutic vaccine [10, 11].

Recently, much advance has been made in the area of HPV therapeutic vaccine research area [2, 12, 13]. Long E7 peptide/Incomplete Freunds adjuvant (IFA) and a nuclear acid vaccine (VGX-3100) have been shown to have therapeutic efficacy against HPV infection related pre-cancerous lesions [1]. However, up to now, HPV therapeutic vaccines are still not able to show efficacy against cervical cancer [14]. Current therapeutic vaccines often fail to generate enough numbers of CTLs, and as the tumour micro-environment is immunosuppressive, this prevents CTLs from killing tumour or viral infected cells [12]. To be more effective, therapeutic vaccines need to

* Correspondence: xiaosongl@yahoo.com
[2]Cancer Research Institute, The First People's Hospital of Foshan, Foshan, Guangdong 528000, China
[3]Inflammation and Healing Research Cluster, University of the Sunshine Coast, Maroochydore DC, QLD 4558, Australia
Full list of author information is available at the end of the article

elicit the right type, and enough numbers of effector cells either through generation of new effector cells or through the activation of endogenous effector cells; these effector cells must then be able to migrate to tumour sites; overcome the immunosuppressive tumour microenvironment and finally kill the viral infected or tumour cells [15–19].

Interleukin 10 (IL-10) is an anti-inflammatory cytokine with the ability to suppress excessive inflammatory responses to both self and foreign antigens, through interacting with IL-10 receptors on the membranes of their target cells [20–22]. Cancer patients often have increased levels of serum IL-10; and increased levels of IL-10 often indicate poor prognosis [23–26]. IL-10 is detected in a variety of freshly excised human tumour samples [26–28]. IL-10 can be secreted by different types of cells, including tumour cells, and hematopoietic cells that infiltrate the tumour tissues. Tumour associated T regulatory cells and tumour associated antigen presentation cells, such as dendritic cells and macrophages, have been shown to produce IL-10 [27]. IL-10 secreting regulatory T cells inhibit vaccine induced CD8+ T cell responses, and can be amplified after therapeutic vaccination [26, 29].

Blocking IL-10 at the time of immunization drastically increases vaccine induced CTLs [30]. Recently, it has been demonstrated that blocking IL-10 concomitantly with immunization using Toll like receptor agonist inhibits tumour growth in a human papillomavirus E7 transformed TC-1 tumour mouse model, similar to a long E7 peptide/IFA vaccine that is effective against HPV infection related pre-cancer [11]. Moreover, it has been shown that immunization and simultaneous IL-10 signalling blockade better control tumour growth in a TC-1 mouse model than immunization without IL-10 signalling blockade [29]. Therefore, a therapeutic vaccine that contains IL-10 signalling inhibitor may be effective against cervical cancer. IL-10 signalling inhibitors have been developed for possible translation this novel immunization strategy into clinical practice [31, 32].

However, IL-10 deficiency in mice results in autoimmune disease in the intestinal tract driven by unimpeded reactivity of effector CD4+ T cells to antigens of intestinal microorganisms [33]. IL-10 deficiency increases hepatic damage, and leads to more severe disease during acute murine cytomegalovirus infection [34]. IL-10 is required for the generation of IL-10 secreting CD4 + T cells in vitro and in vivo [35]. Therefore, blocking IL-10 signalling at the time of immunization may also prevent the generation of antigen induced IL-10 secreting cells and result in unwanted side effects, especially in the intestine. Concerns about the development of autoimmune disease may prevent the inclusion of IL-10 inhibitor as a component of a therapeutic vaccine.

In the current paper, we investigated whether immunizing mice using TLR4 ligand as adjuvant and 2 different antigens (HPV16 E7 peptide, soluble antigen OVA), and simultaneously blocking IL-10 signalling would lead to inflammation in the gut and cause autoimmune disease. Unexpectedly, the numbers of IL-10 producing cells were significantly increased in mice immunized with HPV16 E7 peptide when IL-10 signalling is blocked compared to mice immunized without IL-10 signalling blockade.

Methods

Mice

Six to eigth weeks old, specific pathogen free (SPF) adult female C57BL/6 (H-2^b) mice were ordered from the Animal Resource Centre, Sun Yat-Sen University and kept at the Animal Resource Centre, Sun Yat-Sen University, Guangdong province, China. Experiments in the current paper were approved by and then performed in compliance with the guidelines of Foshan First Peoples Hospital Animal Experimentation Ethics Committee (Ethics Approval Number: FSFH20160316). Mice were sacrificed by neck dislocation after the experiments. Mice were treated with dextran sulfate sodium sodium (DSS) inducing ulcerative colitis as mouse models of intestinal inflammation described elsewhere [30]. Six to eigth weeks old adult female autoimmune prone Non-obese diabetic (NOD)/Lt mice were purchased SPF from the Animal Resource Centre, Perth, Australia. NOD/Lt mice experiments were carried out at Princess Alexandra Hospital Animal House Facilities, University of Queensland. The experiment with NOD mice was approved by and performed in compliance with the guidelines of the University of Queensland Animal Experimentation Ethics Committee. Blood glucose levels of NOD/Lt mice were monitored weekly. Following two consecutive weekly blood glucose readings >12 mmol/l, mice were considered to be diabetic and were sacrificed. Mice were sacrificed by CO_2 inhalation after the experiments.

Peptides and antibodies

Anti-CD45.2-FITC (104); Anti-CD11b-PE (M1/70), Anti-CD4-FITC (RM4–4), anti-CD4-PE (RM 4–5), anti-GITR-PE (RAM34), anti-IL-10 (JES5-16E3), anti-IFNγ-PE (XMG1.2), anti-IL-10-APC (JES5-16E3) were purchased from eBioscience (San Diego, CA, USA). Anti-CD3-PE (17A2), Anti-CD4-APC (RM4–5) mAbs were purchased from BioLegend (San Diego CA). Anti-mouse/Rat Foxp 3 staining kit was purchased from eBioscience (San Diego, CA, USA). Anti-CD3 mAb (CD 3–12) was purchased from GeneTex (Alton Parkway Irvine, CA, USA), anti-Ly-6G (1A8) was purchased from BioLegend (San Diego, CA, USA).

Ovalbumin (OVA), Lipopolysaccharide (LPS), Monophosphoryl Lipid A (MPLA) and Dextran Sulfate

Sodium Salt (DSS) were bought from Sigma. Anti-IL10 receptor (1B1.3a) Monoclonal Antibody (MAb) was ordered from BioXcell, USA and stored at -80 °C till further use.

Long HPV16 E7 peptide GQAEPDRAHYNIVTFCC KCDSTLRLCVQSTHVDIR, HPV16 E7 the MHC class I (H-2 Db) restricted epitope RAHYNIVTF, the MHC class I (H-2 D^b) restricted ovalbumin (OVA) peptide SII FINKLE, and the MHC class II (H-2 Db) restricted peptide ISQAVHAAHAEINEAGR were synthesised and purified by Mimotopes (Melbourne, Australia). The purity of the synthesised peptides were 95% and was determined by reverse-phase HPLC. Peptides were dissolved in 0.5% DMSO in PBS and stored at −20 °C till use.

Production of recombinant VLPs

Papillomavirus virus like particles (VLPs) L1E7 were produced, purified and confirmed as described elsewhere [30, 36].

2.1.4 immunization of mice

Groups of three to six mice were immunized as indicated with a): 50 µg of OVA and 15 µg of LPS subcutaneously (s.c.). with or without Intraperitoneal injection (i.p.) of 500 µg of anti-IL10R antibodies; or b): with 50 µg of long E7 peptide/15 µg of Monophosphoryl Lipid A (MPLA) with 300 µg of anti-IL10R antibodies or control antibodies s.c; or c): with 50 µg of VLPs intramuscularly (i.m.), with or without i.p. injection of 500 µg of anti-IL10R antibodies at 14 days apart.

ELISA for IL10 and IFN-γ cytokines from culture supernatants

ELISA for IL-10 and IFN-γ (ebioscience, USA) was performed according to the manufacturer's recommended procedures and were described elsewhere [37].

ELISPOT

ELISPOT for antigen specific IFNγ CD8 T cell response was performed as previously described [37]. Briefly, single spleen cell suspensions were added to the 96 well plates (Millipore, Bedford, MA) previously coated with anti-IFN-γ (BD Harlingen, San Diego, CA). RAHY NIVTF was added and cells cultured at 37 °C overnight. Biotinylated anti-IFN-γ (BD Harlingen), avidin –horseradish peroxidase (Sigma-Aldrich) were sequentially added before developed with DAB (Sigma-Aldrich). Experiment was stopped by washing with tap water. The results were determined by an ELISPOT reader (AID Autoimmun Diagnosticka GmbH, Strassberg, Germany).

Intracellular staining for IFNγ, IL-10

Single spleen cell suspensions or single lymph node cell suspension obtained from immunized and control mice

were stimulated with PMA and ionomycin for 3–5 h in the presence of protein transport inhibitor monensin (BioLegend). For some experiments, the cells were cultured for 72 h in the presence of 1 µg/ml of OVA, 1 µg/ml of SIINFEKLE or 1 µg/ml of ISQAVHAAHAEI NEAGR and then stimulated with PMA and ionomycin for 3–5 h. After specific or non-specific stimulation, the cells were firstly surface stained with anti-CD3, CD4 or CD8 antibodies before intracellularly stained for IL-10 and IFN-γ, by using commercial Per/Fix reagents (BD Pharmingen) [37].

Isolation and staining of intestinal lymphocytes (IELs)

The intestinal lymphocytes (IELs) were isolated by following Lefrancois's protocol [38]. Briefly, the mice were sacrificed by cervical dislocation and the intestines were harvested and separated from unwanted fat and connective tissue. Fecal matter in the intestinal was expelled by flushing the entire intestine with 40 ml, 4 °C CMF solution. After removing remaining fat and connective tissues and Peyer's patches, the intestines were then cut longitudinally and laterally into ~ 0.5 cm pieces. The intestine pieces were washed with 4 °C CMF solution until supernatants were relatively clear. The intestinal pieces were incubated with 20 ml CMF/FBS/DTE solution at 37 °C with stirring for another 20 min. The intestinal pieces were then transferred to a 50-ml conical centrifuge tube and vortex for 15 s at maximum setting. Intestinal pieces were allowed to settle and supernatant transferred to another 50-ml conical tube, followed by a 10-min incubation on ice. Supernatants contained the IEL and some epithelial cells. The IEL supernatant was then centrifuged at 350 g for 5 min and the supernatant discarded. Counted viable cells were re-suspended in Cell Staining Buffer at 5 × 10^6 cells/ml. Fc receptors were then blocked with 1.0 µg Anti-Mouse CD16/CD32 Purified (clone: 93) for 10 min on ice, then anti-mouse CD45.2 FITC, anti-mouse CD3 PE, anti-mouse CD8 PerCP Cyanine5.5 and anti-mouse CD4 APC added as appropriate and incubated on ice for 20 min in the dark. The cells were acquired on BD FACSCalibur. Flow cytometry data was analyzed by flowjo.

Immunohistochemistry (IHC) for the detection of intestinal infiltrating CD3$^+$ T cells and neutrophils

Intestines from immunized and control mice were excised and cut into pieces as described above. Mouse intestine pieces were fixed in 10% buffered neutral formalin, then processed through graded ethanol and three changes of xylene, before infiltrated with paraffin. Samples were embedded into paraffin blocks and cut into 4 mm sections before mounted onto slides. The Vectastain® ABC kit was used for antibody detection and the methods has been described elsewhere [31]. Briefly,

Anti-CD3 mAb (clone CD3–12) or anti-Ly-6G (clone 1A8) were used to detect T cells and neutrophils. Murine lymph node was used as the positive control for CD3 + T cells staining. Slides from the same series without primary antibody were used as negative controls.

CD3 positive or anti-Ly-6G positive cells were quantified using Image analysis software Image pro Plus 6.0 (IPP). The infiltrating CD3+ T cells or neutrophils was quantified from five high-power fields (HPFs, 200×) and intestinal infiltrating CD3+ T cell or neutrophil numbers were calculated as the ratio of integrated option density IOD /area (IOD/area) [39].

Statistical analysis
Statistical analysis was performed by using the two tailed Student's test, or Log rank test using Prism 4.0 (Graphpad Software, San Diego).

Results
Blocking IL10 signalling at the time of immunization increases the numbers of IL-10 producing cells
We have previously shown that HPV16 early protein E7 long peptide/MPLA immunization and simultaneously blocking IL-10 signalling enhances vaccine induced E7 specific CD8+ T cell responses compared with immunization without IL-10 signalling blockade [11]. We investigated the number of IL-10 secreting CD4 + T cells in HPV16 early protein E7 long peptide/MPLA immunized mice with or without blocking IL-10 signalling. Mice were immunized twice subcutaneously at 2 weeks apart, with long E7 peptide/MPLA with or without administration of anti-IL-10R antibodies subcutaneously. Splenocytes and lymphocytes from draining lymph nodes were stained for CD3, CD4, GITR and IL-10. While the total numbers of splenic cells and draining lymph nodes were increased in IL-10 signalling blocked group, the ratio of CD4+ and CD4 + GITR+ T cells were slightly increased in IL-10 signalling blocked group compared with non-IL-10 signalling blocked group (data not shown). Unexpectedly, the numbers of IL-10 producing CD4+ T cells were significantly increased in the long E7/MPLA immunized and simultaneously IL-10 signalling blocked mice compared to mice immunized without IL-10 signalling blockade (Fig. 1a, b). The numbers of CD4 + GITR+ IL10+ T cells were also significantly increased in IL-10 signalling blocked and long E7 peptide/MPLA immunized mice (Fig. 1e, f) as measured by IL-10 intracellular staining in CD4 + GITR+ T cells. The numbers of IFNγ + IL10 + CD4+ T cells that limit the strength of Th1 responses [38] were also increased in immunized and IL-10 signalling blocked mice (Fig. 1c, d). The numbers of CD4 + IL-10+ cells in the spleen of IL-10 signalling blocked group is also increased compared with IL-10 non-blocked group (Fig. 1g).

We further confirmed this phenomenon by using another antigen ovalbumin (OVA). Similar to papillomavirus (PV) virus like particles (VLPs) and HPV16E7 long peptide immunization, blocking IL-10 with simultaneous OVA/LPS immunization enhanced the vaccine induced antigen specific CD8+ T cell response by ELISPOT, intracellular staining and ELISA (Additional file 1: Figure S1a). To investigate if the numbers of IL-10 secreting CD4+ T cells were increased after OVA/LPS immunization and IL-10 signalling blockade, mice were immunized with OVA/LPS, with or without administration of anti-IL-10R antibodies twice, splenocytes and lymphocytes isolated from draining lymph nodes were stained for IL-10. Similarly, splenic IL-10 secreting CD4+ T cells, CD4 + GITR+ IL10 + T cells, and CD4 + IFNγ + IL-10+ T cells were significantly increased in mice immunized with OVA/LPS plus administration of anti-IL-10R antibodies, compared with mice immunized with OVA/LPS without administration of anti-IL-10R antibodies (Additional file 1: Figure S2).

Blocking IL10 signalling at the time of immunization in mice does not increase the numbers of spleen CD4 + Foxp3+ T cells
We next investigated whether the numbers of Foxp3 + CD4 + T cells are changed after blocking IL-10 signalling at the time of immunization. Mice were immunized with HPV16E7 peptide/MPLA in the presence or absence of anti-IL10R antibodies, and the numbers of CD4 + Foxp3+ T cells from spleen and draining lymph nodes were measured by flow cytometry. The results showed that the numbers of CD4 + Foxp3+ T cells were similar in the draining lymph nodes (Fig. 2a) and spleen (Fig. 2b), whether the mice were immunized simultaneously with or without anti-IL10R antibody administration. Similar results were obtained in mice immunized with OVA/LPS in the presence or absence of anti-IL-10R antibodies (Additional file 1: Figure S3).

Neutralizing IL10 at the time of immunization does not cause pathological changes in intestines
We investigated whether blocking IL-10 signalling at the time of immunization causes inflammation in important tissues and organs. We especially wished to know whether this immunization strategy causes inflammation in the intestine, as IL-10 knockout mice have chronic inflammation in their intestine late in their life. Mice were immunized with long E7 peptide/MPLA twice at 14 days apart, in the presence or absence of anti-IL10R administration. 2 weeks after the final immunization there were no signs of inflammation observed in the heart, brain, kidney, and intestine by eye or under the microscope (data not shown and Fig. 3a) in mice immunized with long E7 peptide/MPLA, long E7 peptide/MPLA/anti-IL10R antibody, long E7 peptide/MPLA/Normal Rat

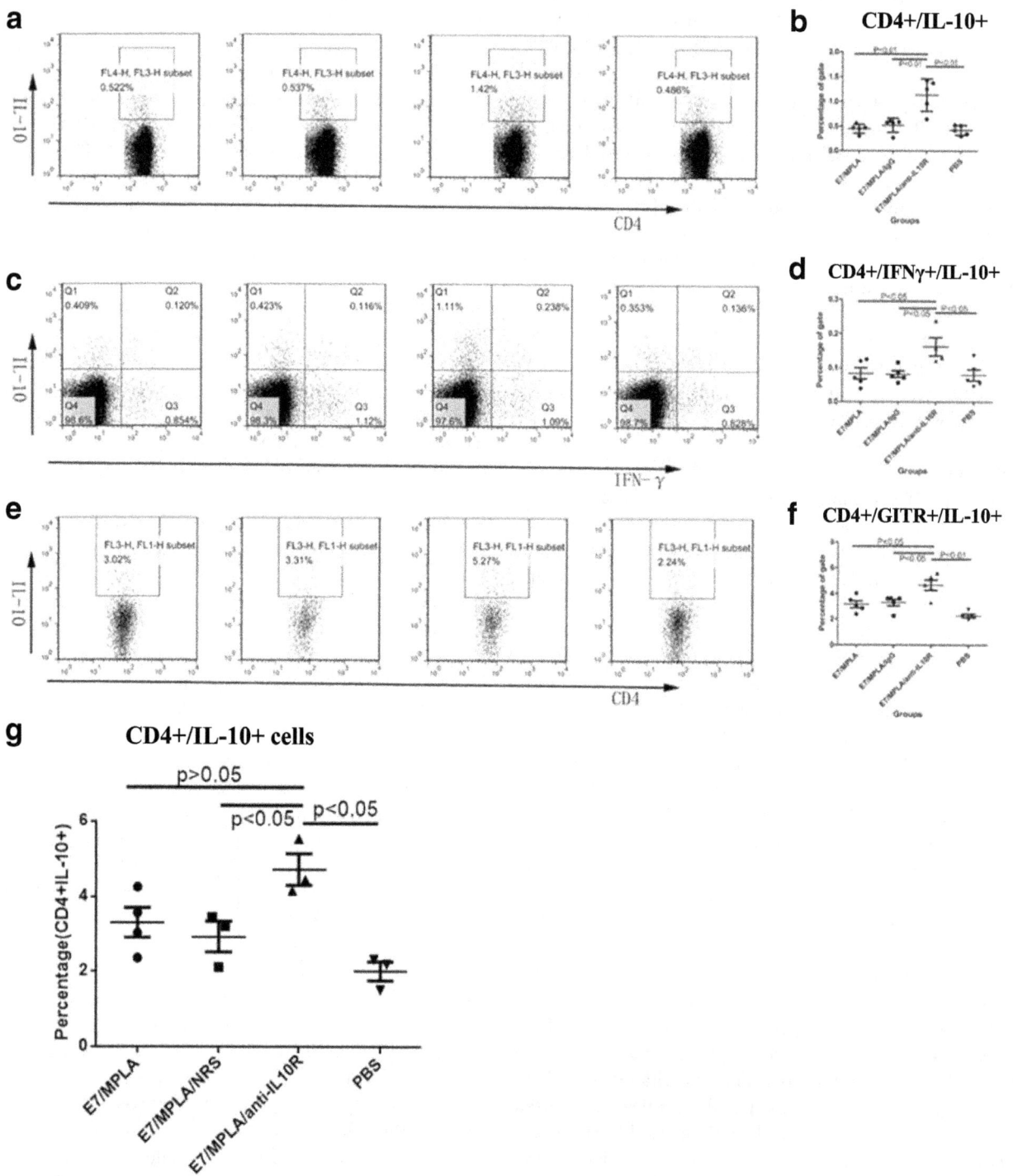

Fig. 1 Blocking IL-10 signalling at the time of long HPV16 E7 peptide/MPLA immunization increases the numbers of IL-10 producing cells. Groups of five C57BL/6 mice were immunized as indicated with 50 µg of E7 peptide/15 µg of Monophosphoryl Lipid A (MPLA), 300 µg of anti-IL10R antibodies or control antibodies s.c on days 0 and 14. Splenocytes and draining lymph node cells from immunized mice were harvested and stimulated with 25 ng/ml PMA and 1 µg/ml ionomycin for 6 h in the presence of monensin on 7 days after final immunization. Cells were surface stained for CD3, CD4, and GITR and intracellular stained for IL-10 and IFN-γ. CD3+ cells were gated. Results for cells of draining lymph nodes were shown. A and B: IL-10 secreting CD3 + CD4+ T cells IL-10 (**a**) FACS plot and (**b**) summarised data showing IL-10 expression by CD3 + CD4+ T cells. C and D: CD3 + CD4+ T cells secreting IL-10 and IFN-γ *dot* plots (**c**) and summarised data from different groups (**d**) E and F: CD4 + GITR+ T cells secreting IL-10: FACS profile (**e**) and summarised data from different groups (**f**). Splenic CD4 + IL-10+ cells were shown in (**g**)

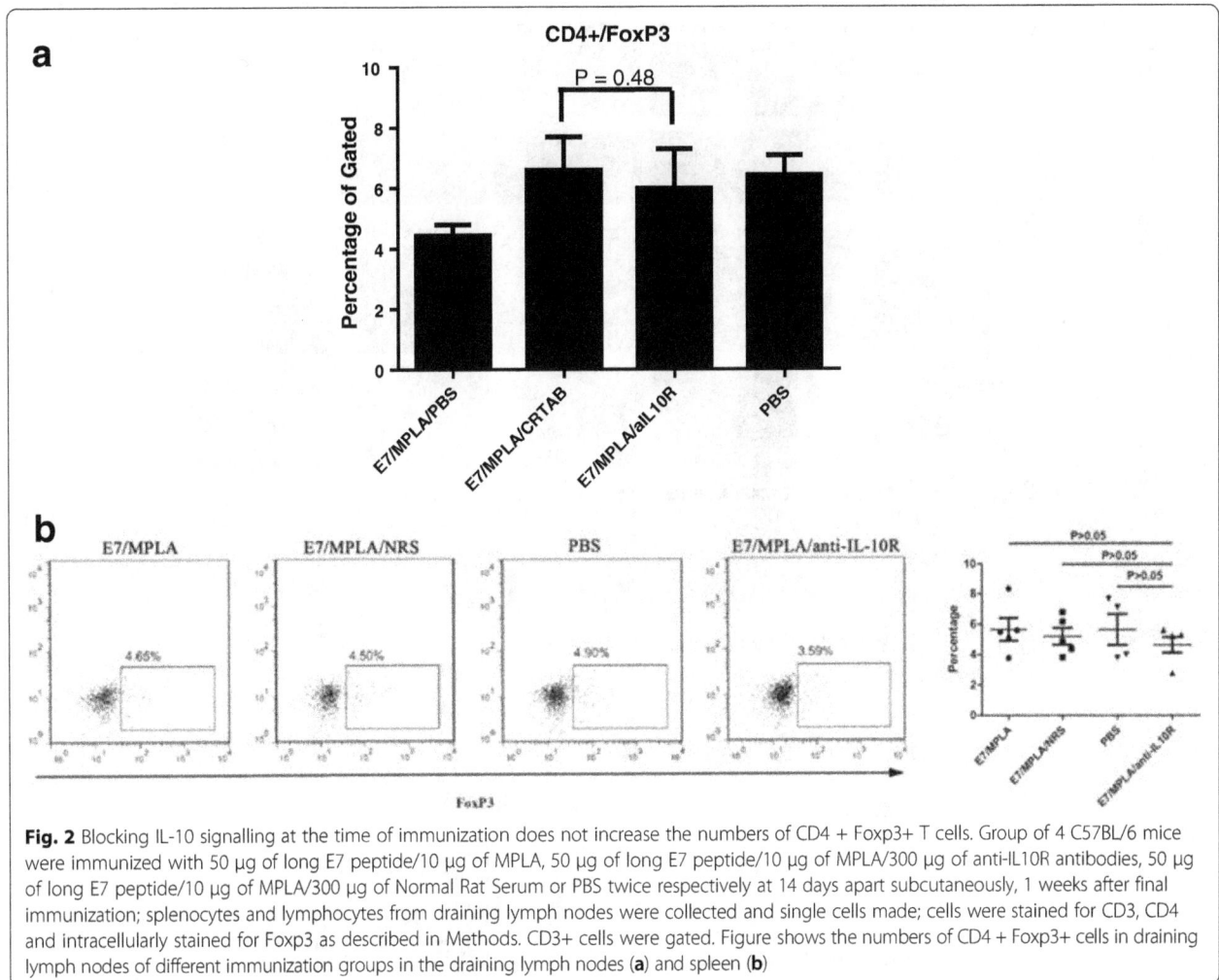

Fig. 2 Blocking IL-10 signalling at the time of immunization does not increase the numbers of CD4 + Foxp3+ T cells. Group of 4 C57BL/6 mice were immunized with 50 μg of long E7 peptide/10 μg of MPLA, 50 μg of long E7 peptide/10 μg of MPLA/300 μg of anti-IL10R antibodies, 50 μg of long E7 peptide/10 μg of MPLA/300 μg of Normal Rat Serum or PBS twice respectively at 14 days apart subcutaneously, 1 weeks after final immunization; splenocytes and lymphocytes from draining lymph nodes were collected and single cells made; cells were stained for CD3, CD4 and intracellularly stained for Foxp3 as described in Methods. CD3+ cells were gated. Figure shows the numbers of CD4 + Foxp3+ cells in draining lymph nodes of different immunization groups in the draining lymph nodes (**a**) and spleen (**b**)

Serum or PBS, while mice with DSS-induced ulcerative colitis had significant infiltration of blood cells in intestine (Fig. 3). Pathological score of intestinal inflammation was determined by a pathologist blinded to which immunization group the mouse was from, using a method published elsewhere [40]. The pathological score was also similar among different immunization groups (Fig. 3). Furthermore, intestinal samples were stained with anti-CD3 (Fig. 3), or with anti-Ly-6G (1A8) (Fig. 3) for T cells and neutrophils; both T cell and neutrophil infiltration were similar among different immunization groups (Fig. 3).

In another experiment intestines from different immunization and control groups, 1 week after final immunization, were cut into pieces and IELs isolated following the procedures described above. The IELs were stained for CD45+ cells, T cells and neutrophils and results were analysed by flow cytometry. The results showed that the numbers of total CD45+ cells, and the numbers of both T cells and neutrophils were similar between mice immunized with long E7 peptide/MPLA,

with or without blocking IL-10 with anti-IL-10R antibodies (Fig. 4).

Neutralizing IL10 at the time of immunization does not increase the incidence of diabetics in NOD mice

We showed that blocking IL-10 at the time of immunization increases vaccine induced CTL responses, whether the antigens is papillomavirus like particles [41]; soluble protein [42] or peptide [40]. As we are interested in applying this novel immunization strategy to clinic, papillomavirus like particles are licensed in 2006, next we investigated whether autoimmune prone NOD mice were more likely to develop diabetes when IL10 signalling was blocked at the time of immunization. NOD mice, which develop diabetes spontaneously, were immunized twice using papillomavirus like particles 14 days apart, with or without neutralizing IL-10 antibody. The incidence of diabetes was similar amongst the immunized, immunized/anti-IL10R antibody, and immunized/Normal Rat Serum (NRS) groups ($p > 0.05$, Log rank test). These results suggest that temporarily blocking IL-

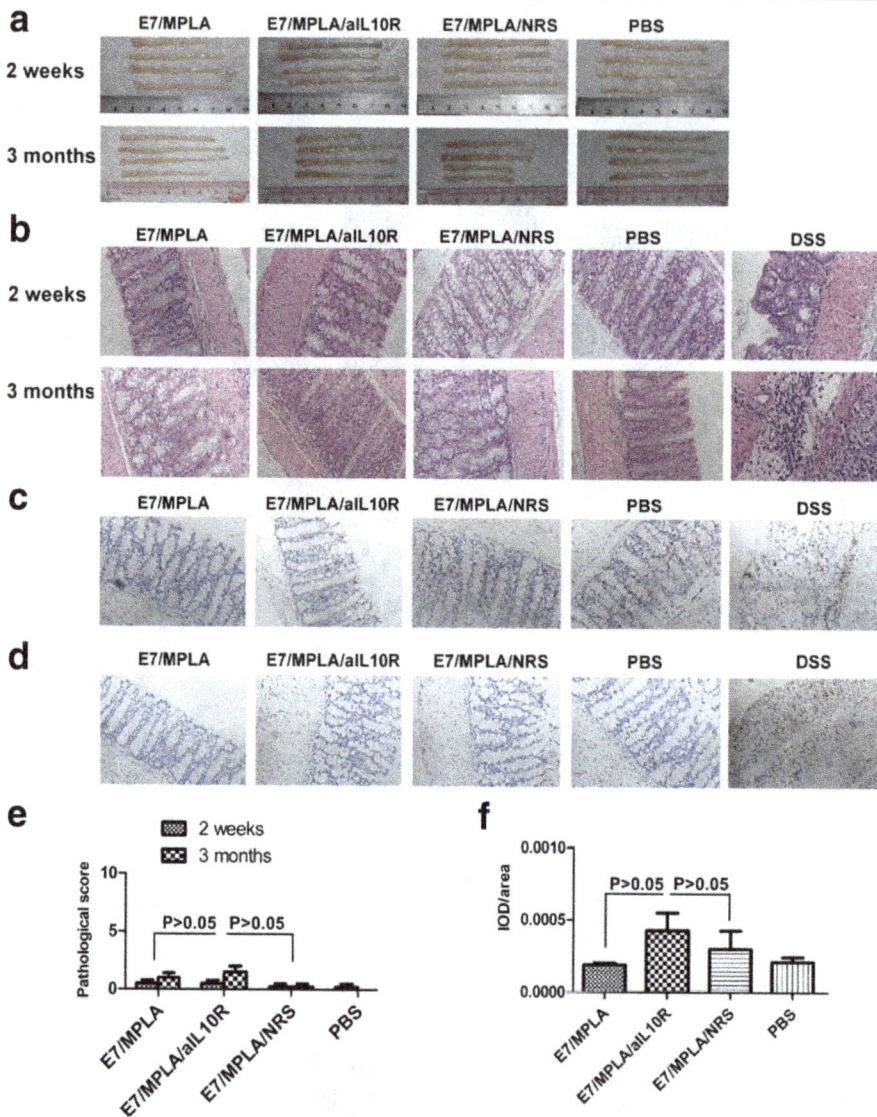

Fig. 3 Neutralizing IL-10 at the time of immunization does not cause inflammation in intestines. Group of 4 C57BL/6 mice were immunized with 50 μg of long E7 peptide/10 μg of MPLA, 50 μg of long E7 peptide/10 μg of MPLA/300 μg of anti-IL10R antibodies, 50 μg of long E7 peptide/10 μg of MPLA/300 μg of Normal Rat Serum or PBS twice at 14 days apart subcutaneously, 2 weeks or 3 months after final immunization. Mouse model of ulcerative colitis was induced by administering 5% DSS in the drinking water for 10 days. Samples of intestines were collected and examined for blood cells infiltration. **a**: Morphology of intestinal tract. **b**: Histology characterization of intestinal tract. Intestinal tract section were stained with hematoxylin/eosion (200 × magnification). **c, d**: Immunohistochemistry characterization of intestinal tract 2 weeks after final immunization. Intestinal tract section were incubated with anti- CD3 (**c**) or anti-Ly-6G mAb (**d**). **e**: Pathological score of intestinal tract. **f**: Expression of CD3 was calculated as integrated option density IOD /area (IOD/area) 2 weeks after final immunization. Results are from pooled two independent experiments (**e, f**)

10 at the time of immunization is safe, and does not increase the incidence of autoimmune disease in autoimmune prone mice (Fig. 5).

Discussion

In the current study, we demonstrated that temporal blocking of IL-10 signalling at the time of immunization does not result in the infiltration of T cells and neutrophils to the intestine. This immunization strategy also does not increases the development of autoimmune disease in NOD mice. We also showed by using two different antigens, OVA and HPV16E7 long peptide as the immunogen, that the numbers of IL-10 producing CD4+ T cells, including CD4 + GITR+ IL10+ cells and CD4 + IL10 + IFNγ + cells are significantly increased in mice immunized with OVA or E7 long peptide simultaneously with IL-10 signalling blockade, than those immunized without IL-10 signalling blockade.

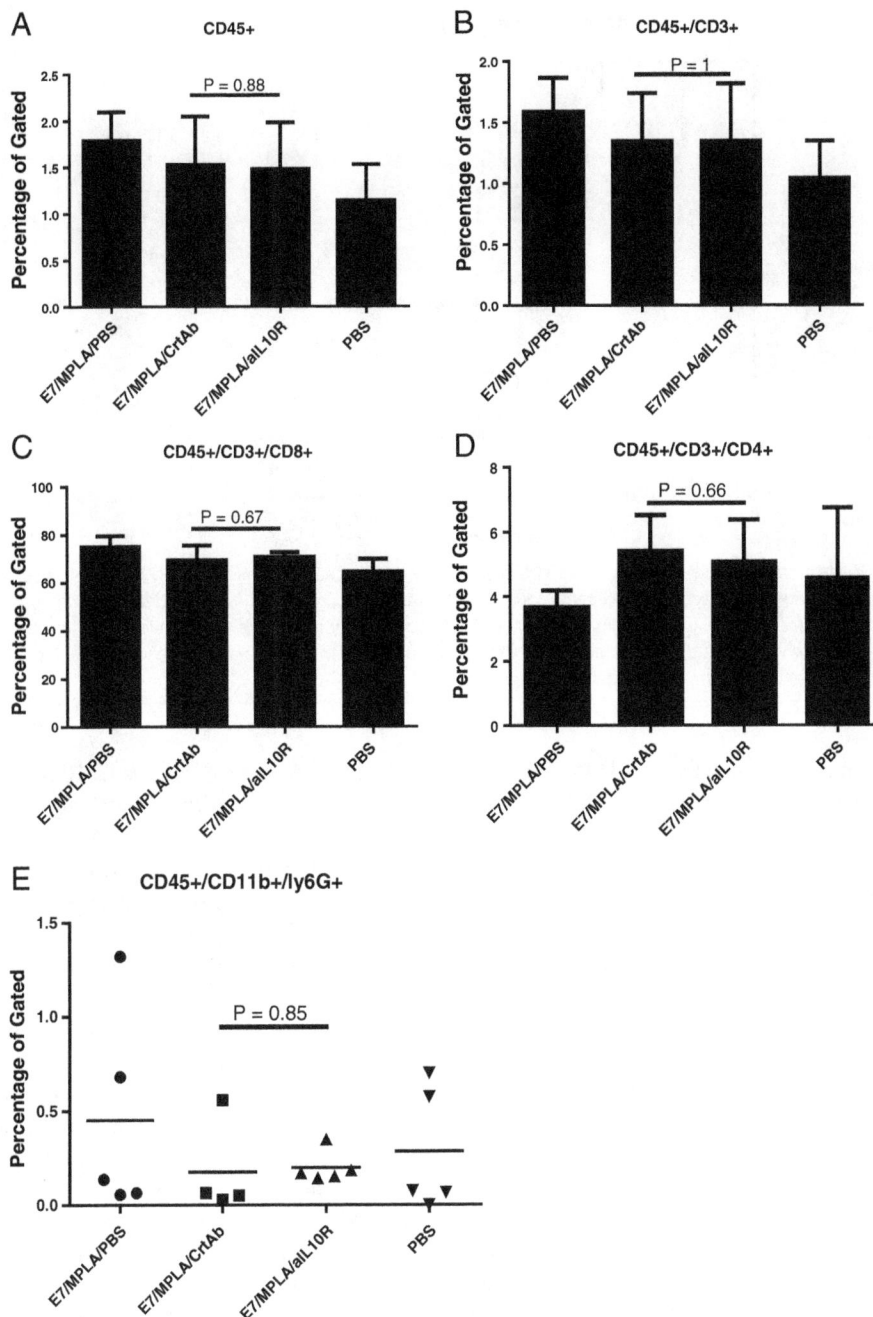

Fig. 4 Neutralizing IL-10 at the time of immunization does not attract T cells and neutrophils to the intestines of immunized mice. Group of 4 C57BL/6 mice were immunized with 50 μg of long E7 peptide/10 μg of MPLA, 50 μg of long E7 peptide/10 μg of MPLA/300 μg of anti-IL10R antibodies, 50 μg of long E7 peptide/10 μg of MPLA/300 μg of Normal Rat Serum or PBS twice at 14 days apart subcutaneously. 1 weeks after final immunization; samples of intestines were collected and examined for blood cells infiltration as described in Methods. CD45+ cells were gated. **a**: Total CD45+ cells, **b**: CD3+ T cells, **c**: CD8+ T cells, **d**: CD4+ T cells, **e**: CD45 + CD11b + Ly6G+ cells

IL-10 signalling blockade at the time of immunization increases vaccine induced cytotoxic T cell responses [9, 43]. The increased CD8+ T cell responses by IL-10 signalling blockade can be achieved by the administration of anti-IL10R antibodies subcutaneously and with different TLRs and Incomplete Freund Adjuvant (IFA)

[9]. In a mouse chronic LCMV infection model, blockade of IL10 increases the efficacy of a therapeutic DNA vaccine by increasing vaccine induced T cell responses and enhancing the clearance of persistent LCMV replication [44–46]. Intra-tumour injection of Toll like receptor 9 ligand CpG, plus anti-IL-10

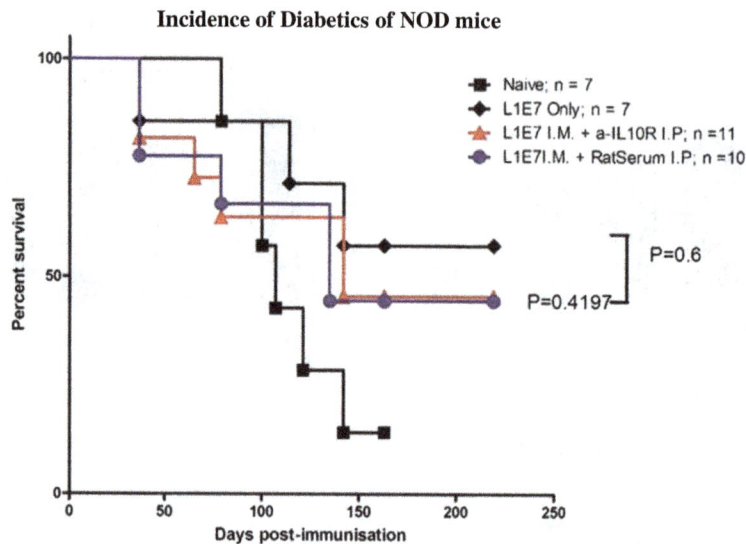

Fig. 5 Neutralizing IL-10 at the time of immunization does not increase the incidence of diabetics in NOD mice. 6–8 weeks old adult female autoimmune prone NOD/Lt mice were divided into different groups. No treatment group (*square*), VLP immunization (*Diamond*), VLP immunization plus Normal Rat Serum (*Down Triangle*), VLP immunization plus anti-IL10R antibody (*Cycle*). Mice were either untreated or immunized twice with 50 μg of papillomvirus like particles with or without 500 μg of anti-IL10R antibody *i.p.* on day 0 and 14. The development of diabetes was monitored weekly. Results are shown of pooled results from two independent experiments

receptor antibody intraperitoneally, leads to tumour rejection in mouse tumour models [47]. Recently, it was shown in a human papillomavirus 16 tumour antigen transformed TC-1 tumour model that immunization plus IL10 signalling blockade prevents TC-1 tumour growth [11], and moreover, this immunization strategy improved the prevention of tumour growth than immunization without IL-10 signalling blockade [29]. Blocking IL-10 at the time of immunization also promotes the generation of more IFNγ producing CD4+ T cells (Fig. S1). Therefore, therapeutic vaccines containing a IL-10 signalling inhibitor may be effective against chronic HPV infection and HPV infection related cancers in human.

IL-10 deficiency leads to autoimmune diseases in the gut [33]. IL-10 deficiency also increases hepatic immunopathology, leading to more severe disease and weight loss during acute murine cytomegalovirus infection [34]. Leishmania major infected IL-10−/− mice developed larger lesions but had fewer parasites due to the increased level of IL-17 [48]. Blocking IL-10 signalling at the time of immunization may therefore have the possibility of inducing autoimmune diseases in immunized patients. Interestingly, our results in NOD mice show that immunization with papillomavirus like particles, a TLR4 receptor stimulator, plus blocking IL-10 signalling does not increase the incidence of diabetes in NOD mice, suggesting this immunization strategy may be safe, as IL-10 signalling is blocked only for a short period. In support of the NOD mice results, we observed that blocking IL-10 signalling at the time of immunization in

C57/BL6 mice induced mores IL-10 secreting CD4+ T cells than immunization without blocking IL-10 signalling. Antigen experienced CD4 + GITR + IL10+, CD4 + IL10 + IFNγ + cells but not CD4 + Foxp3+ T cells (Figs. 1, 2 and Fig. 3) were increased in immunized and IL-10 signalling blocked mice. CD4 + IL-10 + IFNγ + cells are a group of cells which control the Th1 responses. These IL-10 secreting Th1 CD4+ T cells have been identified in parasite infection models [49], with both effector and regulatory functions [50]. Factors influencing IL-10 secretion by IFNγ producing CD4+ T cells include antigen concentration, IL-12 and IL-27 levels, and expression of Notch and inducible costimulatory molecule ligands (ICOS-L) on dendritic cells [50]. The increased numbers of CD4 + GITR + IL10+ T cells and CD4 + IFNγ + IL10+ T cells in immunized and IL-10 signalling blocked mice indicates that the increased IFNγ secreting CD8 + T cell and CD4+ T cell responses are balanced with the increased numbers of IL-10 secreting T cells after vaccination and simultaneously blocking IL-10 signalling. Increased IL-10 levels secreted by CD4+ T cells in vaccinated and IL-10 signalling blocked mice may be beneficial to patients, as increased IL-10 may protect the patients from over reaction to the vaccination. Stronger T cell responses without IL-10 may induce autoimmune diseases in vaccinated patients.

Conclusion

In summary, blocking IL-10 signalling at the time of immunization increases the numbers of IL-10 producing T cells; does not induce unwanted side effects, especially in the intestine of the immunized mice therefore this immunisation strategy may be effective against HPV chronic infection and HPV infection related cancers, with minimal chance of increasing the incidence of auto-immune diseases of immunized patients.

Abbreviations
CTL: Cytotoxic T lymphocyte; HPV: Human papillomavirus; IFA: Incomplete Freunds adjuvant; IL-10: Interleukin 10; LPS: Lipopolysaccharide; MPLA: Monophosphoryl Lipid A; NOD: Non-obese diabetic; OVA: Ovalbumin; TEM: Transmission Electron Microscope; VLPs: Virus like particles

Acknowledgements
The authors would like to thank Diamantina Institute of University of Queensland for performing the NOD mice experiment.

Funding
The current research was supported in part by Science and Technology Research program of Foshan city (No.: 2012AA100461); Foshan City Council Research Platform Fund (No.: 2015AG1003); Science and technology Department of Guangdong province (No.: 2012B03180003), National Natural Science Foundation of China (No: 81,472,451) and Science and Technology Research program of Guangdong province (No: 2016A020213001).

Authors' contributions
GN, ZL, SC1 (Su Chen), JY carried out the experiments in the Manuscript. XL performed the NOD mice experiment. JY, TW, KM, XP, MW, SC1 (Su Chen), SC2participated in the design of the study, analysed the data and critically read and commented on the Manuscript. GN, MW, XL conceived of the study. SC1, ZL, GN, MW, XL write the manuscript. All authors read and approved the final manuscript.

Competing interests
The authors declare that they have no competing interests.

Author details
[1]School of Medical Science, Griffith Health Institute, Griffith University, Gold Coast, QLD 4333, Australia. [2]Cancer Research Institute, The First People's Hospital of Foshan, Foshan, Guangdong 528000, China. [3]Inflammation and Healing Research Cluster, University of the Sunshine Coast, Maroochydore DC, QLD 4558, Australia. [4]Molecular diagnosis and Target Therapy Laboratory, The First Affiliated Hospital of Guangdong Pharmaceutical University, Guangzhou, Guangdong, China.

References
1. de Vos van Steenwijk PJ, Ramwadhdoebe TH, Lowik MJ, van der Minne CE, et al. Cancer Immunol Immunother. 2012;61:1485–92.
2. van Meir H, Kenter GG, Burggraaf J, Kroep JR, Welters MJ, Melief CJ, et al. The need for improvement of the treatment of advanced and metastatic cervical cancer, the rationale for combined chemo-immunotherapy. Anti-cancer agents in medicinal chemistry. 2014;14:190–203.
3. Frazer IH. Prevention of cervical cancer through papillomavirus vaccination. Nat Rev Immunol. 2004;4:46–54.
4. Leggatt GR, Frazer IH. HPV vaccines: the beginning of the end for cervical cancer. Curr Opin Immunol. 2007;19:232–8.
5. Frazer IH. Cervical cancer vaccine development. Sexual health. 2010;7:230–4.
6. Frazer IH. Measuring serum antibody to human papillomavirus following infection or vaccination. Gynecol Oncol. 2010;118:S8–11.
7. Frazer IH, Levin MJ. Paradigm shifting vaccines: prophylactic vaccines against latent varicella-zoster virus infection and against HPV-associated cancer. Curr Opin Virol. 2011;1:268–79.
8. Frazer IH, Leggatt GR, Mattarollo SR. Prevention and treatment of papillomavirus-related cancers through immunization. Annu Rev Immunol. 2011;29:111–38.
9. Chen J, Ni G, Liu XS. Papillomavirus virus like particle-based therapeutic vaccine against human papillomavirus infection related diseases: immunological problems and future directions. Cell Immunol. 2011;269:5–9.
10. Ni G, Wang T, Walton S, Zhu B, Chen S, Wu X, et al. Manipulating IL-10 signalling blockade for better immunotherapy. Cell Immunol. 2015;293:126–9.
11. Chen S, Wang X, Wu X, Wei MQ, Zhang B, Liu X, et al. IL-10 signalling blockade at the time of immunization inhibits Human papillomavirus 16 E7 transformed TC-1 tumour cells growth in mice. Cell Immunol. 2014;290:145–51.
12. van Duikeren S, Fransen MF, Redeker A, Wieles B, Platenburg G, Krebber WJ, et al. Vaccine-induced effector-memory CD8+ T cell responses predict therapeutic efficacy against tumors. J Immunol. 2012;189:3397–403.
13. Melief CJ. Synthetic vaccine for the treatment of lesions caused by high risk human papilloma virus. Cancer J. 2011;17:300–1.
14. Trimble CL, Frazer IH. Development of therapeutic HPV vaccines. Lancet Oncol. 2009;10:975–80.
15. Ding Z, Wei Y. Therapeutic vaccine for melanoma: the untouched grail? Expert review of vaccines. 2007;6:907–11.
16. Eggermont AM. Immunostimulation versus immunosuppression after multiple vaccinations: the woes of therapeutic vaccine development. Clin Cancer Res. 2009;15:6745–7.
17. Gissmann L, Nieto K. The therapeutic vaccine: is it feasible? Arch Med Res. 2009;40:493–8.
18. Gulley JL, Madan RA, Tsang KY, Jochems C, Marte JL, Farsaci B, et al. Immune impact induced by PROSTVAC (PSA-TRICOM), a therapeutic vaccine for prostate cancer. Cancer Immunol Res. 2014;2:133–41.
19. Levy Y, Thiebaut R, Montes M, Lacabaratz C, Sloan L, King B, et al. Dendritic cell-based therapeutic vaccine elicits polyfunctional HIV-specific T-cell immunity associated with control of viral load. Eur J Immunol. 2014;
20. O'Garra A, Vieira PL, Vieira P, Goldfeld AE. IL-10-producing and naturally occurring CD4+ Tregs: limiting collateral damage. J Clin Invest. 2004;114:1372–8.
21. O'Garra A, Vieira P. T(H)1 cells control themselves by producing interleukin-10. Nat Rev Immunol. 2007;7:425–8.
22. O'Garra A, Murphy KM. From IL-10 to IL-12: how pathogens and their products stimulate APCs to induce T(H)1 development. Nat Immunol. 2009;10:929–32.
23. Gabrysova L, Howes A, Saraiva M, O'Garra A. The regulation of IL-10 expression. Curr Top Microbiol Immunol. 2014;380:157–90.
24. Redford PS, Murray PJ, O'Garra A. The role of IL-10 in immune regulation during M. tuberculosis infection. Mucosal Immunol. 2011;4:261–70.
25. Saraiva M, O'Garra A. The regulation of IL-10 production by immune cells. Nat Rev Immunol. 2010;10:170–81.
26. O'Garra A, Barrat FJ, Castro AG, Vicari A, Hawrylowicz C. Strategies for use of IL-10 or its antagonists in human disease. Immunol Rev. 2008;223:114–31.
27. Terai M, Tamura Y, Alexeev V, Ohtsuka E, Berd D, Mastrangelo MJ, et al. Human interleukin 10 receptor 1/IgG1-Fc fusion proteins: immunoadhesins for human IL-10 with therapeutic potential. Cancer Immunol Immunother. 2009;58:1307–17.
28. Mocellin S, Marincola FM, Young HA. Interleukin-10 and the immune response against cancer: a counterpoint. J Leukoc Biol. 2005;78:1043–51.
29. Llopiz D, Aranda F, Diaz-Valdes N, Ruiz M, Infante S, Belsue V, et al. Vaccine-induced but not tumor-derived Interleukin-10 dictates the efficacy of Interleukin-10 blockade in therapeutic vaccination. Oncoimmunology. 2016;5:e1075113.

30. Peng S, Frazer IH, Fernando GJ, Zhou J. Papillomavirus virus-like particles can deliver defined CTL epitopes to the MHC class I pathway. Virology. 1998;240:147–57.

31. Chen S, Ni G, Wu X, Zhu B, Liao Z, Wang Y, et al. Blocking IL-10 signalling at the time of immunization renders the tumour more accessible to T cell infiltration in mice. Cell Immunol. 2016;300:9–17.

32. Ni G, Chen S, Yang Y, Cummins SF, Zhan J, Li Z, et al. Investigation the Possibility of Using Peptides with a Helical Repeating Pattern of Hydro-Phobic and Hydrophilic Residues to Inhibit IL-10. PloS one. 2016;11:e0153939.

33. Rennick DM, Fort MM. Lessons from genetically engineered animal models. XII. IL-10-deficient IL-10-/- mice and intestinal inflammation. Am J Physiol Gastrointest Liver Physiol. 2000;278:G829–33.

34. Gaddi PJ, Crane MJ, Kamanaka M, Flavell RA, Yap GS, Salazar-Mather TP. IL-10 mediated regulation of liver inflammation during acute murine cytomegalovirus infection. PloS one. 2012;7:e42850.

35. Roncarolo MG, Gregori S, Battaglia M, Bacchetta R, Fleischhauer K, Levings MK. Interleukin-10-secreting type 1 regulatory T cells in rodents and humans. Immunol Rev. 2006;212:28–50.

36. Liu XS, Abdul-Jabbar I, Qi YM, Frazer IH, Zhou J. Mucosal immunisation with papillomavirus virus-like particles elicits systemic and mucosal immunity in mice. Virology. 1998;252:39–45.

37. Liu XS, Xu Y, Hardy L, Khammanivong V, Zhao W, Fernando GJ, et al. IL-10 mediates suppression of the CD8 T cell IFN-gamma response to a novel viral epitope in a primed host. J Immunol. 2003;171:4765–72.

38. Jankovic D, Kullberg MC, Feng CG, Goldszmid RS, Collazo CM, Wilson M, et al. Conventional T-bet(+)Foxp3(-) Th1 cells are the major source of host-protective regulatory IL-10 during intracellular protozoan infection. J Exp Med. 2007;204:273–83.

39. Wang Y, Blozis SA, Lederman M, Krieg A, Landay A, Miller CJ. Enhanced antibody responses elicited by a CpG adjuvant do not improve the protective effect of an aldrithiol-2-inactivated simian immunodeficiency virus therapeutic AIDS vaccine. Clin Vaccine Immunol. 2009;16:499–505.

40. Chen X, Li L, Lai Y, Liu Q, Yan J, Tang Y. Characteristics of human papillomaviruses infection in men with genital warts in Shanghai. Oncotarget. 2016;7:53903–10.

41. Liu XS, Dyer J, Leggatt GR, Fernando GJ, Zhong J, Thomas R, et al. Overcoming original antigenic sin to generate new CD8 T cell IFN-gamma responses in an antigen-experienced host. J Immunol. 2006;177:2873–9.

42. Liu XS, Leerberg J, MacDonald K, Leggatt GR, Frazer IH. IFN-gamma promotes generation of IL-10 secreting CD4+ T cells that suppress generation of CD8 responses in an antigen-experienced host. J Immunol. 2009;183:51–8.

43. Chen J, Liu XS. Development and function of IL-10 IFN-gamma-secreting CD4(+) T cells. J Leukoc Biol. 2009;86:1305–10.

44. Brooks DG, Lee AM, Elsaesser H, McGavern DB, Oldstone MB. IL-10 blockade facilitates DNA vaccine-induced T cell responses and enhances clearance of persistent virus infection. J Exp Med. 2008;205(3):533–541.

45. Blackburn SD, Wherry EJ. IL-10, T cell exhaustion and viral persistence. Trends Microbiol. 2007;15:143–6.

46. Wilson EB, Yamada DH, Elsaesser H, Herskovitz J, Deng J, Cheng G, et al. Blockade of chronic type I interferon signaling to control persistent LCMV infection. Science. 2013;340:202–7.

47. Vicari AP, Chiodoni C, Vaure C, Ait-Yahia S, Dercamp C, Matsos F, et al. Reversal of tumor-induced dendritic cell paralysis by CpG immunostimulatory oligonucleotide and anti-interleukin 10 receptor antibody. J Exp Med. 2002;196:541–9.

48. Gonzalez-Lombana C, Gimblet C, Bacellar O, Oliveira WW, Passos S, Carvalho LP, et al. IL-17 mediates immunopathology in the absence of IL-10 following Leishmania major infection. PLoS pathogens. 2013;9:e1003243.

49. Anderson CF, Oukka M, Kuchroo VJ, Sacks D. CD4(+)CD25(-)Foxp3(-) Th1 cells are the source of IL-10-mediated immune suppression in chronic cutaneous leishmaniasis. J Exp Med. 2007;204:285–97.

50. Jankovic D, Kugler DG, Sher A. IL-10 production by CD4+ effector T cells: a mechanism for self-regulation. Mucosal Immunol. 2010;3:239–46.

17

Lung–infiltrating T helper 17 cells as the major source of interleukin-17A production during pulmonary *Cryptococcus neoformans* infection

Elaheh Movahed[1], Yi Ying Cheok[1], Grace Min Yi Tan[1], Chalystha Yie Qin Lee[1], Heng Choon Cheong[1], Rukumani Devi Velayuthan[1], Sun Tee Tay[1], Pei Pei Chong[2], Won Fen Wong[1]* and Chung Yeng Looi[2]

Abstract

Background: IL-17A has emerged as a key player in the pathologies of inflammation, autoimmune disease, and immunity to microbes since its discovery two decades ago. In this study, we aim to elucidate the activity of IL-17A in the protection against *Cryptococcus neoformans*, an opportunistic fungus that causes fatal meningoencephalitis among AIDS patients. For this purpose, we examined if *C. neoformans* infection triggers IL-17A secretion in vivo using wildtype C57BL/6 mice. In addition, an enhanced green fluorescence protein (EGFP) reporter and a knockout (KO) mouse models were used to track the source of IL-17A secretion and explore the protective function of IL-17A, respectively.

Results: Our findings showed that in vivo model of *C. neoformans* infection demonstrated induction of abundant IL-17A secretion. By examining the lung bronchoalveolar lavage fluid (BALF), mediastinal lymph node (mLN) and spleen of the IL-17A–EGFP reporter mice, we showed that intranasal inoculation with *C. neoformans* promoted leukocytes lung infiltration. A large proportion (~ 50%) of the infiltrated CD4+ helper T cell population secreted EGFP, indicating vigorous T$_H$17 activity in the *C. neoformans*–infected lung. The infection study in IL-17A–KO mice, on the other hand, revealed that absence of IL-17A marginally boosted fungal burden in the lung and accelerated the mouse death.

Conclusion: Therefore, our data suggest that IL-17A is released predominantly from T$_H$17 cells in vivo, which plays a supporting role in the protective immunity against *C. neoformans* infection.

Keywords: CD4+ T cells, T$_H$17 cells, Macrophages, IL-17A, *Cryptococcus neoformans*

Background

The opportunistic pathogenic basidiomycete *Cryptococcus neoformans* is an encapsulated yeast commonly found in bird excrement worldwide [1]. The infection is often asymptomatic in healthy individuals but causes severe pulmonary cryptococcosis and life-threatening meningo-encephalitis in immunocompromised patients. *C. neoformans* has gained attention in recent years as it is a major cause of death among patients who have advanced acquired immunodeficiency syndrome (AIDS) [2]. Hence, it is important to study the host interaction with this pathogen

as 30–60% of the patients who have cryptococcal meningitis succumb to cryptococcosis infection within 1 year despite antifungal therapy [3].

The essential role of T cells in the host immune response to *C. neoformans* has been well-studied using T cell depletion mouse model [4–6]. In recent years, T$_H$17, has been implicated in the immune response to fungus such as *Candida albicans* [7, 8]. A different study for *Aspergillus fumigatus* claimed that IL-17A promotes the fungal infection [9]; as such, the nature and role of T$_H$17 cell subset require further investigations. T$_H$17 cell is characterized by its hallmark RORγt transcription factor and IL-17A secretion. Its differentiation from naïve CD4+ T cells is induced in the presence of IL-6 and TGF-β during inflammatory response. IL-23 is another important inducer for IL-17A as

* Correspondence: wonfen@um.edu.my
[1]Department of Medical Microbiology, Faculty of Medicine, University of Malaya, Kuala Lumpur, Malaysia
Full list of author information is available at the end of the article

the IL-17A production was strongly impaired in the IL-23p19 deficient mice [10]. *C. gattii*, a highly virulent cryptococcal species is able to attenuate both T_H1 and T_H17 by suppressing *IL-12* and *IL-23* genes transcription [11].

T_H17 is not the sole source of IL-17A as it can also be released by other cells such as macrophages, NK cells, and neutrophils [12]. In the mice with helper T cell impairment, *C. neoformans* infection caused a compensatory neutrophil response that required IL-17A [13], whereas in neutrophil-depleted mice, *C. neoformans* infection results in increase IL-17A and IL-17A$^+$ $\gamma\delta^+$ T cells [13]. IL-17A elicits inflammatory response by recruiting neutrophils, but does not contribute to classical macrophage activation as seen in pulmonary cryptococcosis induction in the mouse model [14]. IL-17A enhances host defense against lung infection with moderately virulent *C. neoformans* through leukocyte recruitment and activation besides inducing release of IFN-γ [15]. T_H17 cells release a panel of other cytokines in addition to IL-17A such as IL-17F, IL-22, and IL-23. *C. neoformans* produces prostaglandin E2 (PGE2) which inhibits Interferon regulatory factor 4 (IRF4) and IL-17A but not IL-22 [15]. A full picture of regulatory mechanism as to how this subset of T cell interacts and eliminates the fungal infection requires further investigation.

In this study, we examined the association of IL-17A with *C. neoformans* infection by using in vivo infection model. The main focus of our study lies on identifying the source of IL-17A secretion and determining its protective role in *C. neoformans*–infected mice. Using enhanced green fluorescence protein (EGFP) reporter mouse model, we showed that lung infiltrating T_H17 cells are likely the predominant source of IL-17A. Data from a knockout (KO) mouse model supports a protective function of the IL-17A against *C. neoformans* infection.

Results

C. neoformans infection induces IL-17A production in in vivo model

To investigate if *C. neoformans* infection–mediated IL-17A secretion occurs in vivo, C57BL/6 mice were intranasally inoculated with four different strains of *C. neoformans* (H99, S48B, S68B and H4) at 2×10^5 cells for 14 days. These *C. neoformans* strains exhibit distinct virulence properties as shown by different fungal burdens in a pulmonary infection mouse model. Such differences are attributed to variations in their transcriptome profile, ability in polysaccharide capsule formation as well as laccase activity [16]. Serum was collected for Bio-plex Pro Mouse Th17 assay which included the following cytokines: IL-17A, IL-17F, IL-21, IL-22, IL-23, IL-31, IL-33 and MIP-3α (Fig. 1). An elevated serum level of IL-17A was detected in the *C. neoformans*–infected mice (Fig. 1a). We

noted that the serum IL-17A level was correlated with the degree of virulence of different *C. neoformans* strains [16], whereby the highest amount of serum IL-17A was observed in the group of mice infected with the most virulent *C. neoformans* H99 strain (115 ± 12 pg/ml). This was followed by moderate serum IL-17A level observed in the mice infected with less virulent environmental strains, S48S (89 ± 3 pg/ml) and S68B (75 ± 2 pg/ml), and lowest level of serum IL-17A was noted in the mice infected with non-virulent strain H4 (24 ± 1 pg/ml) strains, compared to control uninfected mice (< 20 pg/ml). The level of serum IL-23 was also elevated in all *C. neoformans*–infected mice, i.e. H99 (67 ± 5 pg/ml), S48S (78 ± 3 pg/ml), S68B (36 ± 1 pg/ml) and H4 (47 ± 5 pg/ml) compared to < 20 pg/ml in the mock control (Fig. 1b). This suggests IL-23–IL-17A axis pathway plays a major role in the host immunity against *C. neoformans* infection. On the other hand, the serum IL-17F levels were only scarcely increased in mice infected with *C. neoformans* H99 and S48B strains (Fig. 1c). Whereas no noteworthy induction was observed for other cytokines (IL-21, IL-22, IL-31 and IL-33, and MIP-3α) examined (Fig. 1d, e, f, g, h).

Intranasal *C. neoformans* inoculation causes leukocytes lung infiltration

To examine the importance of IL-17A in providing immunity to *C. neoformans* infection, we utilized a mouse model harboring IRES-EGFP-SV40-polyA signal sequence cassette after the stop codon of *Il-17A* gene in which the EGFP is co-expressed in the IL-17A–producing cells. Mice were intranasally administrated with 20 μl of control PBS or *C. neoformans* (2×10^5 cells) in suspension, and splenic, mediastinal lymph nodes (mLN), bronchoalveolar lavage fluid (BALF) cells were inspected after 4 weeks (Fig. 2). Total numbers of cells were significantly increased in the BALF ($4.8 \times 10^6 \pm 1.0 \times 10^6$ versus $4.6 \times 10^4 \pm 1.0 \times 10^4$ cells) and mLN ($3.0 \times 10^5 \pm 2.0 \times 10^4$ versus $1.5 \times 10^5 \pm 1.9 \times 10^4$ cells) of the *C. neoformans* H99–infected mice versus the control group (Fig. 2a, b). No significant increased numbers of cells were observed in the spleen after intranasal *C. neoformans* H99 infection ($5.6 \times 10^7 \pm 7.1 \times 10^6$ versus $4.7 \times 10^7 \pm 6.1 \times 10^6$) (Fig. 2c).

To examine the types of leukocytes in these tissues, we stained the cells using different markers and analyzed by flow cytometer to identify the following cell types, namely helper T (TCRβ$^+$ CD4$^+$), and cytotoxic T (TCRβ$^+$ CD8$^+$), macrophages (F4/80$^+$ CD11b$^+$ Gr-1$^+$), neutrophils (F4/80$^-$ CD11b$^+$ Gr-1^{high}), and inflammatory monocytes (F4/80$^-$ CD11b$^+$ Gr-1^{medium}) (Additional file 1). In the BALF from the *C. neoformans*–infected mice, active immune response was noted in all types of leukocytes examined, except CD8$^+$ T cells demonstrated an average of 2-fold increment (Fig. 3a). No significant differences of the cell constituents were observed in lymph node (Fig. 3b). In spleen, the

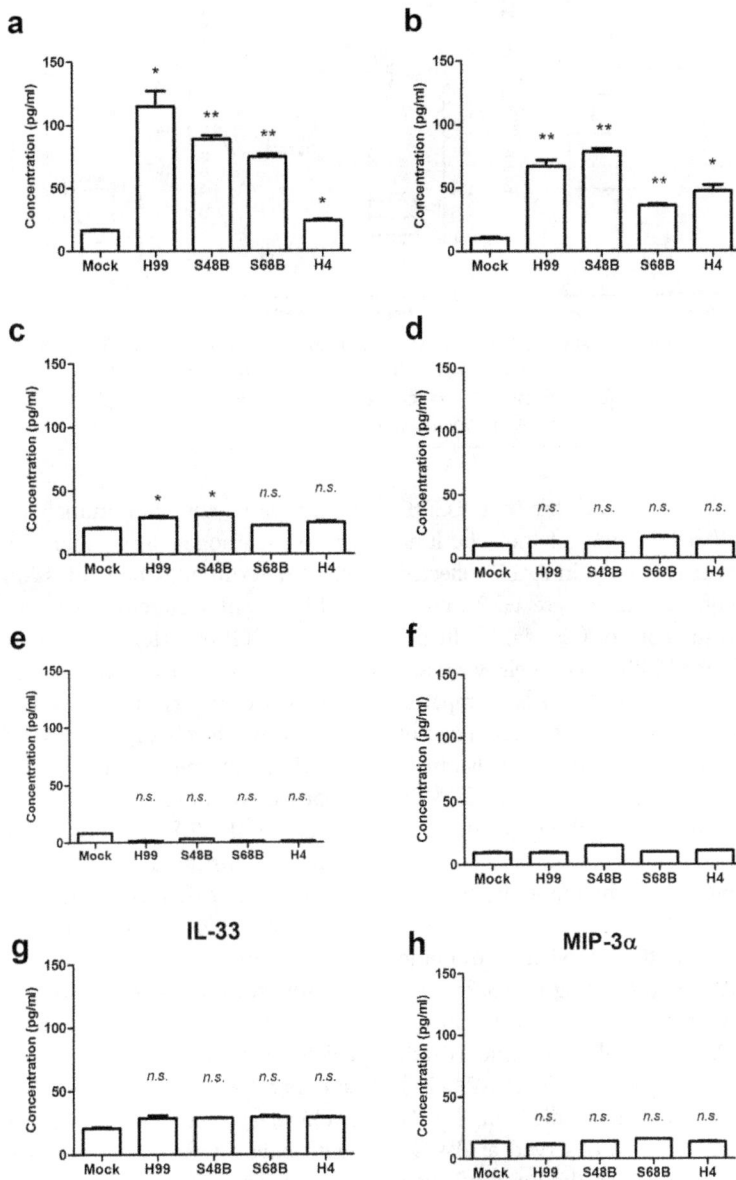

Fig. 1 Elevated serum IL-17A, IL-23 and IL-17F levels in the *C. neoformans*–infected mice. C57BL/6 mice (*n* = 2 per group) were intranasally inoculated with 1×10^5 cells of four different strains of *C. neoformans* (H99, S48B, S68B and H4), serum were collected after 14 days for Bio-plex cytokine array. Mock denotes control mice intranasally administrated with equal volume of PBS. Different cytokines in the T_H17 panel, (**a**) IL-17A, (**b**) IL-17F, (**c**) IL-21, (**d**) IL-22, (**e**) IL-23, (**f**) IL-31, (**g**) IL-33 and (**h**) MIP-3α were measured. Data are representative of two independent experiments. **P* < 0.05, ***P* < 0.01, *n.s.*: not significant or *P* ≥ 0.05, by Student's *t*-test

percentages of innate immune cells i.e. macrophages and neutrophils were increased at approximately 3– to 6–fold (Fig. 3c). On the contrary, percentages of T (both CD4+ and CD8+) cells were slightly reduced at 1.2– to 1.3–fold.

Increased IL-17A–producing T cells in the lung of *C. neoformans H99*-infected mice

In the IL-17A–EGFP reporter mice, IL-17A–producing cells can easily be identified as they display EGFP fluorescence, hence this mouse model was utilized to determine

the main source of IL-17A during *C. neoformans* infection. Our result showed that there was no profound increase of GFP+ cells amongst macrophage or inflammatory monocytes populations in the *C. neoformans*–infected mice (Additional file 2). The percentages of the IL-17A–producing neutrophils were scarcely increased in BALF (from 0.06 ± 0.03% to 1.08 ± 0.97%) and mLN (from 0.06 ± 0.03% to 0.62 ± 0.37), but not in the spleen.

On the contrary, significant increases of GFP+ cells were detected among the T cells (Fig. 4). Major source of

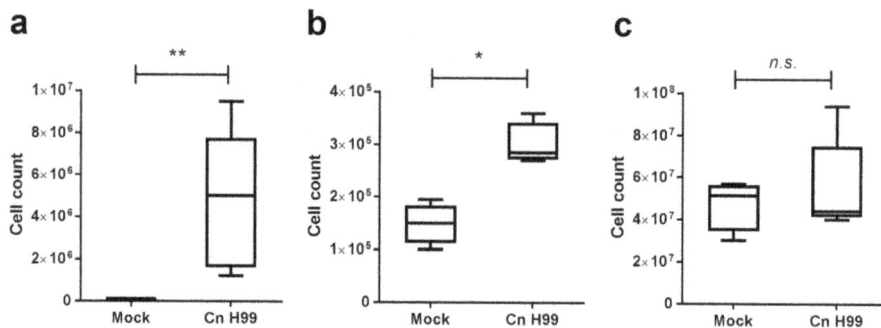

Fig. 2 Increased number of leukocytes in BALF and mLN of the *C. neoformans*–infected mice. IL-17A–EGFP reporter mice ($n = 4$ per group) were uninfected (mock) or intranasally inoculated with 1×10^5 cells with *C. neoformans* H99 strain (Cn H99), BALF, mLN and spleen were collected after 14 days for analysis. Total number of cells in (**a**) BALF, (**b**) mLN and (**c**) spleen were determined by manual cell count using a haemocytometer. *$P < 0.05$, **$P < 0.01$, *n.s.*: not significant or $P \geq 0.05$, by Mann-Whitney U test

IL-17A was derived from TCRβ⁺ CD4⁺ but not TCRβ⁺ CD8⁺ T cells. Almost half ($54.2 \pm 11.6\%$) of the total lung infiltrated TCRβ⁺ CD4⁺ T cells recovered in BALF collected from *C. neoformans* H99-infected mice were GFP⁺, compared to only $4.8 \pm 0.8\%$ in the control (Fig. 4a, b). In the mLN, the percentages of GFP⁺ TCRβ⁺ CD4⁺ cells were approximately 4–fold greater at $21.7 \pm 1.4\%$ cells, compared to $5.1 \pm 0.6\%$ in control mice (Fig. 4a, c). The percentages of GFP⁺ cells among TCRβ⁺ CD4⁺ population were also marginally increased ($17.53 \pm 4.1\%$) among the splenic CD4⁺ T cells compared to $6.1 \pm 0.6\%$ in the control (Fig. 4a, d).

IL-17A provides a supportive role in the immunity to pulmonary *C. neoformans* infection

A knock out mouse model was then applied to examine the protective role of IL-17A to host during *C. neoformans* infection. Intranasal inoculation of *C. neformans* in wildtype C57/BL6 mice and IL-17A–KO resulted in mice death starting from day 26 and 24, respectively. In IL-17A–KO mice, more than 80% (5 out of 6) mice died on day 34 whereas in wildtype control, this was observed at day 40 (Fig. 5a). The amounts of fungal cells in the local infection site (lung) as well as systemic infection (brain) were assessed. CFU counts in the lung derived from IL-17A–KO mice stayed at 657 ± 92, a higher level compared to 473 ± 119 in the wildtype control, whereas CFU count in the brain was 237 ± 39 compared to 133 ± 30 in the control mice (Fig. 5b). Hence, the absence of IL-17A may contribute to accelerated mice death as a result of an increased CFU count. Given that the differences in count were not substantial, further investigation is required to elucidate the factors contributing to the accelerated mouse mortality such as involvements of other types of immune cells and secretions of other cytokines or oxidative stress molecules.

Discussions

Increasing prevalence of mortality attributed to cryptococcal meningitis in the immunocompromised patients underscores the importance of elucidating the host defense–pathogen interaction. In this study, we focused on (i) determining the expression and source of elevated IL-17A from different types of immune cells using a IL-17A–GFP reporter animal model and, (ii) investigating the role of IL-17A in protective immunity using a IL-17A–KO mouse model. Our data demonstrated elevated serum levels of T_H17 cytokines, i.e. IL-17A, IL-17F and IL-23 in the infected wildtype C57BL/6 mice; and proposed the lung–infiltrating T_H17 subset as the major source for IL-17A secretion at the lung upon pulmonary *C. neoformans* infection. In addition, we also showed that the absence of IL-17A resulted in a greater fungal burden and accelerated death of the infected mice, which may suggest a protective role of the potent IL-17A response at an early stage of *C. neoformans* infection.

Previous study suggests neutrophil as the predominant leukocyte in supplying IL-17A [17], however we showed here that the T_H17 cells is the major player in secreting the cytokine, although the percentages of IL-17A–producing neutrophils were also increased. We consider EGFP reporter system as a more superior strategy to detect the intracellular cytokine production compared to fixation and staining method used in previous study. In fact, both neutrophils and T cells could have redundant or compensatory role as the depletion of neutrophils using anti-1A8 treatment in animal model causes an increased intracellular amount of IL-17A among the γδ⁺ T cell population [13].

Most studies thus far pinpoint the association of T_H1-type cytokine responses with protective immunity against pulmonary cryptococcosis [18–20]. The cytokines in response were mainly those of T_H1 subsets (IFN-γ, TNFα, IL-8), whereas moderate increases were also observed in T_H2 (IL-4) and T_H17 cytokines (IL-17A) [21]. A predominant T_H1 and/or T_H17 cytokine profile limits the growth of *C. neoformans* and *C. gattii*, whereas a T_H2 cytokine profile promotes intracellular fungus proliferation [22]. In humans, it has also been reported that

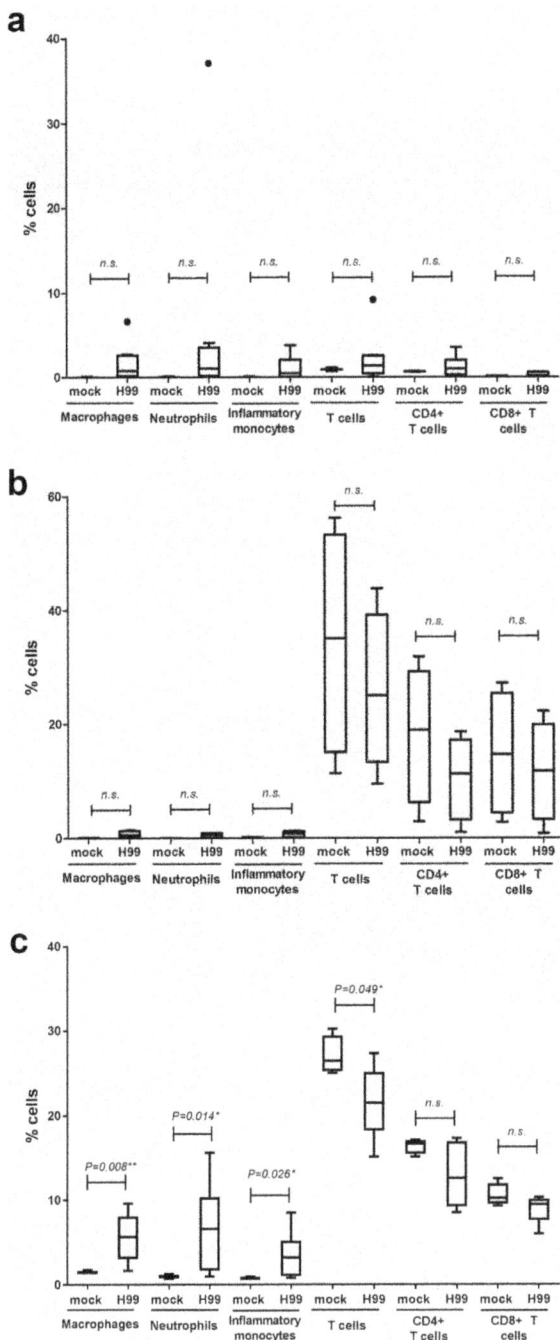

Fig. 3 Percentages of leukocytes in spleen of the *C. neoformans*–infected mice. Box and whiskers plot show the percentages of different leukocytes in the (**a**) BALF, (**b**) mLN, and (**c**) spleen. IL-17A–EGFP reporter mice (*n* = 4 per group) were uninfected (mock) or intranasally inoculated with 1×10^5 cells with *C. neoformans* H99 strain (Cn H99). Number of GFP$^+$ cells among the macrophages (F4/80$^+$ CD11b$^+$ Gr1$^+$)–, neutrophils (F4/80$^-$ CD11b$^+$ Gr-1^{high})–, and inflammatory monocytes (F4/80$^-$ CD11b$^+$ Gr1^{medium})–, T cells (TCRβ$^+$)–, helper T cells (TCRβ$^+$ CD4$^+$), cytotoxic T cells (TCRβ$^+$ CD8$^+$)–gated cell populations. *P < 0.05, **P < 0.01, *n.s.*: not significant or *P* ≥ 0.05, by Mann-Whitney U test

cryptococcal-specific CD4$^+$ T-cell response is predominantly a T$_H$1 type response with minimal involvement of T$_H$2 and T$_H$17 cells [21]. However, patients with higher IFN-γ or TNF-α production showed greater level of IL-17A level in their cerebrospinal fluid (CSF) [21]. These patients demonstrated lower fungal burdens and faster clearance of *C. neoformans* infection, suggesting that both T$_H$1 and T$_H$17 responses cooperatively provide optimal immunity against pulmonary cryptococcosis.

Previous study using IL-17A receptor (IL-17AR) deficient mice reported a slower rate of recovery from pulmonary fungal burden but the overall survival was not deteriorated [17]. By contrast, in this study, our data demonstrated accelerated death of the *C. neoformans*–infected mice. It is important to note that in IL-17AR deficient mouse model, the animal still possesses the ability to produce IL-17A, but signaling through its receptor, IL-17RA, is abrogated. Besides, it has also been shown that absence of IL-17A did not alter survival after 8 weeks of infection [15]. This could be due to differences of cryptococcal stains selected, whereby a highly virulent strain was used in our in vivo infection model compared to a moderate strain, 52D that was used in the previous study. Although previous study highlighted the robust activities of T$_H$1 and T$_H$17 assist in fungal clearance but lacks the efficacy in preventing dissemination of *C. neoformans* in animal infection [23], we report here that a higher fungal dissemination to the brain was observed in the surviving IL-17A–depleted mice. These data highlight that IL-17A participates in providing protective anti-cryptococcal host defenses through the suppression of fungal growth and dispersal.

This observation is also in line with studies on several other fungal species including *C. albicans* and *A. fumigatus* [7, 24, 25]. It was shown that a deficiency in IL-17A response results in increased susceptibility to oropharyngeal and disseminated candidiasis [7, 24]. Decreased neutrophil infiltration, increased fungal burden, and exacerbated pathology were reported upon IL-17A neutralization in *C. albicans* and *A. fumigatus* infections [7, 24, 25]. Toll IL-1R8 (TIR8), another negative regulator of T$_H$17 response, has also been shown to reduce the susceptibility and immunopathology to candidiasis [26]. Some studies, on the contrary, provide evidence that outcome of aspergillosis in human is independent of T$_H$17 responses [9], and the IL-23/IL-17A–driven inflammation could impede antifungal immune resistance and promote infection of *A. fumigatus* [27]. Hence, further investigation is necessary to validate the precise function of T$_H$17 immunity towards fungal infection in humans.

Conclusions

In summary, our data suggest that IL-17A derived from the lung infiltrating T$_H$17 in BALF and mLN, plays a supportive role in rendering protection to pulmonary *C.*

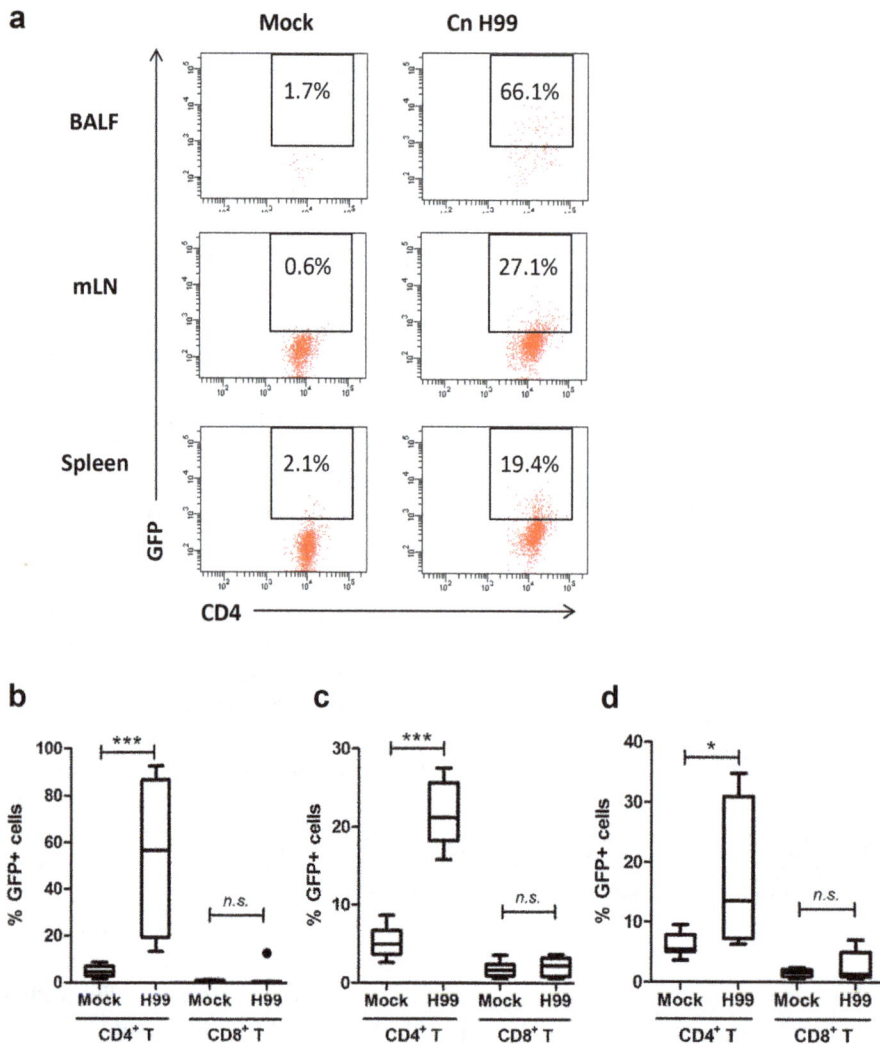

Fig. 4 Production of IL-17A by CD4⁺ T helper cells. IL-17A–EGFP reporter mice (n = 4 per group) were uninfected (mock) or intranasally inoculated with 1×10^5 cells with *C. neoformans* H99 strain (Cn H99), BALF, mLN and spleen were collected after 14 days for analysis. **a** A representative flow cytometrical plot of GFP⁺ cells in BALF, mLN and spleen among CD4⁺–gated T cells. % denotes the percentage of GFP⁺ cells appear inside the gated area. **b–d** Number of GFP⁺ cells among the CD4⁺– or CD8⁺–gated T cell populations in the (**b**) BALF, (**c**) mLN and (**d**) spleen. *P < 0.05, ***P < 0.001, *n.s.*: not significant or $P \geq 0.05$, by Mann-Whitney U test

neoformans infection. Understanding the host immune response during cryptococcal infection is essential for the development of immunomodulatory therapies.

Methods

Fungal and cell culture

C. neoformans var. grubii (serotype A) H99 was obtained from American Type Culture Collection (ATCC). Environmental strains S48B, S68B and H4 were isolated from pigeon droppings, as described [28, 29]. All cells were stored at – 80 °C freezer until usage. To start the culture, a small drop of fungal cell stock was streaked on the Sabouraud's dextrose agar (SDA) and incubated at 37 °C for 48 h. Then, 2 to 3 single colonies from freshly

prepared agar plate were inoculated into Sabouraud's dextrose broth (SDB) and incubated at 37 °C for 48 h.

Animals

Wildtype C57BL/6, IL-17A–EGFP (*C57BL/6-Il-17a*$^{tm1Bc-gen}$*/J*) and IL-17A–KO (STOCK *Il-17a*$^{tm1.1(ire)Stock}$*/J*) mice were obtained from Jackson Laboratory (Bar Harbor, ME). IL-17A–EGFP mice contain an IRES-EGFP-SV40-polyA signal sequence cassette inserted after stop codon of *Il-17a* gene and express EGFP as a marker of IL-17A activity. Whereas IL-17A–KO mice contained abolished IL-17A expression due to insertional mutation of a codon optimized Cre-recombinase and a polyA signal into exon 1 of *Il-17a* gene. Groups of 4 to 6 mice at age 8–12 weeks old were used in the study. All mice were maintained in

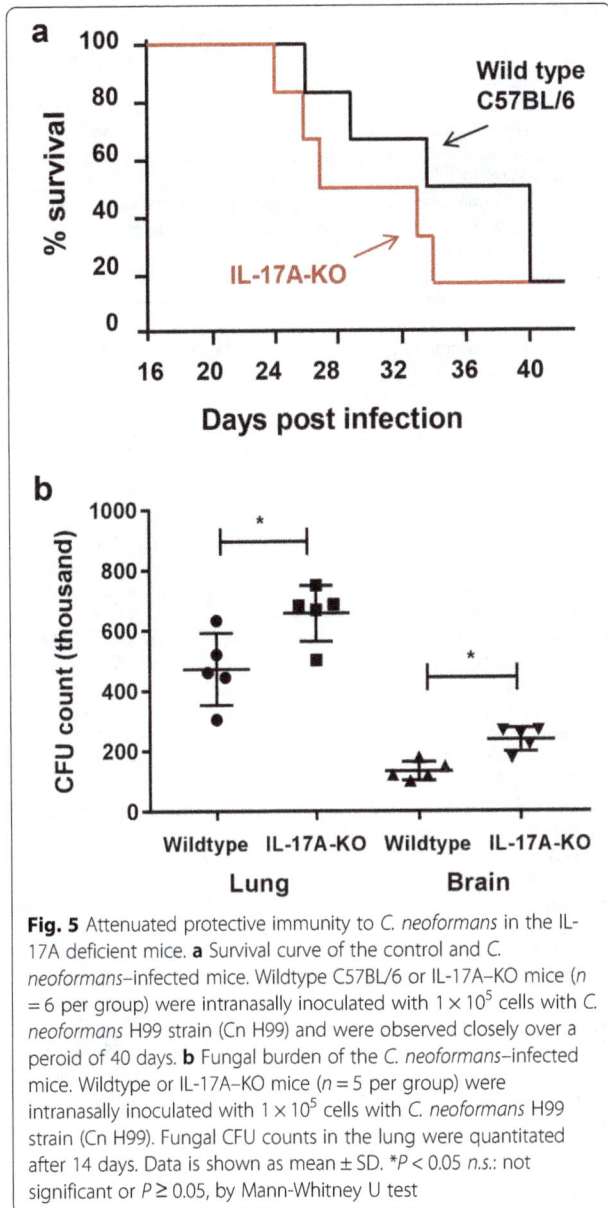

Fig. 5 Attenuated protective immunity to *C. neoformans* in the IL-17A deficient mice. **a** Survival curve of the control and *C. neoformans*–infected mice. Wildtype C57BL/6 or IL-17A–KO mice (*n* = 6 per group) were intranasally inoculated with 1 × 10⁵ cells with *C. neoformans* H99 strain (Cn H99) and were observed closely over a period of 40 days. **b** Fungal burden of the *C. neoformans*–infected mice. Wildtype or IL-17A–KO mice (*n* = 5 per group) were intranasally inoculated with 1 × 10⁵ cells with *C. neoformans* H99 strain (Cn H99). Fungal CFU counts in the lung were quantitated after 14 days. Data is shown as mean ± SD. *$P < 0.05$ n.s.: not significant or $P \geq 0.05$, by Mann-Whitney U test

individually ventilated cages under specific pathogen free condition. Mice were euthanized with CO_2 inhalation when they exhibited overt signs including hunched posture, fur ruffling, weakness, increased respiratory rate and difficulty breathing. This study has been approved by the Faculty of Medicine Ethics Committee for Animal Experimentation at the University of Malaya (Reference number: 2013-12-03/MMB/R/EM).

In vivo infection

Fresh cultures of *C. neoformans* were washed and harvested by centrifugation at 1800×g for 10 min. Cells were adjusted to 10⁷ cells/ml in phosphate buffer saline (PBS) using a hemocytometer. Mice were first anesthetized with intraperitoneal injection of a mixture of

ketamine (90 mg/kg) and xylazine (10 mg/kg) before inoculated with intranasal pipetting of 20 µl (2 × 10⁵ cells) yeast suspension. For survival study, each infected mouse was examined daily from 2 to 6 weeks post infection. For other study, mice were euthanized with CO_2 inhalation at 28 days post-infection and serum was collected from blood. Lung was lavaged with 1.0 ml PBS and BALF was collected. Lung, mLN, spleen and brain were excised for further analysis.

Flow cytometry analysis

Cells collected from BALF, mLN or spleen were adjusted to 1 × 10⁶, washed with PBS-Tween20 with 3% fetal bovine serum, pelleted and stained with antibodies for 30 min. Two sets of antibodies used were (i) anti-TCRβ-PE (H57–597), anti-CD4-PE/Cy7 (GK1.5) and anti-CD8-PerCPCy5.5 (53–6.7), and (ii) anti-CD11b-APC (M1/70), anti-F4/80-PerCPCy5.5 (BM8) and anti-Ly-6G/Ly-6C-PE (Gr-1, RB6-8C5) (Biolegend, San Diego, CA). Cells were washed in PBS-Tween20 and resuspended in 1 ml flow buffer. Cells were analyzed in BD Canto II flow cytometer (BD Biosciences, Franklin Lakes, NJ) and data were processed using FACSDiva (BD Biosciences).

CFU count

Brain and lungs from the mice were excised, weighed and homogenized in 1 ml PBS using glass slides. A total volume of 20 µl of the serially diluted homogenates (at 10, 100 and 1000 folds) were plated on SDA plates in duplicates and cultured at 30 °C for 48 h. Fungal load was quantified using colony forming unit (CFU) per ml by calculating yeast colonies on each plate.

Bioplex assay

Sera from each mouse were collected for measurement of cytokines using Bio-plex Pro Mouse Th17 assay (Bio-rad, CA, USA) which included the following cytokines: IL-17A, IL-17F, IL-21, IL-22, IL-23, IL-31, IL-33 and MIP-3α according to the manufacturer's instructions. The Multiplex bead working solution was diluted from 25× stock solution beads and 50 µl of it was added into each well followed by 50 µl of sample. Each cytokine standards and samples were assayed in duplicate as provided by manufacturer. Samples with microbeads were incubated at room temperature on a magnetic microplate shaker for 30 min. After incubation, Bio-Plex detection antibody working solution was then added, washed 3× with Bio-Plex wash buffer and finally 1× streptavidin-PE was added before reading the plate on the Bio-Plex 200 system (Bio-Rad). Cytokine concentrations from each tissue homogenates were calculated based on each cytokine standard curve.

Statistics

All statistical analyses were performed using GraphPad Prism 6. Analyses between groups were performed using Student's t-test or Mann-Whitney U test, whereby a P value of < 0.05 was considered statistically significant.

Additional files

Additional file 1: Percentages of leukocytes in BALF, mLN and spleen of the C. neoformans–infected mice. Cells were stained with two sets of markers for identification of different cell types. (a) Gate P3: helper T (TCRβ$^+$ CD4$^+$), and gate P4: cytotoxic T (TCRβ$^+$ CD8$^+$). (b) Gate P3: macrophages (F4/80$^+$ CD11b$^+$ Gr-1$^+$), gate P5: neutrophils (F4/80$^-$ CD11b$^+$ Gr-1^{high}), and gate P6: inflammatory monocytes (F4/80$^-$ CD11b$^+$ Gr-1^{medium}). (TIF 544 kb)

Additional file 2: Production of IL-17A by different innate cells after C. neoformans infection. IL-17A–EGFP reporter mice ($n = 4$ per group) were uninfected (mock) or intranasally inoculated with 1×10^5 cells with C. neoformans H99 strain (Cn H99), BALF, mLN and spleen were collected after 14 days for analysis. (a–b) Number of GFP$^+$ cells among the macrophages (F4/80$^+$ CD11b$^+$ Gr1$^+$)–, neutrophils (F4/80$^-$ CD11b$^+$ Gr-1^{high})–, and inflammatory monocytes (F4/80$^-$ CD11b$^+$ Gr1^{medium})–gated cell populations in the (a) BALF and (b) mLN. n.s.: not significant or *$P \geq 0.05$, by Mann-Whitney U-test. (TIF 260 kb)

Abbreviations

BALF: Bronchoalveolar lavage fluid; EGFP: Enhanced green fluorescent protein; IL-17A: Interleukin-17A; KO: Knock out; mLN: Mediastinal lymph node; MOI: Multiplicity of infection; T$_H$17: T helper 17

Acknowledgements

We thank staffs at University of Malaya Animal Experimental Unit for assistance in animal works.

Funding

This work was supported by fund from Institut Mérieux – Malaysian Society of Infectious Diseases and Chemotherapy: MSIDC (IF039–2017) and University of Malaya Research Grant (RG525-13HTM).

Authors' contributions

EM, YYC, GMYT, CYQL, and HCC performed the experiments and analyzed the data. EM, WFW and CYL designed the experiments and wrote the paper. RDV, STT and PPC contributed reagents tools and revised the manuscript. All authors read and approved the final manuscript.

Competing interests

The authors declare that they have no competing interests.

Author details

[1]Department of Medical Microbiology, Faculty of Medicine, University of Malaya, Kuala Lumpur, Malaysia. [2]School of Bioscience, Taylor's University, Subang Jaya, Selangor, Malaysia.

References

1. May RC, Stone NR, Wiesner DL, Bicanic T, Nielsen K. Cryptococcus: from environmental saprophyte to global pathogen. Nat Rev Microbiol. 2016; 14(2):106–17.
2. Mitchell TG, Perfect JR. Cryptococcosis in the era of AIDS--100 years after the discovery of Cryptococcus neoformans. Clin Microbiol Rev. 1995;8(4):515–48.
3. Jarvis JN, Harrison TS. HIV-associated cryptococcal meningitis. Aids. 2007; 21(16):2119–29.
4. Hill JO, Harmsen AG. Intrapulmonary growth and dissemination of an avirulent strain of Cryptococcus neoformans in mice depleted of CD4+ or CD8+ T cells. J Exp Med. 1991;173(3):755–8.
5. Huffnagle GB, Yates JL, Lipscomb MF. Immunity to a pulmonary Cryptococcus neoformans infection requires both CD4+ and CD8+ T cells. J Exp Med. 1991;173(4):793–800.
6. Mody CH, Lipscomb MF, Street NE, Toews GB. Depletion of CD4+ (L3T4+) lymphocytes in vivo impairs murine host defense to Cryptococcus neoformans. J Immunol. 1990;144(4):1472–7.
7. Conti HR, Shen F, Nayyar N, Stocum E, Sun JN, Lindemann MJ, Ho AW, Hai JH, Yu JJ, Jung JW, et al. Th17 cells and IL-17 receptor signaling are essential for mucosal host defense against oral candidiasis. J Exp Med. 2009;206(2):299–311.
8. Vautier S, Sousa Mda G, Brown GD. C-type lectins, fungi and Th17 responses. Cytokine Growth Factor Rev. 2010;21(6):405–12.
9. Chai LY, van de Veerdonk F, Marijnissen RJ, Cheng SC, Khoo AL, Hectors M, Lagrou K, Vonk AG, Maertens J, Joosten LA, et al. Anti-aspergillus human host defence relies on type 1 T helper (Th1), rather than type 17 T helper (Th17), cellular immunity. Immunology. 2010;130(1):46–54.
10. Kleinschek MA, Muller U, Brodie SJ, Stenzel W, Kohler G, Blumenschein WM, Straubinger RK, McClanahan T, Kastelein RA, Alber G. IL-23 enhances the inflammatory cell response in Cryptococcus neoformans infection and induces a cytokine pattern distinct from IL-12. J Immunol. 2006;176(2):1098–106.
11. Angkasekwinai P, Sringkarin N, Supasorn O, Fungkrajai M, Wang YH, Chayakulkeeree M, Ngamskulrungroj P, Angkasekwinai N, Pattanapanyasat K. Cryptococcus gattii infection dampens Th1 and Th17 responses by attenuating dendritic cell function and pulmonary chemokine expression in the immunocompetent hosts. Infect Immun. 2014;82(9):3880–90.
12. Peck A, Mellins ED. Precarious balance: Th17 cells in host defense. Infect Immun. 2010;78(1):32–8.
13. Wiesner DL, Smith KD, Kashem SW, Bohjanen PR, Nielsen K. Different lymphocyte populations direct dichotomous eosinophil or neutrophil responses to pulmonary Cryptococcus infection. J Immunol. 2017;198(4):1627–37.
14. Hardison SE, Wozniak KL, Kolls JK, Wormley FL Jr. Interleukin-17 is not required for classical macrophage activation in a pulmonary mouse model of Cryptococcus neoformans infection. Infect Immun. 2010;78(12):5341–51.
15. Valdez PA, Vithayathil PJ, Janelsins BM, Shaffer AL, Williamson PR, Datta SK. Prostaglandin E2 suppresses antifungal immunity by inhibiting interferon regulatory factor 4 function and interleukin-17 expression in T cells. Immunity. 2012;36(4):668–79.
16. Movahed E, Munusamy K, Tan GM, Looi CY, Tay ST, Wong WF. Genome-wide transcription study of Cryptococcus neoformans H99 clinical strain versus environmental strains. PLoS One. 2015;10(9):e0137457.
17. Wozniak KL, Hardison SE, Kolls JK, Wormley FL. Role of IL-17A on resolution of pulmonary C. neoformans infection. PLoS One. 2011;6(2):e17204.
18. Shoham S, Levitz SM. The immune response to fungal infections. Br J Haematol. 2005;129(5):569–82.
19. Snydman DR, Singh N, Dromer F, Perfect JR, Lortholary O. Cryptococcosis in solid organ transplant recipients: current state of the science. Clin Infect Dis. 2008;47(10):1321–7.
20. Wozniak KL, Ravi S, Macias S, Young ML, Olszewski MA, Steele C, Wormley FL Jr. Insights into the mechanisms of protective immunity against Cryptococcus neoformans infection using a mouse model of pulmonary cryptococcosis. PLoS One. 2009;4(9):e6854.
21. Jarvis JN, Casazza JP, Stone HH, Meintjes G, Lawn SD, Levitz SM, Harrison TS, Koup RA. The phenotype of the Cryptococcus-specific CD4+ memory T-cell response is associated with disease severity and outcome in HIV-associated cryptococcal meningitis. J Infect Dis. 2013;207(12):1817–28.
22. Voelz K, May RC. Cryptococcal interactions with the host immune system. Eukaryot Cell. 2010;9(6):835–46.

23. Zhang Y, Wang F, Tompkins KC, McNamara A, Jain AV, Moore BB, Toews GB, Huffnagle GB, Olszewski MA. Robust Th1 and Th17 immunity supports pulmonary clearance but cannot prevent systemic dissemination of highly virulent Cryptococcus neoformans H99. Am J Pathol. 2009;175(6):2489–500.

24. Huang W, Na L, Fidel PL, Schwarzenberger P. Requirement of interleukin-17A for systemic anti-Candida albicans host defense in mice. J Infect Dis. 2004;190(3):624–31.

25. Werner JL, Metz AE, Horn D, Schoeb TR, Hewitt MM, Schwiebert LM, Faro-Trindade I, Brown GD, Steele C. Requisite role for the dectin-1 β-glucan receptor in pulmonary defense against aspergillus fumigatus. J Immunol. 2009;182(8):4938–46.

26. Bozza S, Zelante T, Moretti S, Bonifazi P, DeLuca A, D'Angelo C, Giovannini G, Garlanda C, Boon L, Bistoni F, et al. Lack of toll IL-1R8 exacerbates Th17 cell responses in fungal infection. J Immunol. 2008;180(6):4022–31.

27. Zelante T, Bozza S, De Luca A, D'Angelo C, Bonifazi P, Moretti S, Giovannini G, Bistoni F, Romani L. Th17 cells in the setting of aspergillus infection and pathology. Med Mycol. 2009;47(Suppl 1):S162–9.

28. Movahed E, Tan GM, Munusamy K, Yeow TC, Tay ST, Wong WF, Looi CY. Triclosan demonstrates synergic effect with amphotericin B and fluconazole and induces apoptosis-like cell death in Cryptococcus neoformans. Front Microbiol. 2016;7:360.

29. Tay ST, Chai HC, Na SL, Hamimah H, Rohani MY, Soo-Hoo TS. The isolation, characterization and antifungal susceptibilities of Cryptococcus neoformans from bird excreta in Klang Valley, Malaysia. Mycopathologia. 2005;159(4):509–13.

18

Anti-SIRT1 autoantibody is elevated in ankylosing spondylitis: a potential disease biomarker

Qiongyi Hu[1†], Yue Sun[1†], Yuan Li[2†], Hui Shi[1], Jialin Teng[1], Honglei Liu[1], Xiaobing Cheng[1], Junna Ye[1], Yutong Su[1], Yufeng Yin[1], Mengru Liu[1], Jiucun Wang[2*] and Chengde Yang[1*]

Abstract

Background: Little is known about the presence of specific autoantibodies in ankylosing spondylitis (AS), an immune-mediated inflammatory disease. The object of this study was to explore potential autoantibody profiles in AS patients.

Results: Levels of anti-SIRT1 autoantibodies were significantly higher in AS ($P < 0.001$) and psoriatic arthritis (PsA) ($P < 0.01$) patients but not rheumatoid arthritis (RA) patients compared with healthy controls. Additionally, titers of anti-NAD-dependent protein deacetylase sirtuin-1(SIRT1) antibodies were significantly higher in AS patients than in RA ($P < 0.05$) and PsA ($P < 0.05$) patients. Moreover, levels of anti-SIRT1 ($P < 0.001$) antibodies were significantly higher during the first year in patients with hip joint involvement. The anti-SIRT1 antibody positivity rate was 18.9% in AS patients.

Conclusions: Our findings indicate that anti-SIRT1 autoantibodies may serve as a marker for diagnosing AS and predicting hip joint involvement at an early stage.

Keywords: AS, Anti-SIRT1 antibodies, Biomarker

Background

Ankylosing spondylitis (AS) is an immune-mediated, insidiously progressive form of seronegative spondyloarthritis (SpA) that is characterized by enthesitis. AS progressively leads to inflammation, bone erosion, new bone formation and ankylosis of sacroiliac, vertebral, and peripheral joints, with the ultimate radiographic appearance of a "bamboo spine" [1]. The pain and ankylosis that occur in this disease may cause considerable disability.

Although the etiology of AS is incompletely understood, familial and genetic factors are thought to be involved [2]. A surge of genome-wide association studies (GWASs) have been performed to identify associations

* Correspondence: jcwang@fudan.edu.cn; yangchengde@sina.com
†Qiongyi Hu, Yue Sun and Yuan Li contributed equally to this work.
²State Key Laboratory of Genetic Engineering and Ministry of Education (MOE) Key Laboratory of Contemporary Anthropology, Collaborative Innovation Center for Genetics and Development, School of Life Sciences, Fudan University, Shanghai 200438, China
¹Department of Rheumatology and Immunology, Ruijin Hospital, Shanghai Jiao Tong University School of Medicine, No. 197 Ruijin Second Road, Shanghai 200025, China

between genetic variants and AS phenotypes, including the human leukocyte antigen allotype B27 (HLA-B27), the major risk factor for AS, as well as non-MHC genetics [2]. By delineating potential immunomodulatory pathways involving regulating innate and acquired immunity, such GWASs have provided considerable evidence for understanding the pathogenesis of AS [3]. The role of HLA-B27 in antigen presentation to T cells has been well established, and the association of *IL-7R*, *ZMIZ1*, *EOMES* and *RUNX3* variants with AS suggests the involvement of CD8+ T cell-mediated immunity [4]. Regardless, elucidating the roles of these factors in the immune system requires further study. Moreover, elevated numbers of Th17 cells and levels of IL-23 expression have been found in the peripheral blood of AS patients, indicating that CD4+ T cell-mediated inflammation contributes to the pathogenesis of AS. In addition to chronic inflammation, cartilage degeneration and new bone formation are key pathogenic features of AS. It has also been suggested that enhanced bone morphogenetic protein (BMP) and Wnt/β-catenin signaling contributes to ankylosis and chondrogenesis in AS [5].

Despite sharing a susceptibility locus HLA genotype with other autoimmune diseases such as systemic lupus erythematosus (SLE) and Sjögren syndrome (SS) [6, 7], it remains controversial whether AS is an autoimmune disease with specific autoantibodies. Nonetheless, specific immune complexes have recently been found to be involved in AS pathogenesis [8], and levels of antibodies against connective, skeletal, and muscular tissue-related antigens [9], PPM1A [10], CD74 [11, 12], leukocytes [13], neutrophils [14], and some collagen proteins [15] are high in AS patients. Furthermore, an increased prevalence of anti-glycan antibody has been noted in AS and psoriatic arthritis (PsA) patients, with rheumatoid arthritis (RA) patients showing even higher prevalence [16]. In another study, AS patients were found to have higher levels of anti-flagellin antibody than a control group, suggesting an immune response to bacterial antigens in AS patients [17]. A comprehensive review on novel diagnostic autoantibodies in AS has been published, and targets of autoantibodies in AS include microbes, inflammatory factors and structural antigens [18]. Although these studies reveal a certain spectrum of autoantibodies in AS, the AS-related antibodies reported to date were based on small-study populations, and further validation is lacking. More evidence is needed to ascertain the autoreactivity associated with AS.

AS is considered an inflammatory rheumatoid disease, yet it differs from other autoimmune diseases with specific autoantibodies such as SLE and SS, and definitive evidence for autoantibodies in AS is lacking. The aim of this study was to explore potential autoantibody profiles in AS patients using a protein microarray expressing 19,349 recombinant human proteins. Autoantibodies targeting NAD-dependent protein deacetylase sirtuin-1 (SIRT1) in the protein microarray were then validated by an ELISA-based method, and significant differences in anti-SIRT1 antibody levels in AS patients with different clinical variables were assessed.

Results

Global properties of observed antibodies in AS
First, we explored global antibody profiles in serum from AS patients using a protein microarray displaying 19,349 immobilized recombinant human proteins. Analysis of the protein array data revealed 56 targets among the 2125 IgG antibodies expressed at levels 4-fold or greater in AS patients compared with healthy donors (Fig. 1a and Additional file 1: Table S1). Interestingly, functional analysis using the PANTHER pathway classification system indicated that the targets are mainly intracellular (Fig. 1b), similar to autoimmune diseases such as SLE. Additionally, the most significant enrichment in the

antibody signature of AS patients was for terms of "catalytic activity" and "binding" (Fig. 1c). Further analysis of biological processes showed that most of these proteins are related to cellular, metabolic, stimulus response and developmental processes (Fig. 1d). Moreover, 13 proteins targeted by IgG antibodies were more than 10-fold higher in AS patients. The functions of 13 proteins were listed in Table 1. SIRT1 was the only antigen for which there was a significant highest level of IgG antibody in serum from AS patients compared to healthy controls. Interestingly, SIRT1 has been demonstrated to regulate bone metabolism; therefore, we concentrated on SIRT1 as a target.

Distinct antibody expression levels in common rheumatic diseases
To confirm the proteomic results, sera from 185 AS patients, 94 RA patients, 12 PsA patients, and 87 healthy controls were collected. The clinical characteristics of the subjects in each group are detailed in Table 2. As shown in Fig. 2, anti-SIRT1 antibody levels were significantly higher in AS patients than in healthy controls ($P < 0.001$). Among the disease controls, anti-SIRT1 antibody levels in AS patients were significantly different from those in RA ($P < 0.05$) and PsA ($P < 0.05$) patients (Fig. 2). Moreover, sera from 35 patients with AS (18.9%) and 18 with RA (19.1%) were positive for IgG antibodies against SIRT1, whereas serum from only 1 patient with PsA (1%) was positive for anti-SIRT1 antibodies.

Anti-SIRT1 antibody levels were higher in female AS patients
As sex hormones contribute to many autoimmune diseases including SLE, SS and AS [19], we compared levels of anti-SIRT1 antibodies between male and female AS patients. Remarkably, levels of IgG antibodies against SIRT1 were significantly higher in sera from female patients compared to male patients (Fig. 3, $P < 0.05$). However, no gender difference for anti-SIRT1 antibody levels was observed among RA and PsA patients (data not shown). These results indicate that sex hormones may modulate the production and secretion of antibodies in AS patients.

Elevated levels of anti-SIRT1 autoantibodies in AS patients with hip joint involvement at the early stage
We next analyzed statistical differences in serum antibody levels in AS patients with different disease variables. As shown in Fig. 4a, levels of anti-SIRT1 antibodies ($P < 0.001$) were significantly higher in patients with hip joint involvement during the first year, though anti-SIRT1 antibody levels were similar among AS patients regardless of disease duration (Fig. 4b). Furthermore, anti-SIRT1 levels were not significantly different

between ESR-positive and -negative patients and did not correlate with ESR levels (Fig. 4c).

Discussion

In this study, we found serum levels of anti-SIRT1 antibodies to be significantly higher in sera from individuals with AS than from individuals with RA or PsA. In addition, levels of anti-SIRT1 antibodies were significantly higher in patients with hip joint involvement during the first year. The anti-SIRT1 antibody positivity rate among AS patients was 18.9%, suggesting that anti-SIRT1 antibody is a potential novel biomarker in AS.

Although the pathogenesis of AS is not fully understood, it is commonly recognized that genetic susceptibility, environmental factors (especially the microbiome) and the immune system may be crucial factors in the development of this disease [20]. Indeed, multiple genetic variations have been found in genes encoding proteins

essential for antigen presentation and macrophage-related phagocytosis, such as *UBE2E3*, *ERAP1* and *FCGR2A* [1]. These data suggest that dysfunctional antigen processing and eradication occurs in AS. To date, a few studies have identified targets of autoantibodies in AS [9–15], though more definite evidence needs to be provided to verify the existence of autoreactivity in AS patients.

As imbalanced ossification is a hallmark in AS, we focused on proteins related to bone metabolism among 13 proteins targeted by IgG antibodies and showing more than 10-fold increase in AS patients. Interestingly, the anti-SIRT1 antibody level was highest in serum from AS patients. SIRT1, a widely distributed class III histone deacetylase, is involved in regulating T cell activation as well as tolerance and inflammation [21, 22]. Additionally, recent studies have indicated a potential role for SIRT1 in regulating bone metabolism [23], and reduced levels of SIRT1 in osteoblasts from patients with

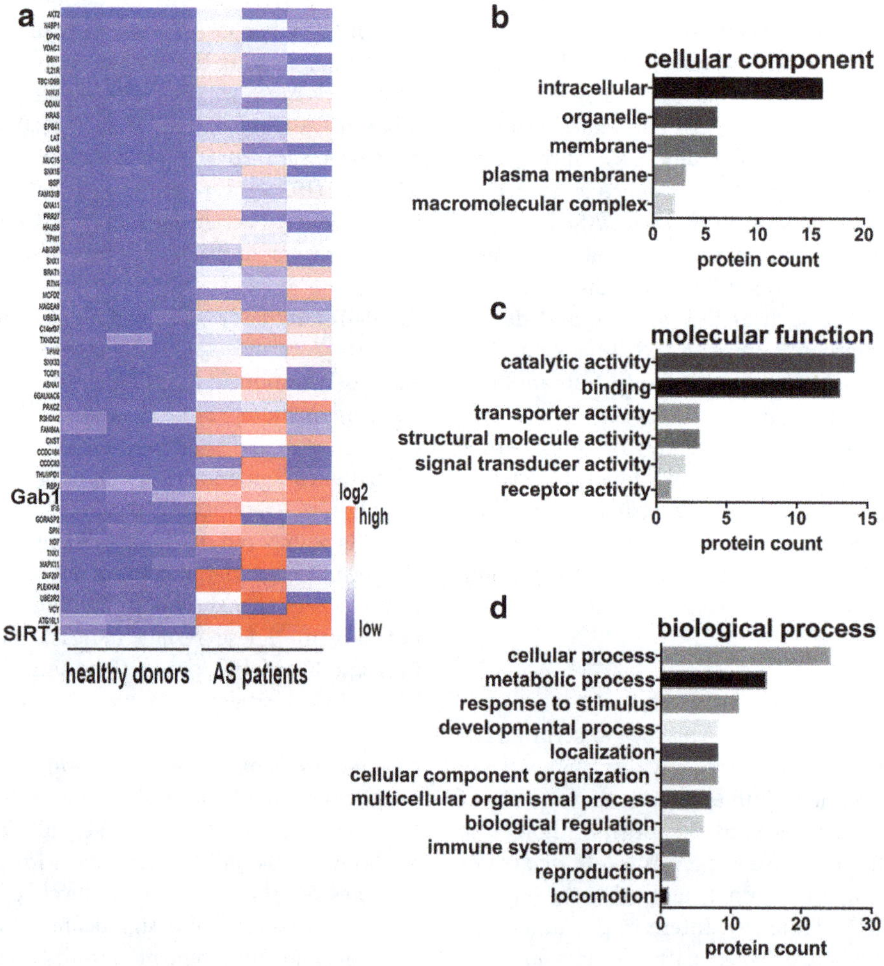

Fig. 1 Proteomic analysis of sera from AS patients. **a**. Heat map representing the 56 protein candidates targeted by IgG antibodies in AS patient sera with 4-fold or greater expression (*P* < 0.05) compared with healthy donors. The classification and clustering of different categories of cellular component (**b**), molecular function (**c**) and biological process (**d**) of all identified proteins were analyzed using PANTHER databases

osteoarthritis, a disorder characterized by inappropriate osteogenesis of bone tissue, lead to increased expression of TGF-β and sclerostin, which regulates bone mineralization via Wnt signaling [24]. Furthermore, MSCs isolated from SIRT1-deficient mice exhibit impaired differentiation into osteoblasts and chondrocytes [25], the major cells involved in the pathogenesis of AS. Moreover, SIRT1 is a negative controller of NF-kB, and well-demonstrated dysregulation of the NF-kB pathway, which is crucial for inflammation and the survival of osteoclasts and osteoblasts, has been reported in AS [26]. In our study, we found elevated levels of anti-SIRT1 antibodies in patients with hip joint involvement during the first year, indicating that SIRT1 may regulate erosive bone destruction in AS. We will explore the pathogenic role of SIRT1 in AS in the future.

PANTHER analysis revealed intracellular proteins to be the main targets of autoantibodies in AS. SIRT1 is mainly a cytoplasmic protein, and the autoreactivity against SIRT1 found in AS serum might reflect failed elimination of these antigens. More research will need to explain the role of these antigens in AS, and we regret the unavailability of spinal samples from AS patients to determine local expression of SIRT1 at affected joints.

Interestingly, our results showed that anti-SIRT1 levels were significantly higher in female patients compared to male patients. For some autoimmune diseases, sex hormones are among the most-studied contributory factors [27]. Unlike other autoimmune diseases with higher prevalence in females, such as SLE, SS and RA, AS is more prevalent in males than in females, and male

patients also have more severe disease than do female patients [28]. It has been reported that testosterone might interact with SIRT1 to protect endothelial cells [29], though it remains to be determined how testosterone regulates SIRT1 and whether it might affect autoantibody production in AS.

Despite the presentation of SIRT1 as a self-antigen in AS, there were no significant differences in antibody levels when comparing diverse groups with low and high ESR or those with different disease durations. This finding indicates that the autoantibodies determined in the current study are irrelevant to inflammation in AS. Considering the functions of SIRT1 in bone formation as well as the positive correlation regarding autoreactivity, our study provides a basis for further research of the pathogenic mechanism of the immune system in AS.

AS has been recognized as a seronegative disease due to the lack of specific autoantibodies, which are the immunologic hallmarks of many autoimmune diseases such as SLE, SS and RA [30]. The present study reveals unique characteristics of AS compared with autoimmune diseases such as RA.

Conclusions

In summary, we found sera from AS patients to be extraordinarily distinct in terms of antibody reactivity toward antigens. In addition to the inflammatory response, autoantibodies produced by dysregulation of the immune system might constitute another feature of AS. Their core signature showed enrichment of a diverse array of proteins

Table 1 Targets of IgG antibodies with 10-fold or greater in AS patients

Name	Fold change	Functions
SIRT1	29.3	NAD-dependent protein deacetylase sirtuin-1
ATG16L1	26.4	Autophagy
VCY	23.0	Spermatogenesis
UBE2R2	20.5	Ubiquitin-conjugating enzyme
PLEKHA8	19.9	Cargo transport protein
ZNF207	16.8	Kinetochore- and microtubule-binding protein
MAPK11	16.3	MAP kinase signal transduction pathway
TNK1	14.9	Negatively regulating RAS-MAPK pathway
ND7	14.7	NADH dehydrogenase subunit 7
SPN	14.3	Regulating multiple T-cell functions
GORASP2	13.1	Golgi reassembly-stacking protein 2
IFI6	11.6	Regulating apoptosis, anti-viral activity
GAB1	11.1	GRB2-associated-binding protein 1
RBPJ	11.0	Playing a central role in Notch signaling
THUMPD1	10.6	tRNA acetylation
CCDC83	10.2	Coiled-coil domain-containing protein
CCDC184	10.1	Coiled-coil domain-containing protein
CNST	10.0	Required for targeting of connexins to the plasma membrane

Table 2 Characteristics of the study cohort

Variable	AS	RA	PsA	HC
Number	185	94	12	87
Age (years) (median)	15–70 (34.6)	14–54 (41.1)	31–62 (45.1)	20–50 (35.2)
Gender ratio (male: female)	139:46	12:82	10:2	66:21
Disease duration (years)	7.4 (0.04–31)	–	–	–
Positive for HLA-B27	94.3%	–	–	–
Hips joint involvement (n, %)	57 (30.8%)	0	0	–
ESR (mm/h) (median)	31.6 ± 42.3	31.2 ± 25.7	32.6 ± 25.9	–

involved in bone metabolism, which may facilitate progression of AS, and included several novel antigens the function of which is not yet understood. These findings provide a framework for better definition of the role of the immune response and autoantibodies in the pathogenesis of AS. Moreover, we report the existence of anti-SIRT1 antibodies in sera from AS patients and the potential of anti-SIRT1 antibodies to serve as a disease biomarker for AS.

Patients and methods
Subjects
The first cohort of patients consisted of 10 treatment-naïve AS patients who fulfilled the modified 1984 New York criteria for AS [31]; 12 sex- and age-matched healthy donors were used as controls. Sera were collected and used for protein array analysis. The clinical characteristics of each group are summarized in Additional file 2: Table S2.

The second cohort of patients and controls consisted of 185 consecutive patients with AS, 94 patients with RA, 12 patients with PsA according to standard diagnostic criteria [32, 33]; 87 sex- and age-matched healthy donors were used as controls. Among the 185 AS

patients and 87 healthy controls, sera from 10 AS patients and 12 healthy controls were used for protein array analysis. Sera from the second cohort were used for ELISA analysis. All of the serum samples were collected at Ruijin Hospital between 2015 and 2016 and stored at – 80 °C until use. The study was performed in accordance with the Declaration of Helsinki and the principles of Good Clinical Practice. Biological samples were obtained under a protocol approved by the Institutional Research Ethics Committee of Ruijin Hospital (ID: 2016–62), Shanghai, China. All participants provided informed consent to participate in the study. Demographic and laboratory data were obtained by the Department of Immunology and Rheumatology.

Serum antibody profiling using a human protein microarray
The human proteome microarray (BC Biotechnology, USA) used in this study is composed of approximately 19,394 unique full-length recombinant proteins printed in duplicate. As a screening procedure, we employed protein array technology to detect new autoantibodies in AS using the first cohort of patients and healthy

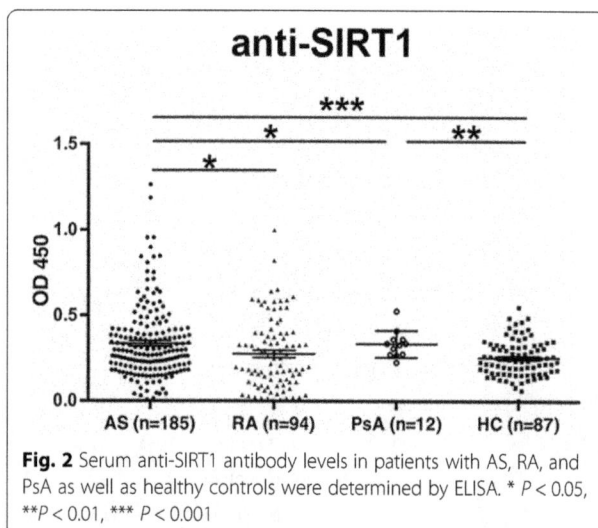
Fig. 2 Serum anti-SIRT1 antibody levels in patients with AS, RA, and PsA as well as healthy controls were determined by ELISA. * $P < 0.05$, **$P < 0.01$, *** $P < 0.001$

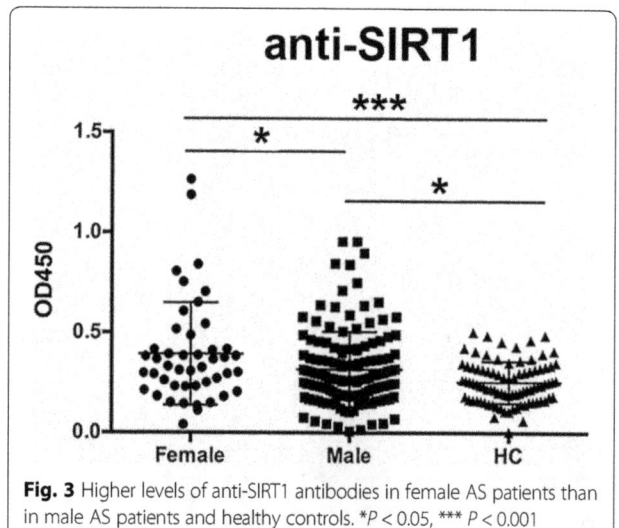
Fig. 3 Higher levels of anti-SIRT1 antibodies in female AS patients than in male AS patients and healthy controls. *$P < 0.05$, *** $P < 0.001$

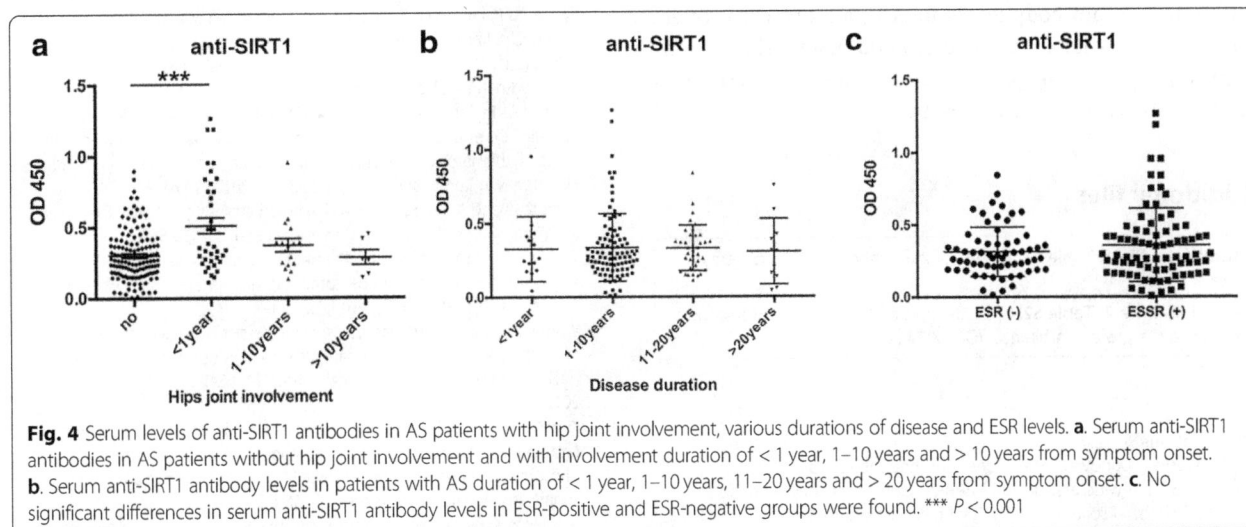

Fig. 4 Serum levels of anti-SIRT1 antibodies in AS patients with hip joint involvement, various durations of disease and ESR levels. **a**. Serum anti-SIRT1 antibodies in AS patients without hip joint involvement and with involvement duration of < 1 year, 1–10 years and > 10 years from symptom onset. **b**. Serum anti-SIRT1 antibody levels in patients with AS duration of < 1 year, 1–10 years, 11–20 years and > 20 years from symptom onset. **c**. No significant differences in serum anti-SIRT1 antibody levels in ESR-positive and ESR-negative groups were found. *** $P < 0.001$

controls. Treatment-naïve patients with AS ($n = 10$) were divided into 3 groups, and sera of every group were mixed for detection. Sex- and age-matched sera from healthy donors ($n = 12$) divided into 3 groups were used as controls.

Human protein microarray data analysis

The protein microarray data analysis was conducted according to the procedure described by Hu et al. [34]. Median foreground and background intensities were obtained for each spot in the protein microarrays using Gene Pix Pro 6.0 Software. To execute background correction and normalize intra-array signal intensity, the raw intensity of each spot was defined as the ratio of the foreground to the background median intensity. To remove the negative effects of non-specific binding and spatial heterogeneity across the protein microarray, "normexp" [35], a background processing approach, was implemented in the R 2.15.1 package for background correction. The P value was calculated for each protein using Fisher's test, and fold change was defined as the mean signal intensity ratio of AS patients to healthy donors.

Identifying proteins differentially recognized by serum autoantibodies

For each protein, spot signals were averaged across the groups. A statistical distribution of the signal intensities among the controls was calculated, from which the signal intensity mean and standard deviation were calculated. According to a previous autoantibody study by Meyer et al. [36], we identified the existence of 2125 proteins targeted by IgG antibodies by defining a cut-off of ≥2 SD from the mean signal intensity of healthy donors and imposing a minimum prevalence of 2/3 for the AS cases and a maximum prevalence of 1/3 for the

healthy donors. After filtering the 2215 protein hits with $P < 0.05$ and fold changes of more than 4, 56 targets were identified as autoantigen candidates. Thus, for every target protein screened, the response of the control population formed a benchmark.

Detection of serum autoantibodies

Serum levels of anti-SIRT1 were measured by ELISA. In brief, 96-well plates were coated with 1 μg/mL SIRT1 (R&D, Canada, USA) at 4 °C overnight. Nonspecific binding was blocked by incubating with PBS containing 5% BSA at 37 °C for 2 h. The wells were then incubated with human serum (1:100) at 37 °C for 2 h and washed five times with PBS plus 0.05% Tween-20. Secondary horseradish peroxidase (HRP)-conjugated goat anti-human IgG monoclonal antibodies (Jackson ImmunoResearch Laboratories, Inc., West Grove, PA, USA) diluted to 1:100,000 were added to each well. After five washes with PBS plus 0.05% Tween 20, 100 μL of tetramethylbenzidine substrate solution (Sigma-Aldrich) was added, and the samples were incubated at room temperature. The reaction was terminated by the addition of 50 μL of 2 N H_2SO_4/well, and optical density (OD) was measured at 450 nm. A cut-off of ≥2 SDs of arbitrary units (AU) from the mean serum level of autoantibodies was used to qualitatively differentiate between positive and negative results.

Statistical analyses

All data were analyzed statistically using SPSS version 20.0 (SPSS Inc., Chicago, IL, USA). Quantitative data are expressed as the mean ± SD. Differences between two groups were calculated using the Mann-Whitney U test or unpaired Student's *t*-test, and differences between three or more groups were analyzed by one-way ANOVA and the Kruskal-Wallis test. Significant differences in antibody levels in AS patients with different clinical variables were evaluated using the Mann-Whitney U test or Kruskal-Wallis test. $P < 0.05$ was considered significantly different.

Additional files

Additional file 1: Table S1. Targets of IgG antibodies in AS patients. (DOCX 16 kb)

Additional file 2: Table S2. Characteristics of AS patients and healthy donors in the protein microarray. (DOCX 14 kb)

Abbreviations

AS: Ankylosing spondylitis; BMP: Bone morphogenetic protein; GWASs: Genome-wide association; HLA-B27: Human leukocyte antigen allotype B27; PsA: Psoriasis arthritis; RA: Rheumatoid arthritis; SIRT1: NAD-dependent protein deacetylase sirtuin-1; SLE: Systemic lupus erythematosus; SpA: Seronegative spondyloarthritis; SS: Sjögren syndrome

Acknowledgements
Not applicable.

Funding
This work was supported by the National Natural Science Foundation of China (81671589, and 81601400), the Shanghai Sailing Program (16YF1407000), the National Basic Research Program (2014CB541801), and International S&T Cooperation Program of China (2013DFA30870). The funding bodies had no role in the study design, data collection or analyses, decision to publish, or preparation of this manuscript.

Authors' contributions

CY and JW designed the research strategy. QH and YS1 wrote the manuscript text and conducted ELISA. YL provided support for the bioinformatics analyses. HS and JT collected the clinical samples and data. HL and XC prepared Figs. 1, 2, 3, 4. JY and YS2 prepared the tables. YY and ML analyzed the data. All authors edited or commented on the manuscript. And all authors read and approved the final manuscript

Competing interests

The authors declare that they have no competing interests.

References

1. Brown MA, Kenna T, Wordsworth BP. Genetics of ankylosing spondylitis--insights into pathogenesis. Nat Rev Rheumatol. 2016;12:81–91.
2. Evans DM, Spencer CC, Pointon JJ, Su Z, Harvey D, Kochan G, et al. Interaction between ERAP1 and HLA-B27 in ankylosing spondylitis implicates peptide handling in the mechanism for HLA-B27 in disease susceptibility. Nat Genet. 2011;43:761–7.
3. Smith JA, Colbert RA. Review: the interleukin-23/interleukin-17 axis in spondyloarthritis pathogenesis: Th17 and beyond. Arthritis Rheumatol. 2014;66:231 41.
4. Benjamin R, Parham P. Guilt by association: HLA-B27 and ankylosing spondylitis. Immunol Today. 1990;11:137–42.
5. Lories R. The balance of tissue repair and remodeling in chronic arthritis. Nat Rev Rheumatol. 2011;7:700–7.
6. Morris DL, Taylor KE, Fernando MM, Nititham J, Alarcon-Riquelme ME, Barcellos LF, et al. Unraveling multiple MHC gene associations with systemic lupus erythematosus: model choice indicates a role for HLA alleles and non-HLA genes in Europeans. Am J Hum Genet. 2012;91:778–93.
7. Fang K, Zhang K, Wang J. Network-assisted analysis of primary Sjogren's syndrome GWAS data in Han Chinese. Sci Rep. 2015;5:18855.
8. Tsui FW, Tsui HW, Las Heras F, Pritzker KP, Inman RD. Serum levels of novel noggin and sclerostin-immune complexes are elevated in ankylosing spondylitis. Ann Rheum Dis. 2014;73:1873–9.
9. Wright C, Sibani S, Trudgian D, Fischer R, Kessler B, LaBaer J, et al. Detection of multiple autoantibodies in patients with ankylosing spondylitis using nucleic acid programmable protein arrays. Mol Cell Proteomics. 2012;11:M9 00384.
10. Kim YG, Sohn DH, Zhao X, Sokolove J, Lindstrom TM, Yoo B, et al. Role of protein phosphatase magnesium-dependent 1A and anti-protein phosphatase magnesium-dependent 1A autoantibodies in ankylosing spondylitis. Arthritis Rheumatol. 2014;66:2793–803.
11. Baraliakos X, Baerlecken N, Witte T, Heldmann F, Braun J. High prevalence of anti-CD74 antibodies specific for the HLA class II-associated invariant chain peptide (CLIP) in patients with axial spondyloarthritis. Ann Rheum Dis. 2014;73:1079–82.
12. Baerlecken NT, Nothdorft S, Stummvoll GH, Sieper J, Rudwaleit M, Reuter S, et al. Autoantibodies against CD74 in spondyloarthritis. Ann Rheum Dis. 2014;73:1211–4.
13. Rosenberg JN, Johnson GD, Holborow EJ. Antinuclear antibodies in ankylosing spondylitis, psoriatic arthritis, and psoriasis. Ann Rheum Dis. 1979;38:526–8.
14. Locht H, Skogh T, Kihlstrom E. Anti-lactoferrin antibodies and other types of anti-neutrophil cytoplasmic antibodies (ANCA) in reactive arthritis and ankylosing spondylitis. Clin Exp Immunol. 1999;117:568–73.
15. Tani Y, Sato H, Hukuda S. Autoantibodies to collagens in Japanese patients with ankylosing spondylitis. Clin Exp Rheumatol. 1997;15:295–7.
16. Aloush V, Dotan I, Ablin JN, Elkayam O. Evaluating IBD-specific antiglycan antibodies in serum of patients with spondyloarthritis and rheumatoid arthritis: are they really specific? Clin Exp Rheumatol. 2018;25. [Epub ahead of print]
17. Wallis D, Asaduzzaman A, Weisman M, Haroon N, Anton A, McGovern D, et al. Elevated serum anti-flagellin antibodies implicate subclinical bowel inflammation in ankylosing spondylitis: an observational study. Arthritis Res Ther. 2013;15:R166.
18. Quaden DH, De Winter LM, Somers V. Detection of novel diagnostic antibodies in ankylosing spondylitis: an overview. Autoimmun Rev. 2016;15:820–32.
19. Fish EN. The X-files in immunity: sex-based differences predispose immune responses. Nat Rev Immunol. 2008;8:737–44.
20. Tam LS, Gu J, Yu D. Pathogenesis of ankylosing spondylitis. Nat Rev Rheumatol. 2010;6:399–405.
21. Kong S, Yeung P, Fang D. The class III histone deacetylase sirtuin 1 in immune suppression and its therapeutic potential in rheumatoid arthritis. J Genet Genomics. 2013;40:347–54.
22. Moon MH, Jeong JK, Lee YJ, Seol JW, Jackson CJ, Park SY. SIRT1, a class III histone deacetylase, regulates TNF-alpha-induced inflammation in human chondrocytes. Osteoarthr Cartil. 2013;21:470–80.
23. Cohen-Kfir E, Artsi H, Levin A, Abramowitz E, Bajayo A, Gurt I, et al. Sirt1 is a regulator of bone mass and a repressor of Sost encoding for sclerostin, a bone formation inhibitor. Endocrinology. 2011;152:4514–24.
24. Abed E, Couchourel D, Delalandre A, Duval N, Pelletier JP, Martel-Pelletier J, et al. Low sirtuin 1 levels in human osteoarthritis subchondral osteoblasts lead to abnormal sclerostin expression which decreases Wnt/beta-catenin activity. Bone. 2014;59:28–36.
25. Simic P, Zainabadi K, Bell E, Sykes DB, Saez B, Lotinun S, et al. SIRT1 regulates differentiation of mesenchymal stem cells by deacetylating beta-catenin. EMBO Mol Med. 2013;5:430–40.
26. Edwards JR, Perrien DS, Fleming N, Nyman JS, Ono K, Connelly L, et al. Silent information regulator (Sir)T1 inhibits NF-kappaB signaling to maintain normal skeletal remodeling. J Bone Miner Res. 2013;28:960–9.
27. Dragin N, Bismuth J, Cizeron-Clairac G, Biferi MG, Berthault C, Serraf A, et al. Estrogen-mediated downregulation of AIRE influences sexual dimorphism in autoimmune diseases. J Clin Invest. 2016;126:1525–37.

28. Taurog JD, Chhabra A, Colbert RA. Ankylosing spondylitis and axial Spondyloarthritis. N Engl J Med. 2016;375:1303.

29. Ota H, Akishita M, Akiyoshi T, Kahyo T, Setou M, Ogawa S, et al. Testosterone deficiency accelerates neuronal and vascular aging of SAMP8 mice: protective role of eNOS and SIRT1. PLoS One. 2012;7:e29598.

30. Ambarus C, Yeremenko N, Tak PP, Baeten D. Pathogenesis of spondyloarthritis: autoimmune or autoinflammatory? Curr Opin Rheumatol. 2012;24:351–8.

31. Rudwaleit M, van der Heijde D, Landewe R, Listing J, Akkoc N, Brandt J, et al. The development of assessment of SpondyloArthritis international society classification criteria for axial spondyloarthritis (part II): validation and final selection. Ann Rheum Dis. 2009;68:777–83.

32. Aletaha D, Neogi T, Silman AJ, Funovits J, Felson DT, Bingham CO 3rd, et al. 2010 rheumatoid arthritis classification criteria: an American College of Rheumatology/European league against rheumatism collaborative initiative. Arthritis Rheum. 2010;62:2569–81.

33. Taylor W, Gladman D, Helliwell P, Marchesoni A, Mease P, Mielants H, et al. Classification criteria for psoriatic arthritis: development of new criteria from a large international study. Arthritis Rheum. 2006;54:2665–73.

34. Hu S, Xie Z, Onishi A, Yu X, Jiang L, Lin J, et al. Profiling the human protein-DNA interactome reveals ERK2 as a transcriptional repressor of interferon signaling. Cell. 2009;139:610–22.

35. Silver JD, Ritchie ME, Smyth GK. Microarray background correction: maximum likelihood estimation for the normal-exponential convolution. Biostatistics. 2009;10:352–63.

36. Meyer S, Woodward M, Hertel C, Vlaicu P, Haque Y, Karner J, et al. AIRE-deficient patients harbor unique high-affinity disease-ameliorating autoantibodies. Cell. 2016;166:582–95.

19

A novel approach for rapid high-throughput selection of recombinant functional rat monoclonal antibodies

Qin Chen[†], Shengping Qiu[†], Huanhuan Li, Chaolong Lin, Yong Luo, Wenfeng Ren, Yidi Zou, Yale Wang, Ninghshao Xia and Chenghao Huang[*]

Abstract

Background: Most monoclonal antibodies against mouse antigens have been derived from rat spleen-mouse myeloma fusions, which are valuable tools for purposes ranging from general laboratory reagents to therapeutic drugs, and yet selecting and expressing them remains a time-consuming and inefficient process. Here, we report a novel approach for the rapid high-throughput selection and expression of recombinant functional rat monoclonal antibodies with different isotypes.

Results: We have developed a robust system for generating rat monoclonal antibodies through several processes involving simultaneously immunizing rats with three different antigens expressing in a mixed cell pools, preparing hybridoma cell pools, in vitro screening and subsequent cloning of the rearranged light and heavy chains into a single expression plasmid using a highly efficient assembly method, which can decrease the time and effort required by multiple immunizations and fusions, traditional clonal selection and expression methods. Using this system, we successfully selected several rat monoclonal antibodies with different IgG isotypes specifically targeting the mouse PD-1, LAG-3 or AFP protein from a single fusion. We applied these recombinant anti-PD-1 monoclonal antibodies (32D6) in immunotherapy for therapeutic purposes that produced the expected results.

Conclusions: This method can be used to facilitate an increased throughput of the entire process from multiplex immunization to acquisition of functional rat monoclonal antibodies and facilitate their expression and feasibility using a single plasmid.

Keywords: Rat monoclonal antibody, Multiplex immunization, High-throughput, Recombinant expression, Immunotherapy study

Background

Mice are generally used to generate hybridoma cells producing monoclonal antibodies (mAbs) against antigens from various species but are seldom used to produce antibodies against mouse antigens due to their tolerance of syngeneic antigens [1, 2]. Rats can provide a large number of spleen B cells that are available for fusion with myeloma cells, which are extremely suitable for generating mAbs against mouse antigens [3]. The ability of rat monoclonal antibodies (RtmAbs) to bind with

high selectivity and affinity to their targets makes them extremely important tools for biomedical research, especially for immune-detection of antigens from a mouse background and for functional evaluation of immunotherapeutic antibodies in immunocompetent mice [4–6]. In addition, RtmAbs possess great performance in recognizing additional epitopes, especially for small and poor immunogenic antigens [7, 8].

The cell fusion technique first reported in 1975 made it possible to generate hybridoma cells producing mAbs [9]. Since then, the methods for mAb production have been improved, and hybridoma technology is now well established [9, 10]. Most RtmAbs have been derived from rat spleen-mouse myeloma fusions using classical

* Correspondence: huangchenghao@xmu.edu.cn
[†]Qin Chen and Shengping Qiu contributed equally to this work.
State Key Laboratory of Molecular Vaccinology and Molecular Diagnostics, National Institute of Diagnostics and Vaccine Development in Infectious Diseases, School of Public Health, Xiamen University, Xiamen 361102, China

hybridoma technology [3, 11]. However, to our knowledge, some of the rat×mouse hybridoma clones grow slowly and would be gradually lost during the clonal selection step due to their instability, and it's also difficult to produce high-quality or large scale RtmAbs from ascites or culture supernatants. Therefore, clonal selecting and expressing RtmAbs requires multiple rounds of clonal selection and continued cell culture, which makes it a time-consuming and inefficient process to obtain the desired RtmAbs [12].

Our aim was to perform rapid high-throughput selection and expression of functional RtmAbs with high affinity and specificity to mouse antigens that could be used as therapeutic mAbs in immunocompetent mouse models and for detecting murine antigens out of a mouse background. To achieve the high-throughput selection of antibodies of a given specificity, we have chosen the injection of pooled cells consisting of three different antigen-expressing cells, which are highly immunogenic and are simple to obtain and use [13]. This procedure may bring about a disadvantage in that the hybridoma cells will be producing antibodies against virtually all cellular antigens and will require several screening steps to select antigen-specific hybridoma cells; however, because only one cycle of screening is needed, this immunization protocol is easy, and multiple immunogens can be easily obtained, which can facilitate the high-throughput immunization process. Moreover, the multiplex immunization strategy, which simultaneously immunised the rat with three different antigens for the purpose of saving time and biological resources, has not been previously reported.

The biggest bottleneck in the screening process of stable and homogenous hybridoma clones is the time-consuming and labour-intensive screening of positive hybridoma cells. To streamline the screening process and avoid the clones missing, these steps were replaced by cloning the rearranged light and heavy chains into a single expression plasmid utilizing the highly efficient Gibson assembly method [14].

Here, we report a robust system for high-throughput generation of recombinant functional RtmAbs through several processes involving simultaneously immunizing rats with three different antigens-of-interest expressing in a mixed cell pools, preparing hybridoma cell pools, in vitro screening of colonized cells using high-throughput cell-based ELISA and subsequently cloning the rearranged light and heavy chains into a single expression plasmid using a highly efficient assembly method, which can successfully select several RtmAbs with different IgG isotypes targeting the mouse PD-1, LAG-3 or AFP protein. We applied the resulting recombinant anti-PD-1 antibodies in immunotherapy to therapeutic purposes that generated the expected results. This method can be used to facilitate an increased throughput and rapid process of enabling the generation of diverse panels of functional recombinant RtmAbs from immunized rats and other hosts.

Results

Overview of a novel approach for the rapid high-throughput selection and expression of recombinant functional RtmAbs.

The schematic illustration of the method is outlined in Fig. 1. This method is based on cell immunization with pooled cells consisting of antigen-expressing cells and standard hybridoma technology with rat spleen-mouse myeloma fusions, which enable researchers to gain easy access to the immunogen and ensures that the fusion process for hybridoma preparation is operating at high efficiency. We can select RtmAbs against different antigens from a single rat immunized with pooled cells consisting of different antigen-expressing cells, either cell surface antigens or secreted antigens. Because of the time-consuming and labour-intensive process of clonal selection that is required for isolation of stable and homogenous hybridoma clones, positive hybridoma clones were first screened through indirect cell-based ELISA and then directly subjected to RT-PCR for amplifying rearranged heavy and light variable regions, which greatly improved the screening efficiency. Then, the amplified heavy and light variable regions were cloned into a single expression plasmid that could express full-length rat antibodies from a single ORF joined by the FMDV 2A self-processing peptide [15]. Thus, a large number of antibodies can be quickly produced by transiently transfecting mammalian cells. The biological activity of recombinant RtmAbs were thereafter validated in vitro and in vivo by functional evaluation.

Immunogen design and verification

Mouse PD-1-, LAG-3-, and AFP-expressing U-2 OS cells (mPD-1 U-2 OS, mLAG-3 U-2 OS and mAFP U-2 OS) were established separately and verified for their antigen expression. Cell surface antigen mPD-1 and mLAG-3 were analysed by flow cytometry, which showed high expression of the corresponding antigen (Fig. 2a). Because mAFP is a secreted protein, cell-based ELISA was established for verifying antigen expression. After specific antibody staining, mPD-1 U-2 OS, mLAG-3 U-2 OS and mAFP U-2 OS showed high expression of the corresponding antigen (Fig. 2b).

Proof of principle: Cloning of the 32D6 RtmAb against mouse PD-1

To highly efficiently clone the heavy and light chain variable region of the RtmAb from hybridoma cells, we designed two sets of specific primers to separately amplify the rat immunoglobulin variable regions of the heavy and light κ chain by analysing 115 signal peptide sequences of the heavy chain and 21 signal peptide sequences of the

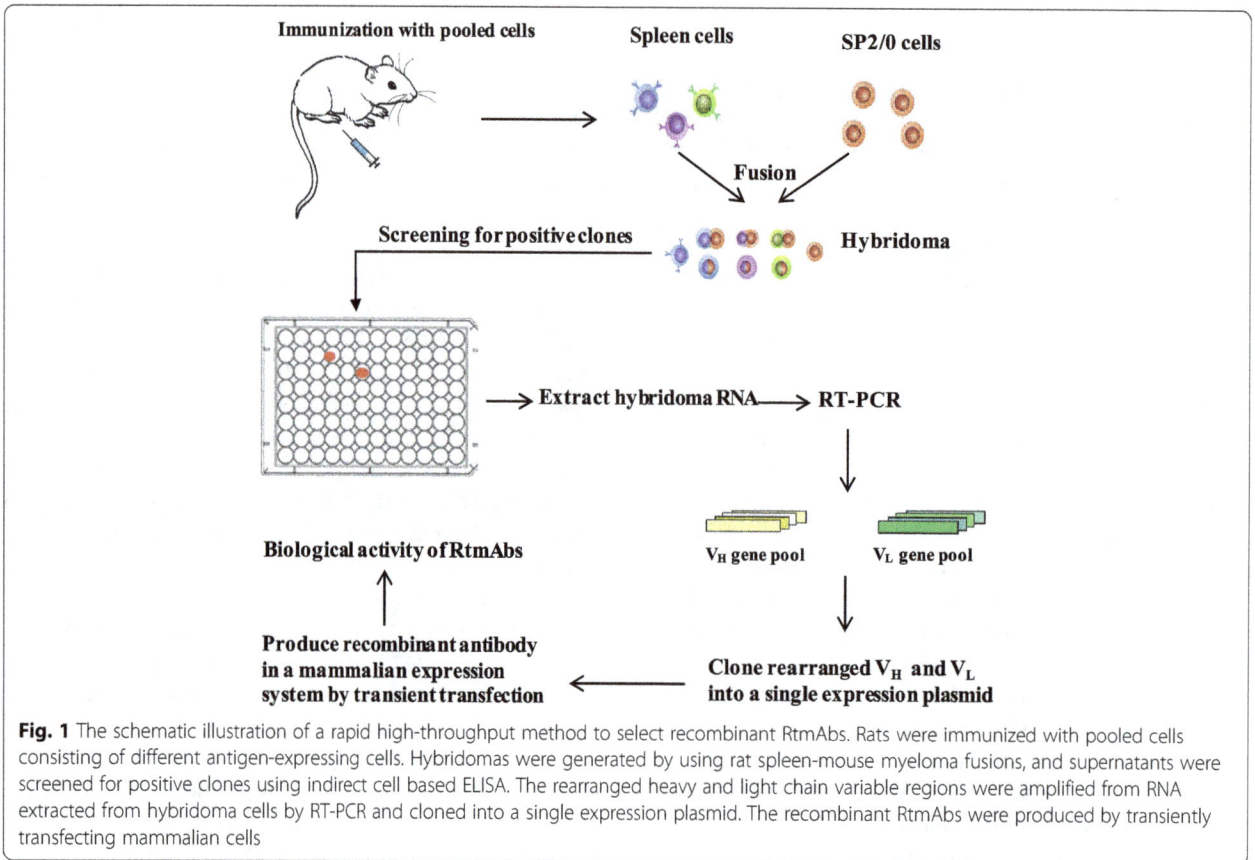

Fig. 1 The schematic illustration of a rapid high-throughput method to select recombinant RtmAbs. Rats were immunized with pooled cells consisting of different antigen-expressing cells. Hybridomas were generated by using rat spleen-mouse myeloma fusions, and supernatants were screened for positive clones using indirect cell based ELISA. The rearranged heavy and light chain variable regions were amplified from RNA extracted from hybridoma cells by RT-PCR and cloned into a single expression plasmid. The recombinant RtmAbs were produced by transiently transfecting mammalian cells

light κ chain retrieved from the IMGT database, which represents 99 and 100% of the signal peptide sequence of the retrieved light and heavy chain. We also designed one universal reverse primer corresponding to the constant region of the heavy chain or the light κ chain, which additionally included a specific sequencing primer for subsequent sequencing (Table 1). Primers to amplify the λ light chains were not included in this study due to a lack of enough signal peptide sequences of the λ chain retrieved from the IMGT database.

By using this method, we cloned the heavy and light chain variable regions of the RtmAbs against mouse PD-1,

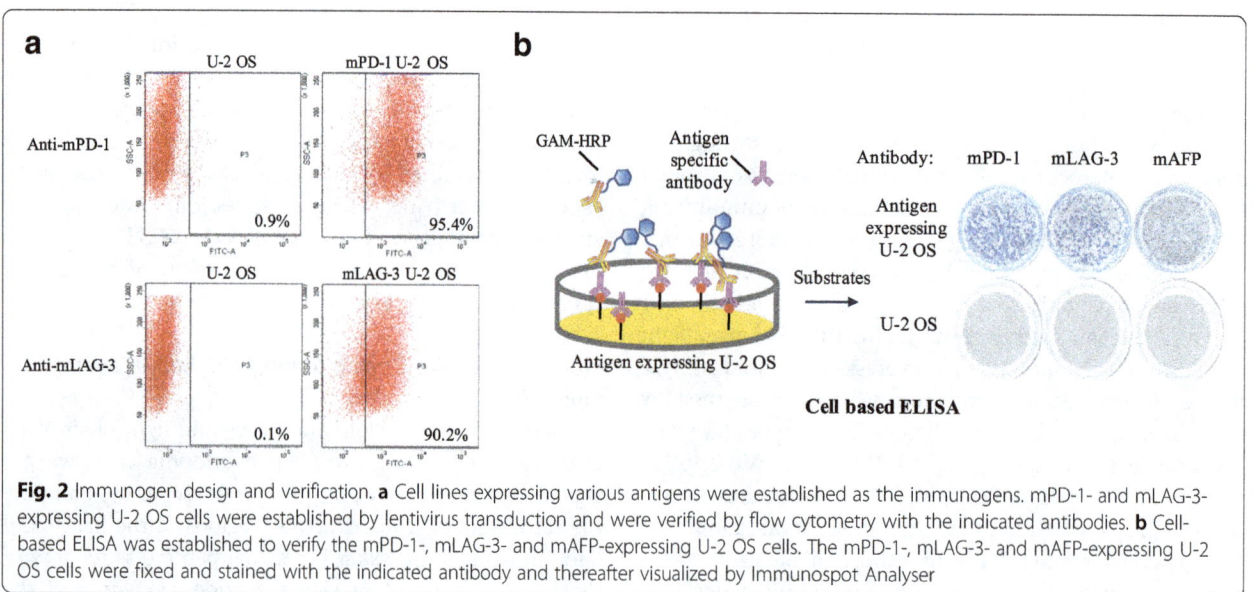

Fig. 2 Immunogen design and verification. **a** Cell lines expressing various antigens were established as the immunogens. mPD-1- and mLAG-3-expressing U-2 OS cells were established by lentivirus transduction and were verified by flow cytometry with the indicated antibodies. **b** Cell-based ELISA was established to verify the mPD-1-, mLAG-3- and mAFP-expressing U-2 OS cells. The mPD-1-, mLAG-3- and mAFP-expressing U-2 OS cells were fixed and stained with the indicated antibody and thereafter visualized by Immunospot Analyser

Table 1 Primers used for the generation of recombinant rat monoclonal antibodies

Reverse primer used for the amplification of heavy chain variable regions	Reverse primer used for the amplification of κ light chain variable regions
R1: AGGATCCAGGRRCCARKGGATAGACAGATG	R2: AGGAGATGGTGGGAAGATGGATACAGTTG
Degenerate primer used for the amplification of heavy chain variable regions	Degenerate primer used for the amplification of κ light chain variable regions
hF:	κF:
1. GCCCGTTTCTGCTAGC ATGTTGGTSCTGMAGTKGGTTTTSGTG	1. GCAATCCAGGTCCA ATGAAAATGACGACACCTGCTCAGTTC
2. GCCCGTTTCTGCTAGC ATGAGACTACTAGGTCTTCTCCTGTGC	2. GCAATCCAGGTCCA ATGAGGGCCCCTTTTCAGTTACTTGGG
3. GCCCGTTTCTGCTAGC ATGGGATGGAGCCAGATCATCCTCTTT	3. GCAATCCAGGTCCA ATGTCTAAAAACTTATTAGAAGTTTCA
4. GCCCGTTTCTGCTAGC ATGGTTTTCGGGCTGATCCTTTTTCTT	4. GCAATCCAGGTCCA ATGGTAAGTCCTGCCCAGTTCCTGTTT
5. GCCCGTTTCTGCTAGC ATGATGGGTTTAGGGGTGATTCTTTTT	5. GCAATCCAGGTCCA ATGATGGCTGCAGTTCAACTCTTAGGG
6. GCCCGTTTCTGCTAGC ATGGGGATTGAGCTGGGTTTTTCTTGTT	6. GCAATCCAGGTCCA ATGAAAGTGCCTGGTAGGCTGCTGGTG
7. GCCCGTTTCTGCTAGC ATGGACTTGCGACTGACTTATGTCTTT	7. GCAATCCAGGTCCA ATGAAGTGGCTGTTAGTCTGTTGGTGC
8. GCCCGTTTCTGCTAGC ATGACTATCCTGGTGCTTCTCCTCTGT	8. GCAATCCAGGTCCA ATGATTCCTGCCCAGTTCCTGTTTCTG
9. GCCCGTTTCTGCTAGC ATGGCTRTCCTGGTGCTGTTGCTCTGC	9. GCAATCCAGGTCCA ATGATGAGTCCTGCCCAGTTCCTGTTT
10. GCCCGTTTCTGCTAGC ATGRAATGSARCTGGRTCWTYYTCTTY	10. GCAATCCAGGTCCA ATGAATTTTCAGGTGCAGGTTTTTAGC
11. GCCCGTTTCTGCTAGC ATGGCTGTCCTGGTGCTGTTGCTCTGC	11. GCAATCCAGGTCCA ATGAAYGTGYCCACTCAACTCCTTGGG
12. GCCCGTTTCTGCTAGC ATGAGARYGYYGRKTCTTCTGTACCTG	12. GCAATCCAGGTCCA ATGGACATGAGGGCCCATRCTCAGTTT
13. GCCCGTTTCTGCTAGC ATGGACWTCAGNCTCAGCTTGGBTTTC	13. GCAATCCAGGTCCA ATGARRKTYSNBVYTSAGYTTYKKGGG
14. GCCCGTTTCTGCTAGC ATGRAGTTGDGSMTRANCTGGRTTTTY	
Primer used for the amplification of heavy and light chains	
F3: CATCTGTCTATCCACTGGCTCCTGGAAC	R3: TGACAGGTGCGCGTTTAGCACG TCATTTACCCGGAGAGTGGGAGAG
F4: CGTGCTAAACGCGCACCTGTCAAAC	R4: TGGACCTGGATTGCTTTCTACATC
F5: CAACTGTATCCATCTTCCCACCATC	R5: GATCCGGCCTTGCCGGC CCTAACACTCATTCCTGTTGAAG

The primers used to amplify the heavy and κ light chain were designed using the genome sequence of the rat immunoglobulin: GenBank: DQ402471.1 for the κ light chain and GenBank: BC095846.1 for the heavy chain. Degenerate base code: M = A + C; R = A + G; W = A + T; S = C + G; Y = C + T; K = G + T; V = A + C + G; B = C + G + T; D = G + A + T; N = C + G + A + T

LAG-3 and AFP. We used a hybridoma (32D6) that secreted a rat anti-PD-1 IgG$_{2a}$ as a proof-of-principle. By using the designed primers, we successfully amplified PCR products from the heavy and light chain variable regions with the expected sizes (Fig. 3a). The expression sequence of the heavy chain or κ light chain of recombinant 32D6 contained a signal peptide, a variable region and a constant region. After sequencing confirmation, the κ light chain and heavy chain with their signal peptides were cloned into an expression plasmid PTT5 driven by the CMV promoter, and containing a joint fragment comprising the furin cleavage site and the 2A sequence. The assembly result in a 6.574-kbp product (Fig. 3b and c).

After transient transfection in HEK 293 cells, the plasmid expressed the recombinant rat anti-PD-1 IgG$_{2a}$ antibody. The supernatant of HEK 293 cells producing the recombinant 32D6 antibody (Rec 32D6) was separated by SDS-PAGE gel and analysed by western blot. The results under reducing conditions showed that the recombinant antibody expression from the expression plasmid had a balanced expression level of the heavy and light chains. Under non-reducing conditions, Rec 32D6 appeared as a single band, which indicated the natural association of the heavy and light chain of Rec 32D6 (Fig. 3d).

An indirect immunofluorescence assay was used to identify the binding specificity of Rec 32D6 and Hybridoma 32D6 (Hyb 32D6) purified from the parental 32D6 hybridoma cells, and the results showed that both Rec 32D6 and Hyb 32D6 could specifically bind to the mPD-1 U-2 OS cells (Fig. 3e).

Biological activity of rec 32D6

Rec 32D6 may differ in several respects from Hyb 32D6 secreted by the hybridoma cells. To prove that they have a comparable performance, the biological activity of Rec 32D6 was first evaluated in parallel with Hyb 32D6 in vitro. Using indirect CEIA to measure the binding activity, a good correlation in determining the reactivity of Rec 32D6 and Hyb 32D6 against the mPD-1 protein was observed. Rec 32D6 showed a slightly higher affinity than Hyb 32D6 (Fig. 4a). Using blocking CEIA to measure the blocking activity of Rec 32D6 for interfering with the interaction between mPD-1 and mPD-L1, Rec 32D6 showed a similar blocking activity to Hyb 32D6 (Fig. 4b).

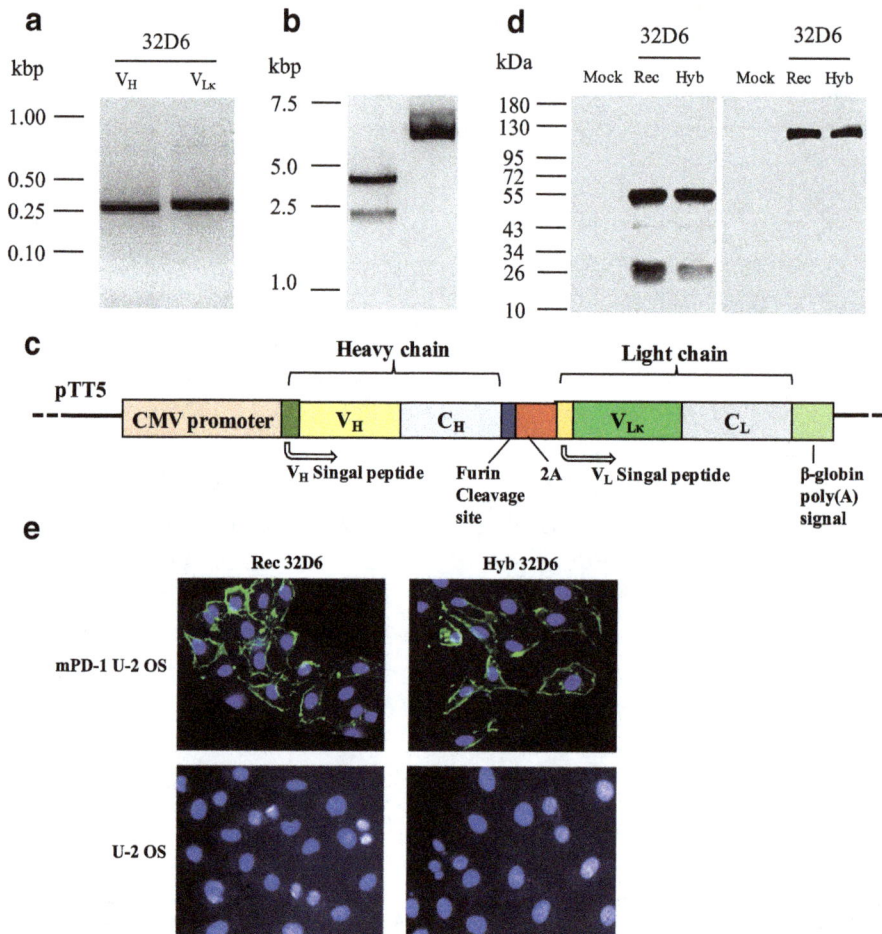

Fig. 3 Cloning of the 32D6 monoclonal antibody against mouse PD-1. **a** RT-PCR amplification of the light chain variable region (VLκ) and heavy chain variable region (VH) from the hybridoma 32D6. **b** Assembly of the 32D6 VH region and VLκ region through a joining fragment resulting in a 6.574-kbp product. **c** Schematic of the plasmid encoding the rat recombinant antibody with the FMDV 2A sequence. **d** Western blot analysis under reducing (left panel) or non-reducing (right panel) conditions: fresh culture medium (Mock), supernatant of cells producing the recombinant 32D6 antibody (Rec 32D6) or the 32D6 monoclonal antibody purified from the parental hybridoma (Hyb 32D6). **e** Immunofluorescence analysis of mPD-1 U-2 OS and U-2 OS cells with Rec 32D6 and Hyb 32D6

The results showed that Rec 32D6 exhibited comparable affinities and full biological activity with Hyb 32D6.

Moreover, we investigated the anti-tumour efficacy of these anti-PD-1 antibodies in a syngeneic tumour model bearing mouse kidney tumours. It was observed that tumour growth was significantly inhibited in both the Rec 32D6 (5/5) and Hyb 32D6 (5/5) treatment groups and there were no toxicities and abnormal weight changes during the treatment (Fig. 4c and d). The results showed that Rec 32D6 exhibited comparable therapeutic efficacy to Hyb 32D6 in vivo.

Selection of multiple RtmAbs with different IgG isotypes from a single fusion

We immunized rats with pooled cells consisting of three different antigen-expressing cells, and the hybridoma supernatants were tested by high-throughput cell-based ELISA to ensure that the secreted antibodies retained specificity for their antigens. After the fusion process, the hybridoma cells were counted and one eighth of them were plated over twenty 96-well plates at a density of 1 cell/well for culture. After clonal expansion for 2 weeks, 1920 supernatants were screened using cell-based ELISA. Of the three different immunized antigens, 20 positive hybridoma supernatants were identified for these three antigens and each of them were subjected to subsequent recombinant construction. Of these 20, 13 were found to weakly cross-react with U-2 OS cells when re-tested by cell based ELISA, but seven recombinant RtmAbs retained high binding specificity to antigen-expressing U-2 OS cells (Additional file 1: Figure S1). These were subjected to isotype phenotyping (Table 2). For each hybridoma, cDNA was synthesized and used to independently amplify both heavy and light chains before joining them into a single expression plasmid.

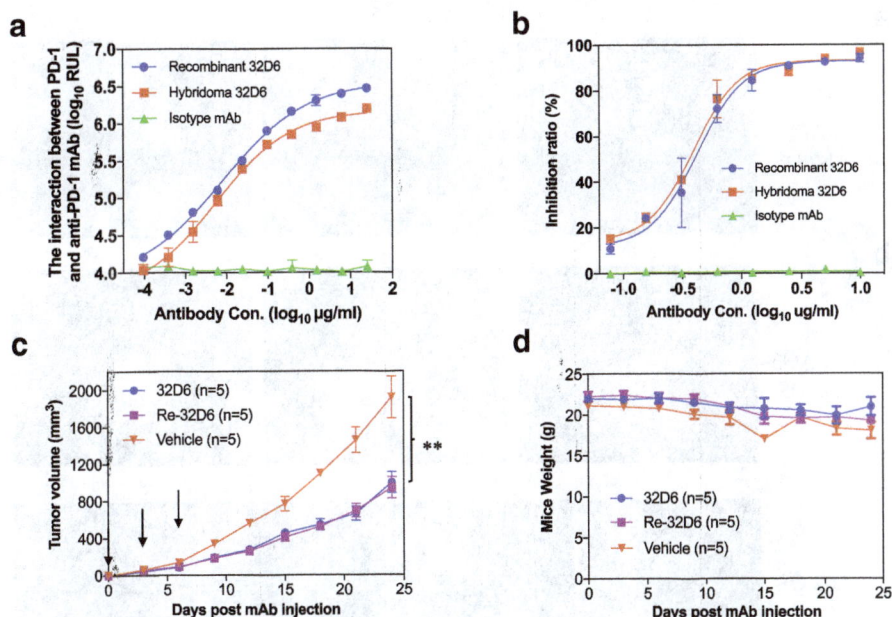

Fig. 4 Biological activity of 32D6 RtmAbs. **a** The reactivity of anti-PD-1 (Rec 32D6 and Hyb 32D6) against his-mPD-1 protein was determined by indirect CEIA. **b** The blocking activity of anti-PD-1 (Rec 32D6 and Hyb 32D6) was determined by a blocking CEIA. **c**, **d** The therapeutic efficacy of anti-PD-1 (Rec 32D6 and Hyb 32D6) was evaluated in a syngeneic tumour model bearing a mouse kidney tumour

Seven hybridoma cells producing functional antibodies with high specificity for which the heavy and light chains were cloned contained a productively rearranged VH and VL region. For antibody subtyping, two recombinant RtmAbs against mouse AFP belonged to the IgG$_1$ isotype, and one recombinant RtmAbs against mouse AFP belonged to the IgG$_{2a}$ isotype. Two recombinant RtmAbs against mouse PD-1 belonged to the IgG$_{2a}$ or IgG$_{2b}$ isotype. Two recombinant RtmAbs against mouse LAG-3 belonged to the IgG$_{2b}$ isotype. All seven RtmAbs were successfully applied in immunofluorescence assays with high binding specificity (Figs. 3e and 5a-c). These data validate that the overall strategy is suitable for high-throughput production of RtmAbs with different IgG isotypes against multiple antigens.

Table 2 A summary of the antibodies selected from a single fusion

Clone	Antigen	Antibody name	Isotype	VH	VL
1.1	mAFP	10B3	IgG1	V1–68 + D1 + J1	V3S19 + J2
1.1	mAFP	10H3	IgG1	V2–41 + D1 + J2	V3S19 + J2
1.1	mAFP	6B8	IgG2a	V2–43 + D1 + J4	V2S23 + J4
2.1	mPD-1	32D6	IgG2a	V1–28 + D5 + J1	V1S13 + J2
2.1	mPD-1	8E2	IgG2b	V7–7 + D1 + J4	V1S19 + J2
3.1	mLAG-3	12D9	IgG2b	V5–50 + D1 + J2	V12S16 + J2
3.1	mLAG-3	1B2	IgG2b	V5–50 + D4 + J2	V14S14 + J2

Discussion

Rat-LOU is excellent for generating mAbs against small and poor immunogenic molecules and yields excellent results against murine antigens. The rat antibodies can be paired with existing antibodies in immunoassays and widely used for therapeutic purposes as cancer immunotherapy.

High-affinity, functionally validated RtmAbs are valuable biomedical reagents, but their acquisition can be time-consuming, labour-intensive and expensive. As far as we know, almost all methods used to produce RtmAbs are based on traditional methods, which are inefficient and inconvenient to obtain the desired RtmAbs. In this study, by immunizing with pooled cells consisting of antigen-expressing cells and quickly cloning the productively rearranged variable antibody regions, we have greatly reduced the time, number of steps, and resources needed to isolate RtmAbs that work in immunotherapy studies and in antigen detection [16]. Importantly, smaller laboratories can benefit from this procedure since only minimal equipment and resources are required.

Compared with traditional methods, our method offers several advantages for producing RtmAbs. The first advantage of this method is cell immunization, which saves not only time and effort but also the amounts of immunogens that are often very valuable or difficult to obtain. We have chosen the injection of whole cells expressing different antigens, which are highly immunogenic and are simple to obtain and use. Although this procedure presents a disadvantage in that hybridomas are produced against virtually all cellular antigens and require several

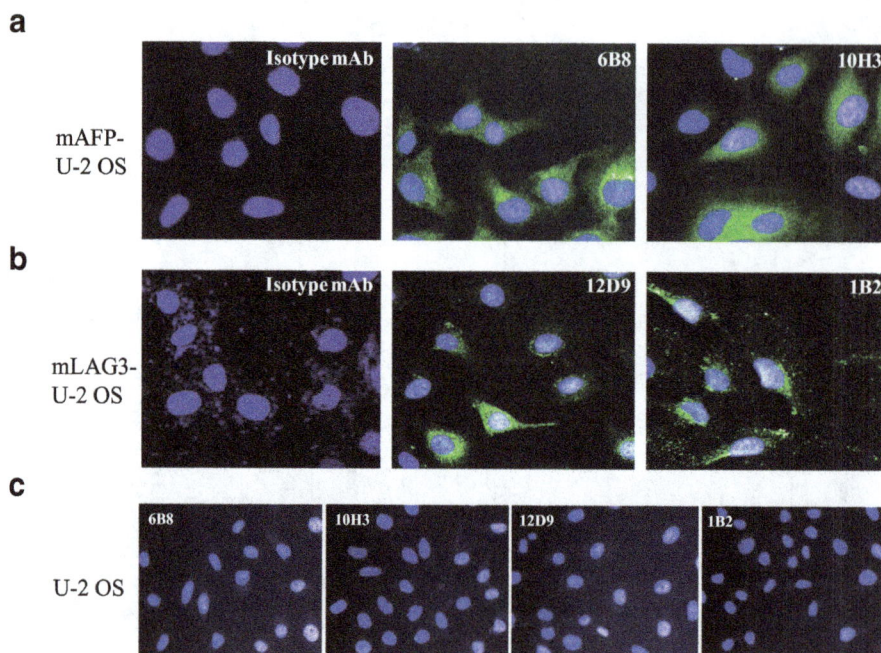

Fig. 5 Immunofluorescence analysis of recombinant anti-mLAG-3 and anti-mAFP antibodies. **a** mLAG-3 U-2 OS cells were stained with rat recombinant 12D9 and 1B2 antibodies. **b** mAFP U-2 OS cells were stained with rat recombinant 6B8 and 10H3 antibodies. **c** U-2 OS cells were stained with rat recombinant 12D9, 1B2, 6B8 and 10H3 antibodies

screening steps to select for anti-antigen-specific hybridoma cells, the immunization protocol is easy and function-blocking antibodies against surface antigens (anti-mPD-1 and anti-mLAG-3) and detection antibodies against cellular antigens (anti-mAFP) can both be readily obtained.

Another advantage of this method is that mouse SP2/0 myeloma cells are used as the fusion partner in this method, and there is absolutely no difficulty in preparing rat×mouse hybridomas. Although reliable rat myeloma cells have already been established, there are still some obstacles in their usage, such as poor cellular adherence, low fusion efficiency and low rates of positive rat×rat hybridomas. Therefore, there might be no advantage compared to the rat×mouse hybridoma method. One potential obstacle of the rat×mouse hybridoma might be mandatory use of nude mice or nude rats for obtaining ascites. In our method, the step involving ascites production is eliminated since the antibody expression sequences of desired antibodies are directly amplified from the positive hybridoma clones.

The third advantage is that we can clone the rat antibody genes out of a positive rat hybridoma clone and use our transient transfection technology to produce the rat antibody for use at any scale [17, 18]. Several molecular cloning steps have been eliminated to significantly enhance precise cloning of the positive hybridoma clones using a well-designed set of degenerate primers and the Gibson assembly method.

A few steps that could use improvement were noted during the optimization process. Given that pooled primers were used, it is possible that nonspecific amplification occurred during the PCR process. To minimize this issue, a specific sequencing primer was added to the 5′ terminus of a set of degenerate forward primers used for the amplification of the heavy and light chain variable regions to correct the obtained sequence by sequencing the PCR products. To streamline the molecular cloning process, multiple ligation and digestion steps were eliminated by utilizing the highly efficient Gibson assembly method. Five PCR fragments, including heavy and light chain variable regions, a joint fragment comprising the furin cleavage site and 2A sequence and the heavy and light chain constant regions, were sequentially cloned into a single vector by homologous recombination.

Because therapeutic human mAbs do not always cross-react with animal tissues, experiments in mice models can be performed using a surrogate antibody [19], which is a mAb directed against the murine antigen. Several surrogate mAbs recognizing mouse antigens have been developed against mouse PD-1 [20] or PD-L1 targets in rats [21], which can be considered as surrogates of Keytruda, Opdivo or Tecentriq. Therefore, we shall detail the procedure we followed to produce and screen RtmAbs against mouse PD-1 that was successful in our hands and that can be adapted for specific therapeutic purposes. Moreover, the RtmAbs recognizing the mouse PD-1 antigen have been chimaerised as rat/mouse mAbs to move closer to the murine system for better immunotherapy [22]. Recent advances in tumour immunology have highlighted the key role of these surrogate antibodies in drug development, raising new hopes for rapid high-throughput production of these valuable reagents [23].

Conclusions

We have reported the development of a novel approach for biomedical scientists that streamlines the production of RtmAbs recognizing mouse antigens. In this paper, we have used this method to raise antibodies against multiple mouse antigens, but it could also be broadly applied to any species that can raise a humoural immune response in rats. As only minimal equipment is required, this technique can also be used by smaller laboratories. Cloning of the rearranged light and heavy chains of selected monoclonal antibodies into a single mammalian expression vector facilitates their distribution, increasing the scope for the creation of valuable antibody resources.

Methods
Cells

FreeStyle 293-F cells (catalogue number: R790–07) were purchased from Invitrogen and maintained in FreeStyle™ 293 Expression Medium containing 10% foetal bovine serum (FBS), 100 U/mL penicillin, and 100 μg/mL streptomycin. Human U-2 OS cells (catalogue number: HTB-96), 293 T cells (catalogue number: CRL-3216) and Renca cells (catalogue number: CRL-2947) were purchased from American Type Culture Collection (ATCC) and maintained in Dulbecco's-modified Eagle's medium (DMEM) containing 10% foetal bovine serum (FBS), 100 U/mL penicillin, and 100 μg/mL streptomycin.

Immunogen preparation

The full-length genes of mouse antigens PD-1, LAG-3, and AFP were amplified and ligated into the pLv vector by the Gibson assembly method. The expression vector for each antigen, together with its packaging plasmids, was transfected into 293 T cells using PEI transfection reagents. Supernatants containing lentivirus were harvested 2 days after transfection, and the U-2 OS cells were transduced with the harvested supernatants in the presence of 6 μg/mL polybrene. Then, 24 h after transduction, the U-2 OS cells were treated with 1 μg/mL puromycin for one week. Mouse PD-1-, LAG-3- and AFP-expressing U-2 OS cells were maintained in DMEM containing 10% FBS and 0.5 μg/mL puromycin. Mouse PD-1- and LAG-3-expressing U-2 OS cells were verified by flow cytometry using commercialized antibodies. Mouse PD-1-, LAG-3- and AFP-expressing U-2 OS cells were verified by cell-based ELISA as previously described [24].

Immunizations

For the preparation of rat monoclonal antibodies, one six-week-old female LOU rat was maintained in individually ventilated cages under specific pathogen free condition and immunized with immunogens at multiple sites by standard vaccination procedures. In brief, the rat received primary immunization with 1×10^6 pooled cells intraperitoneally, consisting of the same amount of PD-1-, LAG-3-, and AFP-expressing U-2 OS cells, and then received immunization (three times) with 6×10^6 pooled cells at two-week intervals. Rats with high serum titres against the indicated immunogens were finally boosted by intra-spleen immunization with 1×10^6 pooled cells 3 days before the hybridoma generation. The use of the rat was approved by the Institutional Animal Care and Use Committee at Xiamen University.

Hybridoma generation

The hybridoma generation procedure followed the protocol reported previously with minor modifications [25]. The immunized rat was firstly euthanized with pentobarbital (200 mg/kg, i.p.), and then followed by spleen dissection and dissociation. The rat splenocytes and mouse SP2/0 myeloma cells were fused at a ratio of 5:1 using PEG 1450 according to a standard protocol. One eighth of the resulting hybridoma cells were plated on twenty 96-well plates at a density of 1 cell/well and initially grown in RPMI 1640 medium supplemented with 20% foetal bovine serum for 24 h. Then, the hybridoma cells were selected with HAT conditioned medium for 2 weeks.

Antibody screening

The supernatant from each well was assayed by cell-based ELISA plated with the indicated immunogens. Briefly, 96-well plates were plated with 10^4 cells/well of a mixed cell pools of three antigen-expressing U-2 OS cells or U-2 OS cells, and the cells were fixed with 1% paraformaldehyde and permeabilized by 0.1% Triton X-100. After washing, the nonspecific binding was blocked with PBS containing 5% BSA, and 50 μl of supernatant was added to the wells for 60 min, followed by washing and reaction with HRP goat anti-rat IgG antibody (Biolegend, San Diego, USA). After the addition of TMB substrate solution for 30 min, the reaction was terminated by addition of an acidic STOP solution. The plates were spin dried and counted using ImmunSpot@S5 UV Analyzer (Cellular Technology Limited). Finally, 20 positive clones secreting antibodies specifically against the indicated immunogens were screened and selected. The isotype phenotyping of antibodies were performed by cell-based ELISA using isotype-specific antibodies. Briefly, after cells plating and fixation, 50 μl of supernatant was added to the wells for 60 min, followed by washing and reaction with HRP goat anti-rat IgM, G1, G2a, G2b and G2c secondary antibody (Invitrogen).

32D6 Colonized culture

For stable and homogenous clonal selection, dilution of 32D6 positive cells to 1 cell/ per well to maximize the proportion of wells that contain one single clone. After colonized culture for 2 weeks, the supernatants were assayed for their reactivity with corresponding antigen. A single clone with high reactivity to PD-1 was picked out for further clonal selection. Three or more cloning procedures were carried out until > 90% of the wells containing single clones are positive for antibody production.

RNA isolation and gene amplification

Twenty positive hybridoma clones were selected for RNA isolation. Total RNA was extracted with TRIzol Reagent (Invitrogen) and was reverse-transcribed into cDNA with random primers by SuperScript® III Reverse Transcriptase (Invitrogen). The cDNA products were then used as the template in PCR amplification with KOD-Plus polymerase (TOYOBO, Japan). The primer sequences designed for amplifying the variable regions of the heavy and light chains are listed in Table 1. The functional rearranged heavy variable region of the positive hybridoma clone was amplified using a set of 14 degenerate forward primers, representing almost all of the signal peptide sequences of the heavy chain, and one universal reverse primer corresponding to the constant region of the heavy chain. Similarly, the functional rearranged light variable region was amplified using a set of 13 degenerate forward primers, representing almost all of the signal peptide sequences of κ light chain, and one universal reverse primer corresponding to the constant region of the κ light chain. The PCR products were separated on a 2% agarose gel. The PCR fragments with approximately 350 bp for the heavy variable region and approximately 320 bp for the light variable region were isolated for further analysis.

Construction of the antibody expression plasmid

Assembly of the rearranged heavy and light variable regions through a joint fragment composed of the constant region of the heavy chain, furin cleavage site and 2A sequence, as well as the constant region of the light chain, was created by the Gibson assembly method with the primers listed in Table 1. The heavy and light variable regions were amplified from the selected cDNA products with forward primer hF1~hF14 with a leading sequence of the heavy chain containing a NheI site and reverse primer R1, and forward primer κF1~ κF13 and reverse primer R2 containing a NaeI site. The constant region of the heavy chain was amplified from rat genomic DNA with primers F3 and R3. The fragments containing the furin cleavage site and 2A sequence were

synthesized and amplified with primers F4 and R4. The constant region of the light chain was amplified from rat genomic DNA with primers F5 and R5. All PCR products were gel-purified and assembled into a NheI and NaeI digested PTT5 vector.

Antibody production

For antibody production from hybridomas, the hybridoma cells were cultured in EX-CELL® 620 HSF Serum-Free Medium (Invitrogen), and the supernatants were collected five days after culture. For recombinant antibody production, the antibody expression plasmid was transfected into FreeStyle 293-F cells using PEI transfection reagents. Supernatants were harvested 5 days after transfection, filtered, concentrated and stored at 4 °C. mAbs were purified by using protein G chromatography according to the manufacturer's instructions. Purified anti-mAFP antibodies (10B3, 10H3 and 6B8), anti-PD-1 antibodies (32D6 and 8E2) and anti-LAG-3 antibodies (12D9 and 1B2) were quantified with a BCA assay and stored at − 20 °C at a concentration of around 0.5 mg/mL in PBS.

Western blotting

mAbs were separated by SDS-PAGE under both reducing and non-reducing conditions and transferred onto a nitrocellulose membrane. After membranes were blocked with 5% BSA for 1 h, they were probed with HRP goat anti-rat IgG antibody (1 μg/mL) overnight at 4 °C, followed by rigorous washing, and finally visualized with the Lumi-Light[PLUS] western blotting substrate (Roche).

Immunostaining

Immunofluorescence staining was performed as previously described [24]. In brief, antigen-expressing U-2 OS cells on glass slides were fixed with 1% paraformaldehyde and permeabilized by 0.1% Triton X-100. After blocked with 5% normal BSA in PBS for 1 h, the slides were stained with antigen-specific antibody (1 μg/mL) overnight at 4 °C, then incubated with FITC conjugated secondary antibody before examination using a fluorescence microscope. The enzyme-linked Immunospot Assay was performed by the same procedure, except for using HRP conjugated secondary antibody before examination using the ImmunSpot@S5 UV Analyzer.

Functional analysis of rat monoclonal antibodies against PD-1

The reactivity of anti-PD-1 RtmAb (32D6) against his-mPD-1 protein was determined by indirect chemiluminescence immunoassay (CEIA). Briefly, 96-well plates were coated with 50 ng/well of his-mPD-1 protein, and nonspecific binding was blocked with PBS containing 20% CBS. Purified hybridoma 32D6 antibody or recombinant 32D6 antibody was first diluted starting from 25 μg/ml in

PBS containing 5% BSA, followed by four-fold serial dilutions with 10 gradients. A 100 μl dilution was added to the wells for 60 min, followed by washing and reaction with HRP goat anti-rat IgG antibody (Biolegend, San Diego, USA). After the addition of Luminol solution for 5 min, the plates were measured with a chemiluminescence reader (Berthod, DE). Control rat isotype IgG added at the same concentration served as a control.

To determine the blocking activity of the 32D6 antibody, a blocking CEIA detecting the interaction between his-PD-1 and biotinylated PD-L1 was developed. Briefly, 96-well plates were coated with 50 ng/well of his-PD-1 protein, and nonspecific binding was blocked with PBS containing 20% CBS. Purified hybridoma 32D6 antibody or recombinant 32D6 antibody was first diluted from 10 μg/ml in PBS containing 5% BSA, followed by two-fold serial dilutions with 8 gradients. Then, a 100 μl dilution or PBS and 100 ng/well biotinylated PD-L1 was added to the wells for 60 min, followed by washing and reaction with HRP goat anti-rat IgG antibody (Biolegend, San Diego, USA). After the addition of Luminol solution for 5 min, the plates were measured with a chemiluminescence reader (Berthod, DE). Control rat isotype IgG added at the same concentration served as a control. The inhibitory ratio was calculated as follows: %inhibitory = $100 \times (1 - $ (average value for each dilution/average value for control)). Each dilution was repeated in triplicate wells and each test was carried out in duplicate or triplicate. The results were interpreted by nonlinear, dose-response regression analysis using GraphPad Prism software.

Animal experiments

Fifteen 6-week-old C57BL/6 female mice were purchased from the Shanghai Slack Laboratory Animal Co., Ltd. and were bred in the Experimental Animal Center of Xiamen University. All mice were maintained in individually ventilated cages under specific pathogen free condition. An inoculum of 10^6 Renca tumour cells was injected s.c. into the flank of mice in 50 μl sterile PBS. Mice were randomized into two treatment groups and one control group ($n = 5$ for each group) on day 8 following tumour inoculation, immediately before treatment. Purified hybridoma 32D6 antibody or recombinant 32D6 antibody was administered via intraperitoneal injection at 200 μg every three days for a consecutive three dosages in total. Tumour growth and body weight were monitored every three days. Eighteen days after the last treatment, mice were euthanized with pentobarbital (200 mg/kg, i.p.). Tumour size was calculated as (length×width^2)/2, and the significant of the difference was analysed between different groups using Fisher's exact test. The use of the mice was approved by the Institutional Animal Care and Use Committee at Xiamen University.

Abbreviations

AFP: Alpha-fetoprotein; CEIA: Chemiluminescence immunoassay; ELISA: Enzyme-linked immunosorbent assay; IgG: Immunoglobulin G; LAG-3: Lymphocyte-activation gene 3; mAb: Monoclonal antibody; PCR: Polymerase chain reaction; PD-1: Programmed cell death-1; PD-L1: Programmed death-ligand 1; RtmAb: Rat monoclonal antibody; RT-PCR: Reverse transcription PCR

Acknowledgements

We thank Qingbing Zheng, Yuanzhi Chen and Quan Yuan for their technical help.

Funding

This work was sponsored by grant 2018ZX10301404–001-002 from the National Science and Technology Major Project and grant 81571990 from the National Natural Science Foundation of China. The funding sources had no role in the study design, data collection or analyses, the decision to publish, or the preparation of this manuscript.

Authors' contributions

CHH and NSX designed the study, QC and SPQ performed all of the experiments except the protein expression, which was performed by CLL, and the antibody screening, which was performed by HHL, YL, WFR, YDZ and YLW. CHH conceived the study and wrote the manuscript. NSX partially drafted the manuscript and revised it critically. All authors read and approved the final manuscript.

Competing interests

The authors declare that they have no competing interests.

References

1. Taggart RT, Samloff IM. Stable antibody-producing murine hybridomas. Science. 1983;219:1228–30.
2. Chiarella P, Fazio VM. Mouse monoclonal antibodies in biological research: strategies for high-throughput production. Biotechnol Lett. 2008;30:1303–10.
3. De Clercq L, Cormont F, Bazin H. Generation of rat-rat hybridomas with the use of the LOU IR983F nonsecreting fusion cell line. Methods Enzymol. 1986;121:234–8.
4. Harada A, Okada S, Saiwai H, Aoki M, Nakamura M, Ohkawa Y. Generation of a rat monoclonal antibody specific for Pax7. Hybridoma (Larchmt). 2009;28:451–3.
5. Yang W, Barth RF, Wu G, Ciesielski MJ, Fenstermaker RA, Moffat BA, et al. Development of a syngeneic rat brain tumor model expressing EGFRvIII and its use for molecular targeting studies with monoclonal antibody L8A4. Clin Cancer Res. 2005;11:341–50.
6. Onizuka S, Tawara I, Shimizu J, Sakaguchi S, Fujita T, Nakayama E. Tumor rejection by in vivo administration of anti-CD25 (interleukin-2 receptor alpha) monoclonal antibody. Cancer Res. 1999;59:3128–33.
7. Rottach A, Kremmer E, Nowak D, Leonhardt H, Cardoso MC. Generation and characterization of a rat monoclonal antibody specific for multiple red fluorescent proteins. Hybridoma (Larchmt). 2008;27:337–43.
8. Maiti PK, Im SH, Souroujon MC, Fuchs S. A monoclonal antibody specific for rat IL-18BP and its application in determining serum IL-18BP. Immunol Lett. 2003;85:65–70.

9. Kohler G, Milstein C. Continuous cultures of fused cells secreting antibody of predefined specificity. Nature. 1975;256:495–7.

10. Galfre G, Milstein C. Preparation of monoclonal antibodies: strategies and procedures. Methods Enzymol. 1981;73:3–46.

11. Kishiro Y, Kagawa M, Naito I, Sado Y. A novel method of preparing rat-monoclonal antibody-producing hybridomas by using rat medial iliac lymph node cells. Cell Struct Funct. 1995;20:151–6.

12. Delcommenne M, Streuli CH. Production of rat monoclonal antibodies specific for mouse integrins. Methods Mol Biol. 1999;129:19–34.

13. Roivainen M, Alakulppi N, Ylipaasto P, Eskelinen M, Paananen A, Airaksinen A, et al. A whole cell immunization-derived monoclonal antibody that protects cells from coxsackievirus A9 infection binds to both cell surface and virions. J Virol Methods. 2005;130:108–16.

14. Krebber A, Bornhauser S, Burmester J, Honegger A, Willuda J, Bosshard HR, et al. Reliable cloning of functional antibody variable domains from hybridomas and spleen cell repertoires employing a reengineered phage display system. J Immunol Methods. 1997;201:35–55.

15. Fang J, Qian JJ, Yi S, Harding TC, Tu GH, VanRoey M, et al. Stable antibody expression at therapeutic levels using the 2A peptide. Nat Biotechnol. 2005; 23:584–90.

16. Crosnier C, Staudt N, Wright GJ. A rapid and scalable method for selecting recombinant mouse monoclonal antibodies. BMC Biol. 2010;8:76.

17. Spidel JL, Vaessen B, Chan YY, Grasso L, Kline JB. Rapid high-throughput cloning and stable expression of antibodies in HEK293 cells. J Immunol Methods. 2016;439:50–8.

18. Smith K, Garman L, Wrammert J, Zheng NY, Capra JD, Ahmed R, et al. Rapid generation of fully human monoclonal antibodies specific to a vaccinating antigen. Nat Protoc. 2009;4:372–84.

19. Loisel S, Ohresser M, Pallardy M, Dayde D, Berthou C, Cartron G, et al. Relevance, advantages and limitations of animal models used in the development of monoclonal antibodies for cancer treatment. Crit Rev Oncol Hematol. 2007;62:34–42.

20. Woo SR, Turnis ME, Goldberg MV, Bankoti J, Selby M, Nirschl CJ, et al. Immune inhibitory molecules LAG-3 and PD-1 synergistically regulate T-cell function to promote tumoral immune escape. Cancer Res. 2012;72:917–27.

21. Zhang L, Gajewski TF, Kline J. PD-1/PD-L1 interactions inhibit antitumor immune responses in a murine acute myeloid leukemia model. Blood. 2009; 114:1545–52.

22. Shen J, Zhu Z. Catumaxomab, a rat/murine hybrid trifunctional bispecific monoclonal antibody for the treatment of cancer. Curr Opin Mol Ther. 2008; 10:273–84.

23. Moynihan KD, Opel CF, Szeto GL, Tzeng A, Zhu EF, Engreitz JM, et al. Eradication of large established tumors in mice by combination immunotherapy that engages innate and adaptive immune responses. Nat Med. 2016;22:1402–10.

24. Luo Y, Xiong D, Li HH, Qiu SP, Lin CL, Chen Q, et al. Development of an HSV-1 neutralization test with a glycoprotein D specific antibody for measurement of neutralizing antibody titer in human sera. Virol J. 2016;13:44.

25. Huang CH, Yuan Q, Chen PJ, Zhang YL, Chen CR, Zheng QB, et al. Influence of mutations in hepatitis B virus surface protein on viral antigenicity and phenotype in occult HBV strains from blood donors. J Hepatol. 2012;57:720–9.

Permissions

All chapters in this book were first published in IMMUNOLOGY, by BioMed Central; hereby published with permission under the Creative Commons Attribution License or equivalent. Every chapter published in this book has been scrutinized by our experts. Their significance has been extensively debated. The topics covered herein carry significant findings which will fuel the growth of the discipline. They may even be implemented as practical applications or may be referred to as a beginning point for another development.

The contributors of this book come from diverse backgrounds, making this book a truly international effort. This book will bring forth new frontiers with its revolutionizing research information and detailed analysis of the nascent developments around the world.

We would like to thank all the contributing authors for lending their expertise to make the book truly unique. They have played a crucial role in the development of this book. Without their invaluable contributions this book wouldn't have been possible. They have made vital efforts to compile up to date information on the varied aspects of this subject to make this book a valuable addition to the collection of many professionals and students.

This book was conceptualized with the vision of imparting up-to-date information and advanced data in this field. To ensure the same, a matchless editorial board was set up. Every individual on the board went through rigorous rounds of assessment to prove their worth. After which they invested a large part of their time researching and compiling the most relevant data for our readers.

The editorial board has been involved in producing this book since its inception. They have spent rigorous hours researching and exploring the diverse topics which have resulted in the successful publishing of this book. They have passed on their knowledge of decades through this book. To expedite this challenging task, the publisher supported the team at every step. A small team of assistant editors was also appointed to further simplify the editing procedure and attain best results for the readers.

Apart from the editorial board, the designing team has also invested a significant amount of their time in understanding the subject and creating the most relevant covers. They scrutinized every image to scout for the most suitable representation of the subject and create an appropriate cover for the book.

The publishing team has been an ardent support to the editorial, designing and production team. Their endless efforts to recruit the best for this project, has resulted in the accomplishment of this book. They are a veteran in the field of academics and their pool of knowledge is as vast as their experience in printing. Their expertise and guidance has proved useful at every step. Their uncompromising quality standards have made this book an exceptional effort. Their encouragement from time to time has been an inspiration for everyone.

The publisher and the editorial board hope that this book will prove to be a valuable piece of knowledge for researchers, students, practitioners and scholars across the globe.

List of Contributors

Elma Kadić, Ying Huo and Ilona Kariv
Department of Pharmacology, Cellular Pharmacology, Merck and Co. Inc, 33 Avenue Louis Pasteur, Boston 02115, MA, USA

Raymond J. Moniz
Department of Biology-Discovery, Immunooncology, Merck and Co. Inc, Boston, MA, USA

An Chi
Department of Chemistry, Capabilities Enhancement, Merck and Co. Inc, Boston, MA, USA

Arianna Palladini, Pier-Luigi Lollini and Patrizia Nanni
Department of Experimental, Diagnostic and Specialty Medicine (DIMES), University of Bologna, Viale Filopanti 22, 40126 Bologna, Italy

Lorena Landuzzi
Laboratory of Experimental Oncology, Rizzoli Orthopaedic Institute, Via di Barbiano 1/10, 40136 Bologna, Italy

Manoochehr Karami
Social Determinants of Health Research Center, Hamadan University of Medical Sciences, Hamadan, Iran
Department of Epidemiology, School of Public Health, Hamadan University of Medical Sciences, Hamadan, Iran

Pegah Ameri and Zeinab Berangi
Department of Epidemiology, School of Public Health, Hamadan University of Medical Sciences, Hamadan, Iran

Jalal Bathaei, Ali Zahiri and Hussein Erfani
Deputy for Health, Hamadan University of Medical Sciences, Hamadan, Iran

Tahereh Pashaei
Social Determinants of Health Research Center, Kurdistan University of Medical Sciences, Sanandaj, Iran

Seyed Mohsen Zahraei
Center for Communicable Diseases Control, Ministry of Health, Tehran, Iran

Koen Ponnet
Department of Communication Studies, Ghent University, Ghent, Belgium
Faculty of Social Sciences, University of Antwerp, Antwerp, Belgium

Ying Zhang, Xiaolong Zhang, Yun Liao, Yongrong Wang, Shengjie Ouyang, Yanchun Che, Jing Pu, Zhanlong He and Qihan Li
Yunnan Key Laboratory of Vaccine Research and Development on Severe Infectious Diseases, Institute of Medical Biology, Chinese Academy of Medical Sciences and Peking Union Medical College, No. 935 Jiaoling Road, Kunming, Yunnan 650118, China

Jing Tang
Yunnan Key Laboratory of Vaccine Research and Development on Severe Infectious Diseases, Institute of Medical Biology, Chinese Academy of Medical Sciences and Peking Union Medical College, No. 935 Jiaoling Road, Kunming, Yunnan 650118, China
National Institutes for Food and Drug Control, Beijing, China

Miao Xu, Qi Shen and Qiang Ye
National Institutes for Food and Drug Control, Beijing, China

Puyuan Xing, Hongyu Wang, Sheng Yang, Yan Su and Yuankai Shi
Department of Medical Oncology, Beijing Key Laboratory of Clinical Study on Anticancer Molecular Targeted Drugs, National Cancer Center/Cancer Hospital, Chinese Academy of Medical Sciences & Peking Union Medical College, Beijing 100021, China

Xiaohong Han
Department of Medical Oncology, Beijing Key Laboratory of Clinical Study on Anticancer Molecular Targeted Drugs, National Cancer Center/ Cancer Hospital, Chinese Academy of Medical Sciences & Peking Union Medical College, Beijing 100021, China
Department of Clinical Laboratory, National Cancer Center/Cancer Hospital, Chinese Academy of Medical Sciences & Peking Union Medical College, Beijing 100021, China

Maria Kuznetsova, Julia Lopatnikova, Julia Khantakova and Sergey Sennikov
Federal State Budgetary Scientific Institution "Research Institute of Fundamental and Clinical Immunology", Yadrintsevskaya str., 14, Novosibirsk 630099, Russia

Rinat Maksyutov
State Research Center of Virology and Biotechnology "VECTOR", Koltsovo, Novosibirsk Region 630559, Russia

Amir Maksyutov
State Research Center of Virology and Biotechnology "VECTOR", Koltsovo, Novosibirsk Region 630559, Russia
Federal State Budgetary Scientific Institution "Research Institute of Fundamental and Clinical Immunology", Yadrintsevskaya str., 14, Novosibirsk 630099, Russia

Gerard Pasternak and Aleksandra Lewandowicz-Uszyńska
3rd Department and Clinic of Paediatrics, Immunology and Rheumatology of Developmental Age, Wroclaw Medical University, L. Pasteura 1, Wroclaw 50-367, Poland
Department of Immunology and Paediatrics, Provincial Hospital J. Gromkowski, Koszarowa 5, Wroclaw 51-149, Poland

Katarzyna Pentoś
Institute of Agricultural Engineering, Wroclaw University of Environmental and Life Sciences, J.Chełmońskiego 37/41, Wroclaw 51-630, Poland

Jinjing Tan and Meng Gu
Department of Cellular and Molecular Biology, Beijing Chest Hospital, Capital Medical University/ Beijing Tuberculosis and Thoracic Tumor Research Institute, Beijing 101149, China

Wentao Yue
Department of Cellular and Molecular Biology, Beijing Chest Hospital, Capital Medical University/ Beijing Tuberculosis and Thoracic Tumor Research Institute, Beijing 101149, China
Central Laboratory, Beijing Obstetrics and Gynecology Hospital, Capital Medical University, Chaoyang, Beijing 100026, China

Xiaoguang Wu
Department of Tuberculosis, Beijing Chest Hospital, Capital Medical University, Beijing 101149, China

Suting Chen and Hairong Huang
National Clinical Laboratory on Tuberculosis, Beijing Key laboratory on Drug-resistant Tuberculosis Research, Beijing Chest Hospital, Capital Medical University/ Beijing Tuberculosis and Thoracic Tumor Institute, Beijing 101149, China

Rajae El Aouad and Fouad Seghrouchni
Laboratory of Cellular Immunology, National Institute of Hygiene, 27, Avenue Ibn Batouta, PB 769, 11400 Rabat, Morocco

Karima Sahmoudi
Laboratory of Cellular Immunology, National Institute of Hygiene, 27, Avenue Ibn Batouta, PB 769, 11400 Rabat, Morocco
Faculty of Sciences, University Mohammed V Agdal, Rabat, Morocco

Abderrahmane Sadak
Faculty of Sciences, University Mohammed V Agdal, Rabat, Morocco

Hassan Abbassi and Mohamed Nouredine El Alami
Department of ENT, Maxillo- facial, Reconstructive and Plastic Surgery, University Hospital Hassan II, Fes, Morocco

Nada Bouklata
National Reference Laboratory of Mycobacteriology, the National Institute of Hygiene, Rabat, Morocco

Christopher Burant
Case Western Reserve University School of Nursing, Cleveland, USA

W. Henry Boom and David H. Canaday
TB Research Unit and Division of Infectious Diseases, Case Western Reserve University, University Hospitals of Cleveland and Cleveland VA, Cleveland, OH, USA

Jingsong Cao and Jianhua Xiao
Institute of Pathogenic Biology, Medical College, Hunan Provincial Key Laboratory for Special Pathogens Prevention and Control; Hunan Province Cooperative Innovation Center for Molecular Target New Drug Study, University of South China, Hengyang, Hunan 421001, China

Luogen Liu and Yunsheng Zhang
Clinical research center, Institute of Pathogenic Biology, Medical College, The Second Affiliated Hospital, University of South China, Hengyang, Hunan 421001, China

Yi Wang
Clinical research center, Institute of Pathogenic Biology, Medical College, The Second Affiliated Hospital, University of South China, Hengyang, Hunan 421001, China
Urinary surgery, The Second Affiliated Hospital, University of South China, Hengyang, Hunan 421001, China

Cristina Vazquez-Mateo, Justin Collins, Michelle Fleury and Hans Dooms
Department of Medicine, Arthritis Center/Rheumatology Section, Boston University School of Medicine, 72 East Concord Street, E519, Boston, MA 02118, USA

Brittany A. Goods
Department of Biological Engineering, Koch Institute for Integrative Cancer Research at the Massachusetts Institute of Technology, Cambridge, MA 02139, USA

J. Christopher Love
Department of Biological Engineering, Koch Institute for Integrative Cancer Research at the Massachusetts Institute of Technology, Cambridge, MA 02139, USA

Department of Chemical Engineering, Koch Institute for Integrative Cancer Research at the Massachusetts Institute of Technology, Cambridge, MA 02139, USA
The Broad Institute of the Massachusetts Institute of Technology and Harvard, Cambridge, MA 02142, USA

Jacqueline M. Vahey
Department of Electrical Engineering and Computer Science, Massachusetts Institute of Technology, Cambridge, MA 02139, USA

Arthur F. Steinschneider, Michael H. Askenase and Lauren Sansing
Department of Neurology, Yale School of Medicine, New Haven, CT 06520, USA

Louisa Kühne, Bettina Jung, Helen Poth, Antonia Schuster, Simone Wurm, Bernhard Banas and Tobias Bergler
Department of Nephrology, University Hospital Regensburg, Franz-Josef-Strauß Allee 11, D-93053 Regensburg, Germany

Petra Ruemmele
Department of Pathology, University Hospital Erlangen, Erlangen, Germany

Javier Sánchez Ramírez, Yanelys Morera Díaz, Mónica Bequet-Romero and Marta Ayala Avila
Department of Pharmaceuticals, Center for Genetic Engineering and Biotechnology (CIGB), Playa Cubanacán, Havana 10600, Cuba

Francisco Hernández-Bernal, Yenima Martín Bauta and Cimara H.Bermúdez Badell
Department of Clinical Research, CIGB, Playa Cubanacán, Havana 10600, Cuba

Katty-Hind Selman-Housein Bernal and Josué de la Torre Pupo
Center of Medical and Surgical Research (CIMEQ), Playa, Siboney, Havana 12100, Cuba

Ana de la Torre Santos
"Celestino Hernández Robau" Hospital, Santa Clara 50100, Cuba

Eduardo Rafael Santiesteban Álvarez
"José Ramón López Tabranes" Hospital, Matanzas 40100, Cuba

John Sidney, Ravi Kolla and Alessandro Sette
La Jolla Institute for Allergy and Immunology, La Jolla, CA 92130, USA

Jose Luis Vela, Dave Friedrich, Matthias von Herrath and Johnna D. Wesley
Novo Nordisk Research Center Seattle, Inc., 530 Fairview Ave N, Seattle, WA 98109, USA

Guoying Ni and and Ming Q. Wei
School of Medical Science, Griffith Health Institute, Griffith University, Gold Coast, QLD 4333, Australia

Zaowen Liao and Shu Chen
Cancer Research Institute, The First People's Hospital of Foshan, Foshan, Guangdong 528000, China

Xiaosong Liu
Cancer Research Institute, The First People's Hospital of Foshan, Foshan, Guangdong 528000, China
Inflammation and Healing Research Cluster, University of the Sunshine Coast, Maroochydore DC, QLD 4558, Australia
Molecular diagnosis and Target Therapy Laboratory, The First Affiliated Hospital of Guangdong Pharmaceutical University, Guangzhou, Guangdong, China

Tianfang Wang, Kate Mounsey and Shelley Cavezza
Inflammation and Healing Research Cluster, University of the Sunshine Coast, Maroochydore DC, QLD 4558, Australia

Jianwei Yuan and Xuan Pan
Molecular diagnosis and Target Therapy Laboratory, The First Affiliated Hospital of Guangdong Pharmaceutical University, Guangzhou, Guangdong, China

Elaheh Movahed, Yi Ying Cheok, Grace Min Yi Tan, Chalystha Yie Qin Lee, Heng Choon Cheong, Rukumani Devi Velayuthan, Sun Tee Tay and Won Fen Wong
Department of Medical Microbiology, Faculty of Medicine, University of Malaya, Kuala Lumpur, Malaysia

Pei Pei Chong and Chung Yeng Looi
School of Bioscience, Taylor's University, Subang Jaya, Selangor, Malaysia

Qiongyi Hu, Yue Sun, Hui Shi, Jialin Teng, Honglei Liu, Xiaobing Cheng, Junna Ye, Yutong Su, Yufeng Yin, Mengru Liu and Chengde Yang
Department of Rheumatology and Immunology, Ruijin Hospital, Shanghai Jiao Tong University School of Medicine, No. 197 Ruijin Second Road, Shanghai 200025, China

Yuan Li and Jiucun Wang
State Key Laboratory of Genetic Engineering and Ministry of Education (MOE) Key Laboratory of Contemporary Anthropology, Collaborative Innovation Center for Genetics and Development, School of Life Sciences, Fudan University, Shanghai 200438, China

Qin Chen, Shengping Qiu, Huanhuan Li, Chaolong Lin, Yong Luo, Wenfeng Ren, Yidi Zou, Yale Wang, Ninghshao Xia and Chenghao Huang
State Key Laboratory of Molecular Vaccinology and Molecular Diagnostics, National Institute of Diagnostics and Vaccine Development in Infectious Diseases, School of Public Health, Xiamen University, Xiamen 361102, China

Index

www.ingramcontent.com/pod-product-compliance
Lightning Source LLC
Chambersburg PA
CBHW082028190326
41458CB00010B/3303